STP 1438

Stainless Steels for Medical and Surgical Applications

Gary L. Winters and Michael J. Nutt, editors

ASTM Stock Number: STP1438

ASTM International
100 Barr Harbor Drive
PO Box C700
West Conshohocken, PA 19428-2959

Printed in the U.S.A.

Library of Congress Cataloging-in-Publication Data
ISBN: 0-8031-3459-2

Symposium on Stainless Steels for Medical and Surgical Applications (2002 : Pittsburgh, Pa.)
    Stainless steels for medical and surgical applications / Gary L. Winters and Michael J.
Nutt [editors].
      p. cm.—(STP; 1438)
    "ASTM Stock Number: STP1438."
    Includes bibliographical references and indexes.
    Contains papers presented at the Symposium on Stainless Steels for Medical and Surgical
Applications held in Pittsburgh, Pa., on May 6 and 7, 2002.
    ISBN 0-8031-3459-2
    1. Medical instruments and apparatus—Congresses. 2. Medical instruments and
apparatus—Design and construction—Handbooks, manuals, etc. 3. Medical instruments and
apparatus industry—Technological innovations—Congresses. 4. Steel,
Stainless—Congresses. 5. Corrosion resistant alloys—Congresses. I. Winters, Gary L. II.
Nutt, Michael J. III. Title. IV. ASTM special technical publication ; 1438.

  R856.A2S96 2002
  681'.761—dc21

                                     2003040381

Photocopy Rights

Peer Review Policy

Each paper published in this volume was evaluated by two peer reviewers and at least one editor.
The authors addressed all of the reviewers' comments to the satisfaction of both the technical
editor(s) and the ASTM International Committee on Publications.

To make technical information available as quickly as possible, the peer-reviewed papers in this
publication were prepared "camera-ready" as submitted by the authors.

The quality of the papers in this publication reflects not only the obvious efforts of the authors and
the technical editor(s), but also the work of the peer reviewers. In keeping with long-standing
publication practices, ASTM International maintains the anonymity of the peer reviewers. The ASTM
International Committee on Publications acknowledges with appreciation their dedication and
contribution of time and effort on behalf of ASTM International.

Printed in (to come)
(to come)

Foreword

This publication, *Stainless Steels for Medical and Surgical Applications,* contains papers presented at the symposium of the same name, held in Pittsburgh, Pennsylvania, on May 6 and 7, 2002. The symposium was sponsored by ASTM Committee F04 on Medical and Surgical Materials and Devices. Gary L. Winters of Cedar Creek, Texas, and Michael J. Nutt of Spinal Innovations, in Bartlett, Tennessee, presided as symposium chairmen and are editors of the resulting publication.

The editors would like to express their appreciation for the help provided by Markus Windler from Sulzer Orthopaedics, Winterthur, Switzerland, in promoting initially the need for such a symposium and in encouraging participation by several European research groups.

We, of course, want to thank all the authors who contributed to the research presented at the symposium and, in particular, we would like to thank the presenters, some of whom made the effort and sacrifice to travel to the United States from Brazil, France, Germany, Sweden, Switzerland, and the United Kingdom in order to attend the symposium.

We would also like to express our thanks to the ASTM staff that helped make the symposium and publication possible: most notably Dorothy Fitzpatrick for her help with the symposium planning and Maria Langiewicz for the handling of manuscript submission and review. We are also indebted to all the reviewers who volunteered their time and expertise for their careful consideration and critique of the manuscripts.

Gary L. Winters
Cedar Creek, Texas, USA

Michael J. Nutt
Spinal Innovations,
Bartlett, Tennessee, USA

Contents

OVERVIEW   ix

ALLOY DESIGN, MECHANICAL PROPERTIES

**Characterization of Sandvik Bioline High-N—A Comparison of Standard Grades
F1314 and F1586**—CHRISTINA HARALDSSON AND STEPHEN COWEN   3

X 15 T.N:™ A New Martensitic Stainless Steel for Surgical Instruments—
NICOLAS PEROT, JEAN-YVES MORAUX, JEAN-PAUL DICHTEL, AND BRUNO BOUCHER   13

Development of a Platinum-Enhanced Radiopaque Stainless Steel (PERSS®)—
CHARLES H. CRAIG, HERBERT R. RADISCH, JR., THOMAS A. TROZERA, PAUL C. TURNER,
R. DALE GOVIER, EDWARD J. VESELY, JR., NEV A. GOKCEN, CLIFFORD M. FRIEND,
AND MICHAEL R. EDWARDS   28

**Mechanical and Corrosion Properties of Forged Hip Stems Made of High-Nitrogen
Stainless Steel**—MARKUS WINDLER AND RAINER STEGER   39

Metallurgical and Mechanical Evaluation of 316L Stainless Steel Orthopaedic Cable—
JOHN A. DISEGI AND LYLE D. ZARDIACKAS   50

PROCESSING, QUALITY ASSURANCE CONCERNS, AND MRI TESTING

**Processing Platinum Enhanced Radiopaque Stainless Steel (PERSS®) for Use as
Balloon-Expandable Coronary Stents**—J. ZACHARY DENNIS, CHARLES H. CRAIG,
HERBERT R. RADISCH, JR., EDWARD J. PANNEK, JR., PAUL C. TURNER, ALBERT G. HICKS,
MATTHEW JENUSAITIS, NEV A. GOKCEN, CLIFFORD M. FRIEND, AND MICHAEL R. EDWARDS   61

Quality Aspects of High-Nitrogen Stainless Steel for Surgical Implants—
MARKUS WINDLER, RAINER STEGER, AND GARY L. WINTERS   72

MRI Safety and Compatibility of Implants and Medical Devices—TERRY O. WOODS   82

Corrosion

Fatigue of Small Bone Fragment Fixation Plates Made from Low-Nickel Steel—
LUKAS ESCHBACH, GIANNI BIGOLIN, WERNER HIRSIGER, AND BEAT GASSER   93

**Comparison of Anodic Polarization and Galvanic Corrosion of a Low-Nickel Stainless
Steel to 316LS and 22Cr-13Ni-5Mn Stainless Steels—**LYLE D. ZARDIACKAS,
SCOTT WILLIAMSON, MICHAEL ROACH, AND JAY-ANTHONY BOGAN   107

**Fatigue Behavior and In-Vitro Biocompatibility of the Ni-Free Austenitic
High-Nitrogen Steel X13CrMnMoN18-14-3—**ILIA TIKHOVSKI, HOLGER BRAUER,
MARTINA MÖLDERS, MARTIN WIEMANN, DIETER BINGMANN, AND ALFONS FISCHER   119

Influence of Macrophage Cells on 316L Stainless Steel Corrosion—SUZANNE H. PARKER,
HSIN-YI LIN, LYLE D. ZARDIACKAS, AND JOEL D. BUMGARDNER   137

**Comparison of Notch Sensitivity and Stress Corrosion Cracking of a Low-Nickel
Stainless Steel to 316LS and 22Cr-13Ni-5Mn Stainless Steels—**
LYLE D. ZARDIACKAS, MICHAEL ROACH, SCOTT WILLIAMSON, AND JAY-ANTHONY BOGAN   154

**Comparative Electrochemical Studies of F 1586-95 and F 138-92 Stainless Steels in
Sodium Chloride, pH = 4.0 Medium—**RUTH F. V. VILLAMIL,
ARNALDO H. P. DE ANDRADE, CELSO A. BARBOSA, ALEXANDRE SOKOLOWSKI,
AND SILVIA M. L. AGOSTINHO   168

**Corrosion Behavior of Platinum-Enhanced Radiopaque Stainless Steel (PERSS®) for
Dilation-Balloon Expandable Coronary Stents—**BERNARD S. COVINO, JR.,
CHARLES H. CRAIG, STEPHEN D. CRAMER, SOPHIE J. BULLARD,
MARGARET ZIOMEK-MOROZ, PAUL D. JABLONSKI, PAUL C. TURNER,
HERBERT R. RADISCH, JR., NEV A. GOKCEN, CLIFFORD M. FRIEND,
AND MICHAEL R. EDWARDS   176

**Comparison of Corrosion Fatigue of BioDur® 108 to 316L S.S.
and 22Cr-13Ni-5Mn S.S.—**LYLE D. ZARDIACKAS, MICHAEL ROACH,
SCOTT WILLIAMSON, AND JAY-ANTHONY BOGAN   194

Wear and Corrosion-Related Wear

Investigation into Wear-Induced Corrosion of Orthopaedic Implant Materials—
MARKUS WINDLER, JULIE E. MACDOUGALL, AND ROLF SCHENK   211

**Results of In-Vitro Studies about the Mechanism of Wear in the Stem-Cement
Interface of THR—**DIETER WIRZ, BRUNO ZURFLUH, BEAT GÖPFERT, FENG LI,
WILLI FRICK, AND ERWIN W. MORSCHER   222

**Fretting and Anodic Current of the Taper Interface of Stainless Steel Hip
Stems/Cobalt-Chromium Femoral Heads—**MENGKE ZHU AND MARKUS WINDLER   235

CLINICAL EXPERIENCE

The Cemented MS-30 Stem in Total Hip Replacement, Matte versus Polished Surface:
Minimum of Five Years of Clinical and Radiographic Results of a Prospective
Study—BERNHARD BERLI, REINHARD ELKE, ERWIN W. MORSCHER   249

Corrosion Products Generated from Mechanically Assisted Crevice Corrosion of
Stainless Steel Orthopaedic Implants—ROBERT M. URBAN, JOSHUA J. JACOBS,
JEREMY L. GILBERT, ANASTASIA K. SKIPOR, NADIM J. HALLAB, KATALIN MIKECZ,
TIBOR T. GLANT, J. LAWRENCE MARSH, AND JORGE O. GALANTE   262

Author Index   273

Subject Index   275

Overview

The Symposium on Stainless Steels for Medical and Surgical Applications undertook to bring together, at one time, current research and development, recent clinical experience, and the substantial history of stainless steels in medical applications. This was done with the expressed purpose of bringing the attendees and participants of the symposium up to date on the current status of the latest technologies and to provide the most current information. Ultimately, this new information may stimulate further research and technical developments in the application of stainless steels for implantable medical devices and surgical instruments.

This Special Technical Publication (STP) furthers the aims of the symposium by documenting the entirety of the body of research that was presented in 20-minute synopses during the symposium. This information, which has not been previously published, is to be made available not only to the attendees and participants of the symposium, but also to the general public. In this manner, the information in the symposium can be distributed more widely and be more helpful in furthering research and technical developments in the application of stainless steels for implantable medical devices and surgical instruments.

This publication will be helpful to individuals engaged in the development of stainless steels for implant applications, or instrument applications in particular. It will also be of interest to other individuals, who are developing, making, or using implantable medical devices and/or surgical instruments in general. This publication may make both of these groups aware of alloys, testing, or applications that they had not previously considered.

This new information can stimulate new research or technical innovations. This information can also be used by individuals to contact researchers or producers with similar interests. Finally, this information may become part of the justifications for device approval by regulatory bodies, and for creation of material specifications by standards writing bodies, which can benefit producers, users, and regulatory bodies.

This publication addresses some of the issues in the medical uses of stainless steels, such as corrosion, wear, biological response, radiopacity, and the high cost of medical products. New alloys are discussed as solutions to some of these issues by offering more biocompatible, higher quality, radiopaque, or low cost alternatives for orthopaedic implants and stents. Several corrosion papers address this key concern for all medical devices. Some of these papers offer creative options for this field. Finally, there are other papers that deal with such timely issues as injuries due to the interaction of implants and MRI examinations.

This symposium covered a wide range of topics on stainless steels, with most of the presentations dealing with narrow segments of a specific topic. Therefore, a single theme of the presentations may be that work on stainless steels for medical uses continues and that stainless steels may be part of the answers for some of the issues facing the surgical community today, such as biological response, corrosion resistance, mechanical performance, quality, and cost.

Certainly, iron-base alloy systems offer excellent opportunities as implant and instrumentation alloys in the medical field to satisfy special needs such as radiopacity, wear resistance, superior mechanical properties, or freedom from allergic responses. As such, work should continue on increasing the corrosion resistance and mechanical properties of stainless steels, as well as the product forms and applications, while decreasing cost and any negative biological responses.

Gary L. Winters
Cedar Creek, Texas

Michael J. Nutt
Spinal Innovations
Bartlett, Tennessee

Alloy Design, Mechanical Properties

Christina Haraldsson[1] and Stephen Cowen[2]

Characterization of Sandvik Bioline High-N - A Comparison of Standard Grades F1314 and F1586

Reference: Haraldsson, C. and Cowen, S. " **Characterization of Sandvik Bioline High-N - A Comparison of Standard Grades F1314 and F1586,**" *Stainless Steels for Medical and Surgical Applications, ASTM STP 1438*, G. L. Winters and M. J. Nutt, Eds., ASTM International, West Conshohocken, PA, 2003.

Abstract: ASTM standard grades for surgical implants F1314 and F1586 are both N-strengthened austenitic stainless steels with high resistance to pitting corrosion. The latter is generally used in Europe while the former is preferred in the United States. In the present study, Sandvik grade Bioline High-N, conforming to ASTM F1586, has been characterized with respect to microstructure, mechanical properties, corrosion resistance and inclusion content and compared with ASTM F1314-material.

In the present comparison it has been shown that Bioline High-N[3] compared to ASTM F1314 material has similar or slightly superior mechanical properties, pitting corrosion resistance and nonmetallic inclusion content. All these properties are of critical importance for medical implant material.

Keywords: Stainless steel, implant materials, nonmetallic inclusions, pitting corrosion resistance, mechanical properties, microstructure

---

[1] Research Engineer, Product Development, Metallurgical Research, AB Sandvik Steel, SE-811 81 Sandviken, Sweden.

[2] General Manager, Sandvik Metinox, Long Acre Way, Holbrook Sheffield S20 3FS, U.K.

[3] Bioline High-N is a registered trademark of AB Sandvik Steel, Sandviken, Sweden.

Introduction

Stainless steel is a widely used material for orthopedic implants due to its competitive price level, wide availability of product forms and relative ease of manufacture. The most common grade of stainless steel used for implants conforms to ASTM specification for Wrought 18 Chromium-14 Nickel-2.5 Molybdenum Stainless Steel Bar and Wire for Surgical Implants (UNS S31673), (F138).

Whilst ASTM F138 has excellent benefits in a wide range of medical implant applications, it does have certain limitations with regard to ultimate tensile strength and corrosion resistance. In specific permanent load bearing orthopedic devices, such as hips, knees and shoulders, and in products for trauma fixation such as intermedullary nails and screws, it is often the case that additional strength, enhanced fatigue properties and better corrosion resistance are required for optimum prosthetic performance and patient benefit.

Materials conforming to both ASTM Specification for Wrought Nitrogen Strengthened-22 Chromium-12.5 Nickel-5 Manganese-2.5 Molybdenum Stainless Steel Bar and Wire for Surgical Implants (F1314) and ASTM Specification for Wrought Nitrogen Strengthened-21 Chromium-10 Nickel-3 Manganese-2.5 Molybdenum Stainless Steel Bar for Surgical Implants (F1586) have additional benefits that make their usage in certain applications more favorable than material conforming to ASTM F138. The base for Bioline High-N material (conforming to ASTM F1586) is a fully austenitic 316 material. Alloying with higher levels of Nitrogen (0.25 – 0.50%) in combination with increased levels of Chromium (19.5 – 22.0%) and small additions of Niobium (0.25 – 0.80%) facilitates solid solution strengthening within the material which in turn delivers higher mechanical strength and enhanced resistance to pitting corrosion. This is achieved without the need for additional Nickel that would increase the cost of the material [1].

In the present study Sandvik Bioline High-N, conforming to ASTM F1586, has been characterized with respect to microstructure, mechanical properties, corrosion resistance and nonmetallic inclusion content and compared with ASTM F1314-material. In cases where experimental results are missing for the ASTM F1314-material the standard requirements have been substituted.

Materials

Nitrogen-strengthened austenitic stainless steels conforming to ASTM F1314 and F1586 are very similar in composition (Table 1). Historically the latter has generally been used in Europe while the former has been more predominant in the United States.

Regarding chemical composition the most significant differences between F1314 and F1586 is the Vanadium (V) addition in the F1314 material, its lower levels of Niobium (Nb) and also the higher Nickel (Ni) level (Table 1). F1586 allows up to 0.08% carbon, which is well above the maximum level for ASTM F1314 (Table 1). But, to avoid carbide precipitation the carbon content in F1586 is generally kept well below the maximum level that reduces the difference in carbon content between the two materials. Vanadium and Niobium both have a stronger tendency to form carbides compared to

Chromium (Cr). This prevents the precipitation of the detrimental chromium carbides within the material. The affinity to carbon, nitrogen, oxygen and sulfur for different elements are schematically shown (Figure 1)[2]. This must be seen as a general ranking since neither the temperature nor the elements' differing solubility in different phases are considered.

Table 1 – *Chemical compositions (weight-%)*

Element	ASTM F1586	Bioline High-N[1]	ASTM F1314
Carbon	0.08 max	0.06 max	0.030 max
Manganese	2.00 – 4.25	4.0	4.00 – 6.00
Phosphorus	0.025 max	0.025 max	0.025 max
Sulfur	0.01 max	0.003 max	0.010 max
Silicon	0.75 max	0.60 max	0.75 max
Chromium	19.5 –22.0	20.5	20.50 – 23.50
Nickel	9.0 – 11.0	9.5	11.50 – 13.50
Molybdenum	2.0 – 3.0	2.4	2.00 – 3.00
Nitrogen	0.25 – 0.5	0.4	0.20 – 0.40
Niobium	0.25 – 0.8	0.3	0.10 – 0.30
Vanadium			0.10 – 0.30
Copper	0.25 max		0.50 max
Iron	Balance		balance

[1] Nominal composition

C:	Fe Mn Cr WMoV	TaNbTiZr			
N:	Fe MnWMoCrNb SiVCaCeTa Al Ti Zr				
O:	Fe	CrNb MnVC Si Ta Ti AlZrMgCeCa			
S:	Fe Cr Nb Ta Mn Ti Al	Zr Mg		Ca Ce	

Increasing affinity

Figure 1 - *Ranking of the alloying elements affinity to C, N, O and S*

V is a rather strong ferrite former. Patti and Schiller [3] have suggested a factor of 5 in the Cr-equivalent that should be compared with their suggestion of a factor 1.75 for Nb, formula (2). The reason for the somewhat higher Ni level in the F1314 material compared to the F1586 might hence be to keep the material fully austenitic, formula (1)

$$Ni_{equ} = Ni + Co + 0.5 \cdot Mn + 0.3 \cdot Cu + 30 \cdot C + 25 \cdot N \qquad (1)$$
$$Cr_{equ} = Cr + 2 \cdot Si + 1.5 \cdot Mo + 5 \cdot V + 5.5 \cdot Al + 1.75 \cdot Nb + 1.5 \cdot Ti + 0.75 \cdot W \qquad (2)$$

Experimental

Microstructure

Microstructural investigations were performed in a Leica DMR light optical microscope (LOM) using specimens electrolytically etched in 40% NaOH at 3V for approximately 10s.

Nonmetallic Inclusions

The inclusion content has been determined on longitudinal samples. Both the ASTM Test Methods for Determining the Inclusion Content of Steel (E45) Method A and the Swedish Standard Steel-Method for assessment of the content of nonmetallic inclusions (SS 11 11 16) have been used.

The inclusion assessment using method ASTM E45-A is described as the rating number of the largest detected inclusion according to a comparative chart. Several inclusions of the same largest size, or just one single inclusion, generate the same results i.e. the inclusion frequency is not considered here. The standard specification requirements for ASTM F1314 and F1586 respectively are given in (Table 2). It can be noted that F1314 allows a somewhat higher inclusion rating for both BT and CT, otherwise the requirements are identical.

Table 2 – *Maximum inclusion ratings according to ASTM E45-A*

	AT	AH	BT	BH	CT	CH	DT	DH
ASTM F1586	1.5	1.5	2.0	1.5	2.0	1.5	2.5	1.5
ASTM F1314	1.5	1.5	2.5	1.5	2.5	1.5	2.5	1.5

A comparative measurement has been performed using the Swedish standard SS 11 11 16. The difference between this and the former measurement is that the Swedish standard takes into account every inclusion larger than a specific size and not just the largest one. This results in an inclusion frequency expressed as the number of inclusions/cm^2 in different size classes. The minimum inclusion size included is 3 μm and the following terminology is used.

Inclusion type
B= Brittle inclusions
C= Brittle-ductile inclusions
D= Undeformed inclusions

Inclusion width
T = thin   3-6 microns
M= medium   6-11 microns
H = heavy   11-22 microns

Corrosion Resistance

The pitting corrosion resistance has been tested in accordance with Method A in ASTM Test Methods for Pitting and Crevice Corrosion Resistance of Stainless Steels and Related Alloys by Use of Ferric Chloride Solution (G48).
A comparison of the pitting resistance equivalent, PRE, has been completed using formula (3)[4]

$$PRE = Cr + 3.3 \cdot Mo + 16 \cdot N \tag{3}$$

At the Royal Institute of Technology an electrochemical study of the resistance to localized corrosion has been performed on ASTM F138 and F1586 (Bioline High-N) [5]. The investigations were performed on annealed material at 25°C with a scanning rate 10mV/min in a phosphate buffered saline (PBS) solution and in a very aggressive simulated crevice solution designed to cause crevice corrosion by a high concentration of chlorides and a low pH value. The composition of the two solutions is given below (Table 3).

Table 3 - *Compositions of the PBS and simulated crevice solutions*

	PBS solution	Simulated crevice solution
NaCl	8.77 g/L	146.25 g/L
Na_2HPO_4	1.42 g/L	1.42 g/L
KH_2PO_4	2.72 g/L	2.72 g/L
PH	7	0.85

Results

Microstructure

The microstructure in both F1314 and F1586 material is austenitic without any traces of ferrite when examined in x100 magnification. Oblong primary precipitates rich in niobium and nitrogen can be seen rather frequently in both materials. In the F1314 material the precipitates generally seem to have sharper corners (Figures 2 and 3). In material of type F1586 the precipitate has been identified as Z-phase [6, 7] with the nominal chemical formula $Cr_2Nb_2N_2$ [8]. Trials to dissolve the Z-phase in Bioline High-N by heat treatment have been performed in the range 900-1200°C without success.

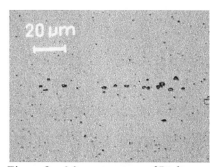

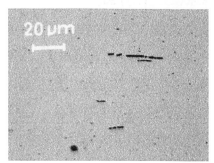

Figure 2 – *Microstructure of Bioline High-N*

Figure 3 - *Microstructure of F1314-material*

Nonmetallic Inclusions

The ASTM E45 results (Table 4) show that both materials fully conform to the standard specifications. From the results it can be seen that neither of the materials has any A-type inclusions due to very low S-content. In the investigated F1314 material, only B-type inclusions were found, whereas Bioline High-N has inclusions of both type B and C, although the C-type dominates. This is due to differences in the method of deoxidization used. Both materials have inclusions of type D – the investigated F1314 material with somewhat higher ratings compared to Bioline High-N. For F1586 the ASTM ratings presented are average values for 17 heats, approximate heat weight 60 tonnes, investigated as billets of dimension 120x120mm square. The F1314 material was investigated as bar samples of diameters 8 and 11 mm. It should be noted that the heavier deformation of the F1314 material might have caused the D-type inclusions to crush and form inclusions of type B.

Table 4 – *Inclusion rating according to ASTM E45 method A, plate III.*

	AT	AH	BT	BH	CT	CH	DT	DH
Bioline High-N[1]	0,0	0,0	0,1	0,0	1,0	0,9	0,9	0,1
F1314-material[2]	0,0	0,0	0,9	0,0	0,0	0,0	1,3	0,1

[1] Average of 17 heats
[2] Average of 2 heats

The inclusion frequency assessment (Table 5) clearly shows that Bioline High-N has a much lower total number of inclusions in the investigated size range, 3-22 μm, compared to the investigated F1314-material. The calculated area-% of inclusions is an average of 0.0080% for Bioline High-N, compared to 0.0140% for the investigated F1314 material.

Table 5 – *Inclusion content according to SS 11 11 16 as No. of inclusions/cm²*

	BT	BM	BH	CT	CM	CH	DT	DM	DH
Bioline High-N[1]	0	0	0	6	4	2	129	10	0
F1314-material[2]	95	0	0	0	0	0	575	90	7

[1] Average of 9 heats
[2] Average of 2 heats

Corrosion

The ASTM G48 test was performed on double samples of both the F1586 and F1314 material. The samples were prepared in the same way and tested at the same time under similar conditions. The results (Table 6) show that the materials have about the same resistance to localized corrosion, F1586 being slightly superior.

Table 6 – *Calculated PRE-values and CPT-values from ASTM G48 test*

	PRE	Specimen I	Specimen II	Average
Bioline High-N	34,8	40°	50°C	45°C
ASTM F1314	33,0	40°	40°C	40°C

Polarization curves obtained from the four cyclic potentiodynamic measurement runs of Bioline High-N in PBS solution (Figure 4) show rather small deviations between the separate runs [9].

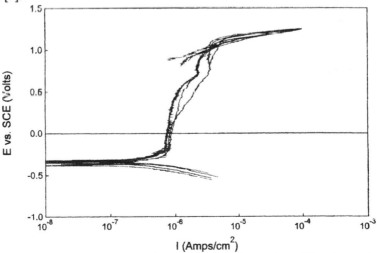

Figure 4 - *Cyclic polarization curves for Bioline High-N obtained in PBS solution, four separate runs. Scan rate 10mV/min*

The pitting potential and the protection potential in PBS solution were determined to 1.10 V/SCE and 1.04 V/SCE respectively to be compared with 0.36 V/SCE respectively - 0.16 V/SCE for F138 material (Table 7) [10]. The results suggest that Bioline High-N has a very low tendency to pitting initiation due to a high pitting potential as well as a strong ability to re-passivate if the passive film is damaged due to its high protection potential.

Table 7 – *Results from cyclic potentiodynamic polarization measurements with regard to Bioline High-N*

	PBS-solution	Simulated crevice solution
Pitting potential	1.10 V/SCE	0.9 V/SCE
Protection potential	1.04 V/SCE	0.8 V/SCE

The results from the cyclic potentiodynamic polarization in the simulated crevice solution resulted, as expected, is somewhat lower values for both the pitting and the protection potential (Table 7) [10]. Despite the much higher aggressiveness of the simulated crevice solution only a slight decrease in both the pitting and protection potential was achieved, indicating excellent resistance to localized corrosion.

Mechanical Properties

For the F1314 material standard data has been used due to no actual test result being available.

Table 8 – *Mechanical requirements according to material specifications*

	ASTM F1314	ASTM F1586		Bioline High-N[1]
Annealed				
Yield strength Rp 0,2/ MPa	380	430		525
UTS Rm / MPa	690	740		862
Elongation A / %	35	35		39
Cold-worked		Medium hard	Hard	
Yield strength Rp 0,2/ MPa	862	700	1000	2
UTS Rm / MPa	1035	1000	1100	2
Elongation A / %	12	20	10	2

[1] Typical values
[2] See Figure 5

When comparing the minimum material requirements ASTM F1586 have higher overall mechanical properties in the fully annealed condition when compared to the F1314 material (Table 8). When the two materials' minimum requirements are compared in the cold worked or hardened condition both the UTS and 0.2% proof stress figures for the F1586 material exhibit higher properties combined with higher values of elongation (for the same UTS level) than for the F1314 material (Table 8).

Bioline High-N therefore, exhibits high strength with good ductility, making it an obvious choice for medical implant devices. Further study has also revealed that High-N material performs in a very linear manner under cold working and a graph of tensile strength vs. reduction of area during cold work can be seen in Figure 5.

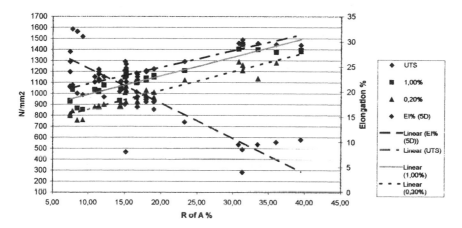

Figure 5 – *Tensile strength vs. reduction of area during cold working of Bioline High-N.*

Conclusion

Bioline High-N has been characterized and compared to both ASTM F1586 and F1314 standards. Chemical composition, microstructure, nonmetallic inclusion, corrosion resistance and mechanical properties have been compared.

The microstructure in both materials is austenitic with precipitates of a niobium rich nitride. According to minimum requirements for mechanical strength in ASTM specifications F1314 and F1586, the latter is slightly superior.

Nonmetallic inclusion evaluation has been performed both according to ASTM E45 method A and as a frequency analysis on both material grades. Bioline High-N has consistently been shown to be well within the demanding requirements of F1586, demands which are somewhat harder to fulfil when compared to F1314.

The pitting corrosion resistance has been found to be very good due to high Cr, Mo and N-levels. The critical pitting potential (CPT), determined by ASTM G48-test has shown a somewhat better result for Bioline High-N compared to the investigated F1314 material.

It has been found that Bioline High-N conforming to ASTM F1586 exhibits lower nonmetallic inclusion levels, somewhat superior pitting corrosion resistance with higher levels of mechanical strength when compared to material meeting the requirements of the F1314 specification.

References

[1] Leclerc, M.F., "Corrosion; 3rd edition"; Eds Shrier,L.L; Jarman, R.A. and Burnstein, G.T.; pp. 164-180; Butterworth-Heinemann Ltd, Oxford, England, (1994).

[2] Hillert, M., Compendium in "Phase Transformation, basic course part II" page Fe20 ("Fasomvandlingar, grundkurs del II") Stockholm 1986, Royal Institute of Materials Science and Technology.

[3] Patti,G. and Schiller,P., Journal of Nuclear Material, Vol. 141/143, 1986, pp.417-426.

[4] Lorentz, K. and Medawar, G., "Über das korrosionsverhalten austenitisscher Chrom-Nickel-molybdän-Stähle mit und ohne Stickstoffzusatz unter besonderer Berücksichtigung ihrer Beanspruchbarkeit in Chloridhaltigen Lösungen." Thyssen Forschung, 1, 1969, pp.97-108.

[5] Pan, J., Karlén, C., and Ulfvin, C., "Electrochemical Study of Resistance to Localized Corrosion of Stainless Steels for Biomaterial Applications," Journal of The Electrochemical Society, Vol.147 (3), 2000, pp. 1021-1025.

[6] Robinson, P.W., and Jack, D.H., "Precipitation of Z-phase in a high-nitrogen stainless steel," New Developments in Stainless Steel Technology, ASM, Metals Park OH 1985, pp. 71-76.

[7] Örnhagen, C., Nilsson, J.-O., and Vannevik, H., "Characterization of a nitrogen-rich austenitic stainless steel used for osteosynthesis devises," Journal of Biomedical Materials Research, Vol.31,1996, pp. 97-103.

[8] Andrews, K.W., Dyson, D.J., and Keown, S.R., "The interpretation of Electron Diffraction patterns," Adan Hilger, London, England, 1971.

[9] Hjalmarsson, C., "Comparative study of local corrosion resistance for implant grade stainless steels using electrochemical methods," MSc Thesis at the Royal Institute of Technology, Division of Corrosion Science, 1997.

Nicolas Perot,[1] Jean-Yves Moraux,[1] Jean-Paul Dichtel,[2] and Bruno Boucher[3]

X 15 T.N™ : A new Martensitic Stainless Steel for Surgical Instruments

Reference: Perot, N., Moraux, J.Y., Dichtel, J.P., and Boucher, B., " **X 15 T.N™: A new Martensitic Stainless Steel for Surgical Instruments,"** *Stainless Steels for Medical and Surgical Applications, ASTM STP 1438,* G. L. Winters, and M. J. Nutt, Eds., ASTM International, West Conshohocken, PA, 2003.

Abstract: The edge retention and wear resistance of steels are dependant upon hardness and structure. Until now, two main principles have been adopted to increase the hardness of martensitic stainless steels:
1. Either through the introduction of a structural hardening mechanism into low carbon martensitic grades such as, AISI 630 and XM 16,
2. Or by increasing the carbon content of the martensite and subsequently strengthening it through the presence of primary carbides.
The first option has not allowed to date, the mass production of steels with hardness levels greater than 52/54 HRC. Furthermore, the absence of carbides deleteriously affects cutting quality. The second option has two distinct disadvantages directly linked to the presence of large carbides, which render the steel brittle and reduce corrosion resistance, through chromium depletion of the matrix in the immediate vicinity of the carbides.
In X 15 T.N™, (UNS S 42025) nitrogen is used as a partial substitute for carbon, causing hardening by interstitial insertion as well as by the formation of fine nitrides and carbonitrides. In this way, a hardness level (58/60 HRC) is obtained equivalent to a high carbon martensitic steel without chromium depletion, thereby giving a substantial improvement in corrosion resistance, i.e. equivalent or superior to AISI 630 and XM 16.

Keywords: medical instruments, hardness, corrosion resistance, cutting, wear resistance, nitrogen alloyed steel, martensitic steel

[1]Market Manager and Chief Metallurgist, respectively, Aubert & Duval Holding, 33 av du Maine, 75755 Paris cedex 15 (France).
[2]Engineer, Aubert & Duval Alliages BP63, 92233 Gennevilliers cedex (France).
[3]President, Forecreu America, 37-35 W. Belmont Av, Chicago, IL, 60618 (USA).

Foreword

Medical instruments are used in a vast field of applications, and properties required from stainless steel grades are widely diversified. For many applications, the selected grade has to simultaneously satisfy the following basic characteristics
1.High hardness for wear resistance.
2.Good shape keeping edge retention for cutting tools, profile keeping for screw drivers.
3.Satisfactory corrosion resistance against cleaning and disinfecting products.
In addition, grades have to posses good fatigue and tenacity properties to avoid premature rupture resulting from high usage. Included in this category are cutting tools in general and ancillary instruments, such as drills, rasps, screwdrivers

Some Examples of Existing Grades (Table 1)

Steel Type AISI 420B: 13% chromium and 0.3% carbon

A 52 HRc hardness combined with chromium carbide in the structure gives this grade very good wear resistance as well as good edge retention. The main disadvantage is poor corrosion resistance. The nominal 13% chromium content is close to the minimum content to insure passive film formation. The matrix chromium content is lowered by the precipitation of $Cr_{23}C_6$ type carbides in the hardened and tempered condition.

Steel Type AISI 431: 17% chromium, 2% nickel and 0.16% carbon

A higher chromium content ensures a better corrosion resistance, but a lower hardness of 43 HRc (47HRc can be reached on small parts).

Steel Type AISI 440C: 17% chromium, 1% carbon and addition of molybdenum

Due to its high carbon content, 60 HRC hardness can be reached, its structure being made mostly of $Cr_{23}C_6$ type carbides. These characteristics allow extremely good edge retention, but, unfortunately, these carbides weaken the Chromium matrix and give this grade very poor corrosion resistance and fracture toughness.

Precipitation Hardening Martensitic Steels such as AISI 630, XM 16

These grades offer better corrosion resistance because nickel is added to the base composition which contains high chromium and low carbon content. Hardening is obtained through fine precipitation of intermetallic compounds : Precipitation Hardening (PH steels). The main advantage is that the 17% of chromium is solely dedicated to corrosion resistance, optimizing it. However, hardness is limited to 47HRC, and the absence of carbides negatively affects the tools' edge retention.

Table 1- *Typical Composition of some Martensitic Stainless steels (%)*

	C	Cr	Mn	Si	S	P	Ni	Mo	V	OTHER	Hardness HRC Max.
AISI XM 16	< 0.03	12	< 0.5	< 0.5	< 0.015	< 0.015	8.5	-	-	+Cu+Ti+ Cb	52
AISI 420 B	0.3	13	< 1.0	< 1.0	< 0.030	< 0.040	-	-	-	-	52
"42010" (T.R)	0.2	14.5	< 1.0	< 1.0	< 0.030	< 0.040	0.7	0.8	-	-	51
AISI 431	0.16	16.5	< 1.0	< 1.0	< 0.030	< 0.040	-	-	-	-	43-47
AISI 630	< 0.07	17	< 1.0	< .0	< 0.030	< 0.040	4	-	-	+Cu+Cb	44
AISI 440 C	1.0	17	< 1.0	< 1.0	< 0.030	< 0.040	-	0.5	-	-	60
X 15 T.N	0.40	15.5	< 0.6	< 0.6	< 0.005	< 0.020	-	2.0	0.3	N: 0.2%	59

Existing steels available offer a dilemma, either a high carbon level offering good mechanical properties and poor corrosion resistance, or low carbon level improving corrosion but lowering mechanical properties. X 15 T.N was designed to address this dilemma and offer a good compromise between hardness, corrosion resistance and mechanical behavior.

Composition

Typical Chemical Composition is as follows: 0.40% carbon, 15.5% chromium, 2.00% molybdenum, 0.30% vanadium, and **0.20% nitrogen**.

Numerical simulation, using the most recent thermodynamic data, was used to optimize chemical composition (Figure 1). This was necessary to obtain a stabilized martensitic composition that contained a high nitrogen content. For reasons of cost and manufacturing capabilities reasons, we chose to use only conventional melting processes. For these reasons, powder metallurgy technology or high pressure remelting such as Pressurized Electro Slag Remelting (PESR) were not taken into consideration. The final composition is based on the achievable properties and structure following a easy heat-treatment.

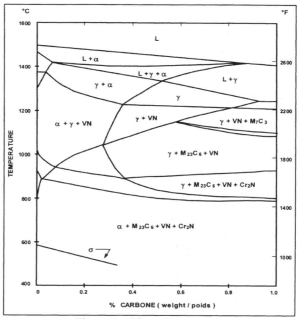

Figure 1 - *Phase Diagram*

It is possible to summarize the optimized balance as follows:

Carbon: This level, combined with le nitrogen content, is adequate for obtaining a high hardness without an excessive number of carbides after hardening and tempering.

Chromium: This level allows, in relation to the carbon content, the formation of a passive layer to ensure high corrosion resistance.

Molybdenum: The addition of molybdenum provides a more stable passive layer for improved corrosion resistance, especially in a chloride environment.

Vanadium: Added to allow the formation of vanadium nitride/carbonitride for improved cutting edge capabilities. Moreover, it allows secondary hardening that can be used with some special heat treatments for parts designed to receive a Physical Vapor Deposition (PVD) type coating.

Nitrogen: Added to replace part of the carbon, to insure proper hardening response and improved corrosion resistance.

Nickel: None added to X 15 T.N.

Micrographs of AISI 440C and X 15 T.N, shown in figure 2, clearly illustrate the improvements brought by X 15 T.N as regards morphology, size and carbide density.

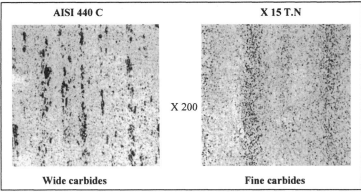

Figure 2 – *Comparison of Structures*

Melting Route

The melting and refining route (Figure 3) starts with an arc furnace primary melting operation followed by Argon Oxygen Decarburization (AOD) refining. At that stage, the nominal composition of the steel is established. At a later stage, an Electro Slag Remelting (ESR) operation is performed with a slag that is formulated for this grade. ESR lowers the sulfur content for increased corrosion resistance, uniformly distributes the nitrogen content and provides microstructural homogeneity. Finally, the nonmetallic inclusion content is lowered thereby increasing toughness and fatigue characteristics. Afterwards, X 15 T.N is converted by forging, hot-rolling and sometime cold-working, to manufacture bars, rods and sheets.

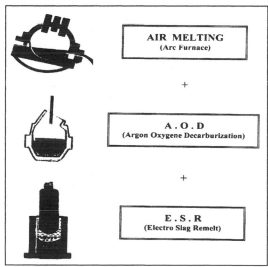

Figure 3 – *Melting Route*

Heat Treatment and Resultant Mechanical Characteristics

Continuous Transformation Temperature (CCT) diagram (Figure 4) and tempering curve (Figure 5), illustrate perfectly the heat treatment possibilities for the grade. For medical instrument applications, best performances are obtained through two different quenching and tempering treatments to which a useful annealing treatment can be added if the instrument is made from a forging.

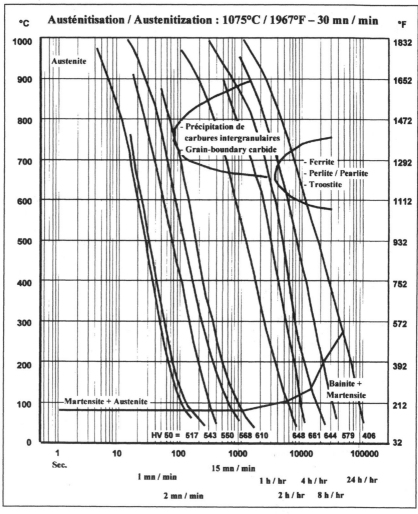

Figure 4 - *Continuous Transformation Temperature (CTT) diagram*

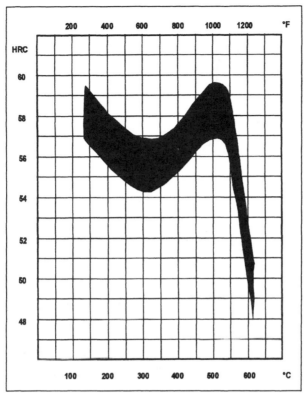

Figure 5 - *Tempering Curve (austenization between*
980°C/1800°F and 1077°C/1970°F)

Annealing

The annealing treatment state is given by the following :
1. Heat up to 840°C/1544°F
2. Slowly cool in furnace or under ashes.
A hardness of approximately 207 HB will be obtained.

Heat Treatment for HRc ≥ 58 : Dedicated for Maximum Hardness (Figure 6)

Typical mechanical properties:

UTS   : 336KSI / 2320MPa   Charpy V-Notch Impact Strenght: 7.5 ft.lb /10J
$YS_{0.2\%}$: 265KSI / 1825MPa K_1C : 12.7KSI$\sqrt{in}$ / 14MPa$\sqrt{m}$
Elongation: 4%
Fatigue limit (rotating bending) 10^7cycles : 135KSI / 928MPa

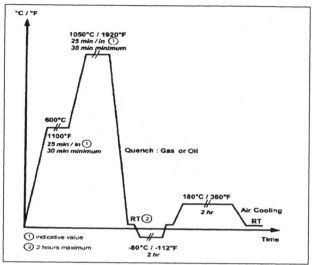

Figure 6 - *Thermal cycle for HRc ≥ 58*

Heat Treatment for HRC ≥ 55 : Dedicated for Easy Heat Treatment (Figure 7)

Typical mechanical properties:

UTS   : 313KSI / 2160MPa   Charpy V-Notch Impact Strenght: 7.5 ft.lb /10J
$YS_{0.2\%}$: 233KSI / 1610MPa K_1C : 18.2KSI$\sqrt{in}$ / 20MPa$\sqrt{m}$
Elongation : 4%
Fatigue limit (rotating bending) 10^7cycles : 125KSI / 865Mpa

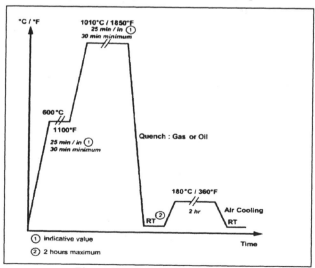

Figure 7 - *Thermal cycle for HRC ≥ 55*

A close look at these properties illustrates :
1. Low nonmetallic inclusion content and a fine carbide distribution provides high resistance to crack initiation and outstanding fatigue behavior.
2. The caracteristics of nitrogenized martensitic steel is a low toughness. This is the result of the intensity of internal stress created by the very high supersaturation of the martensite of these grades in nitrogen and carbon.
This property, seen only in highly nitrogen enriched martensitic steel, brings to the designer the assurance of having a durable instrument as long as he avoids local stress concentration resulting from inadequate design (sharp angle) and/or poor surface finish (machining grooves). A good surface finish improves tenacity and at the same time increases corrosion resistance.

Corrosion Resistance

Salt Spray Test

The closest "real life" environment test to grade corrosion performance is also the most simple: the grade either corrodes or it does not corrode after a given exposure time. Charts of comparative tests between 440C AISI, XM 16, AISI 630 and X 15 TN are shown in Figure 8. They illustrate the drastically superior behavior of X 15 TN.

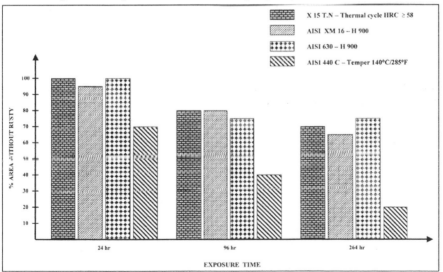

Figure 8 – *Salt Spray Test*

X 15 T.N performs at least as well as precipitation hardening grades, such as AISI 630 and XM 16, in spite of a much higher hardness, respectively 15 and 7 HRC higher.
For a similar hardness, (59/60 HRc) results on the X 15 TN are far better than AISI 440C.

After prolonged exposure, observed rusting of X 15 TN is superficial and can be removed with a light rubbing with sand paper whereas, 440C has deep corrosion pits (Figure 9)

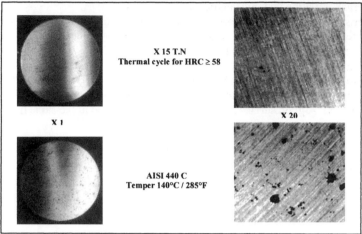

Figure 9 - *Comparison after soft polishing*

These tests were performed according to NFX 41-002 standard on polished samples. Tests conducted on rough machined surfaces show a slower rusting acceleration on AISI 630 and 440C than on X 15 TN and AISI XM 16. Tests run according to ASTM B 117 and DIN 50021 reach the same conclusion.

Potentio-Kinetic Tests

Potentiokinetic tests allow the evaluation of passive layer behavior and the corrosion risks in various grade-environment combinations.

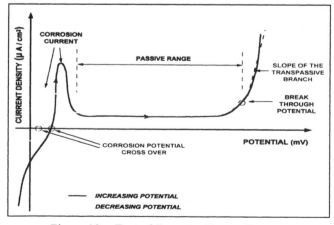

Figure 10 – *Typical Potentio-Kinetic Curve*

The typical feature of potential-current diagrams, and the terms generally used, are shown in Figure 10.

Tests in Sulfuric Acid Solution

Tests were made at a temperature of 20°C/68°F in a 1% sulfuric acid solution, argon saturated, typical environment to test general corrosion. Two potential closed loops were made (Figure 11 and Table 2). Current levels at the corrosion peak allow us to evaluate clearly the behavior of the three grades tested.

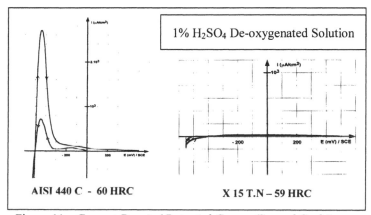

Figure 11 - *Current Density/ Potential Curves (Second Cycle)*

Current levels at the corrosion peak allow us to evaluate clearly the behavior of the three grades tested.

Table 2 - *Corrosion Current at the Peak*

Cycle		Current Density (µA/cm²)		
		AISI 420B 52HRC	**AISI 440C** 60HRC	**X 15 T.N** 59HRC
First	Increasing potential	2400	1100	400
	Decreasing potential	10	500	<6*
Second	Increasing potential	2700	2700	<6*
	Decreasing potential	20	700	<6*

*limite measurement.

Corrosion currents observed on X 15 TN are much lower by a large margin than those of AISI 440C. They are also better than AISI 420 that, furthermore, has a lower hardness.

Tests in 0.9%NaCl Solution, (37°C/98.6°F, Aerated Condition)

Tests made on X 15 T.N at a 59 HRC hardness show a good behavior in this chloride environment and confirm salt spray test results (Figure 12).

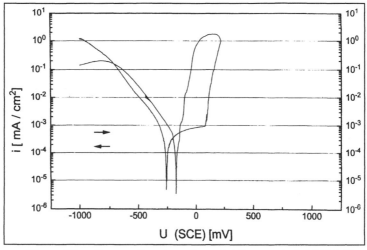

Figure 12 - *Current Density – Potential Curves in 0.9 % NaCl*
Oxygenated Solution (37°C / 98.6°F)

Drill Penetration and Cutting Tests

Drilling Test in bone

Conditions

Drills	: 3.2 mm gray drills
Depth of holes	: 15mm
Speed	: 500 rpm
Cutting Fluid	: Dry
Feed	: 25.5 mm/min.
Tool life End Point	: 0.030" or 300 hole limit

Test Result

X15TN (59HRc)	220 holes - 0.032" wear
AISI 630 (H900)	10 holes - 0.032"wear
AISI XM16 (H900)	35 holes – 0.030"wear

Cutting Test on C.A.T.R.A. Machine

Most tests to qualify cutting behavior of instruments are made with prototype parts put on test bed which simulate the conditions of use. Then it is difficult to match the data of different laboratories. In an over hand the knife industry is using the C.A.T.R.A. machine from British Cutlery Association. During this test, the maximum thickness which a cutting device is able to cut is measured. All test parameters are fixed: paper quality, speed and load.
The decreasing of the maximum thickness reached is recorded test after test without edge sharpening. A second way is to record the total thickness of paper cut after a fixed number of tests.

In the Figure 13 we compare data for steels including AISI 440Amod. (0.55%C, 15%Cr), AISI 420HC (0.42%C, 13%Cr) and X 15TN for 50 mm/sec cutting speed and 45 N load.

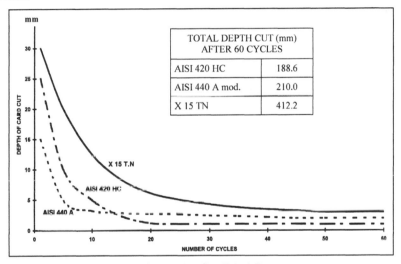

TOTAL DEPTH CUT (mm) AFTER 60 CYCLES	
AISI 420 HC	188.6
AISI 440 A mod.	210.0
X 15 TN	412.2

Figure 13 : C A T R A Test

Workability

Hot Working is easy in the temperature range of 2140/1830°F (1170/1000°C).

Cold Forming characteristics, in operations such as rolling, extrusion, drawing, ... are similar to a number of other martensitic stainless steels of 400 series.

Machinability, in annealed condition, is close to AISI 420 or 431.

For Cleaning/Passivation, the HNO_3-$Na_2Cr_2O_7.2H_2O$ solution, generally used with martensitic steels is appropriate.
Welding is possible, either without filler metal or if needed with AISI 430 filler welding wire.

Applications

As of today X 15 TN has found application as (Figure 14)

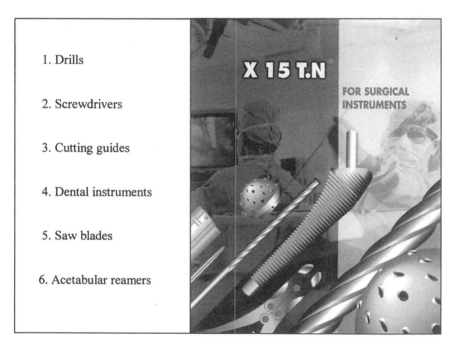

1. Drills

2. Screwdrivers

3. Cutting guides

4. Dental instruments

5. Saw blades

6. Acetabular reamers

Figure 14

1. Disposable drills for trauma and femoral reamers used to implement hip prothesis.
2. Screwdrivers generally used to fix trauma devices and spine systems
3. Cutting guides used during knee operations in order to guide the saw which permit to remorve the appropriate part of bone
4. Dental instruments such as microdrills
5. Saw blade used together with cutting guides during knee operations
6. Acetabular reamers used to remorve the cartilage before fixing the acetabular cup linked to the head of the hip prothesis.

Conclusions

The composition choices made when developing X15T.N have allowed us to respond in a balanced way to various and sometimes conflicting property requirements. X15TN has a similar hardness to that of AISI 440C, and due to its fine and homogeneous structure it exhibits good edge retension. Its corrosion resistance is greatly enhanced. Moreover, X 15T.N offers a better toughness/fatigue than AISI 440C.Compared to XM 16 or 630, heat treatment is not as easy for X 15 T.N and toughness is at a small disadvantage, but cutting properties and wear resistance are greatly superior, while corrosion characteristics are comparable. Machining is comparable to other martensitic stainless steel e.g. AISI 420-431 and 440C.X 15 T.N is registered as UNS S 42025 and an introductory paper was presented at the revision of ASTM F 899, 1995 edition.

Charles H. Craig,[1] Herbert R. Radisch, Jr.,[1] Thomas A. Trozera,[2] Paul C. Turner,[3] R. Dale Govier,[3] Edward J. Vesely, Jr.,[4] Nev A. Gokcen,[5] Clifford M. Friend,[6] and Michael R. Edwards[6]

Development of a Platinum-Enhanced Radiopaque Stainless Steel (PERSS®)[7]

Reference: Craig, C. H., Radisch, H. R., Jr., Trozera, T. A., Turner, P. C., Govier, R. D., Vesely, E. J., Jr., Gokcen, N. A., Friend, C. M., and Edwards, M. R., **"Development of a Platinum Enhanced Radiopaque Stainless Steel (PERSS®),"** *Stainless Steels for Medical and Surgical Applications, ASTM STP 1438,* G. L. Winters and M. J. Nutt, Eds., ASTM International, West Conshohocken, PA, 2003.

Abstract: Balloon-expandable coronary stents may be made of stainless steel conforming to ASTM or ISO specifications, referred to by ASTM as UNS S31673 alloys. A need exists for an alloy with enhanced radiopacity to make stents more visible radiographically and more effective clinically. A research program was initiated with the objectives of enhancing fluoroscopic radiopacity while maintaining adherence to the ASTM and ISO specifications. These objectives were ultimately achieved by adding a noble metal, platinum, to UNS S31673 by vacuum induction melting a commercially-available alloy. Freedom of the resulting microstructure from formation of harmful topologically close packed phases was ensured by use of phase computation methodology (New PHACOMP), and confirmed by X-ray diffraction and transmission electron microscopy. Platinum was chosen since it is over twice as dense as nickel and, with approximately half its effect as an austenitizer, allows nickel content to be reduced to a minimum level.

Keywords: stainless steel, platinum, coronary stent, radiopacity, New PHACOMP

Introduction

Balloon-expandable coronary stents may be made of a low-carbon, austenitic, non-magnetic, implant grade stainless steel that is similar to AISI/ANSI 316L. Bar and wire are described in ASTM Specification for Wrought 18 Chromium-14 Nickel- 2.5

---

[1] Research & Development (R&D) Engineer and Vice President for R&D, respectively, Boston Scientific Corporation/Interventional Technologies, 3574 Ruffin Rd., San Diego, CA, 92123.

[2] Consultant, 437 Pine Needles Dr., Del Mar, CA, 92014.

[3] Associate Director for Thermal Treatment Technologies and Chemist respectively, Albany Research Center, U.S. Department of Energy, 1450 Queen Ave., SW, Albany, OR, 97321.

[4] Consultant, 387 River Bend Dr., Huntsville, AL, 35824.

[5] Consultant, 385 Palos Verdes Dr. W, Palos Verdes Estates, CA, 90274.

[6] Professor and Head, and Senior Lecturer, respectively, Department of Materials and Medical Sciences, Cranfield Postgraduate Medical School, Shrivenham, Swindon SN6 8LA, United Kingdom.

[7] Registered trademark: Boston Scientific Corporation/Interventional Technologies, San Diego, CA.

Molybdenum Stainless Steel Bar and Wire for Surgical Implants (UNS S31673), F138, while sheet and strip are described in ASTM Specification for Wrought 18 Chromium-14 Nickel- 2.5 Molybdenum Stainless Steel Sheet and Strip for Surgical Implants (UNS S31673), F139. In composition and properties, F138 and F139 alloys parallel Composition D of Part 1 (Wrought stainless steel) of International Standard ISO 5832-1 (Implants for surgery – metallic materials). Low carbon content is stipulated to assure freedom from intergranular corrosion susceptibility; F138 and F139 also require these alloys to meet corrosion susceptibility tests. Pitting resistance is ensured by controlling chromium and molybdenum weight percent, w, by the formula

$$Composition\ (C) = w\ Cr + 3.3\ w\ Mo \geq 26. \tag{1}$$

Concerns for both corrosion and fatigue resistance are addressed by maintaining a fine-grained structure that is free from ferrite and low in nonmetallic inclusions.

Tubular, mesh-type coronary stents made from these alloys are placed through non-invasive procedures inside diseased arteries that have been identified as areas where blood flow is restricted. The stent is mounted on a balloon catheter that may have gold or platinum marker bands at each end, which will increase radiographic visibility by increasing overall fluorescent radiopacity of the stent and deployment system, enabling precise placement of the stent within the artery. Once coronary stents are deployed and their deployment systems are removed, including marker bands, stents with poor radiopacity can no longer be visualized radiographically. This represents a problem if it is found that the stent needs further dilatation.

The design of the coronary stent is such that it is at its minimum diameter, in a compressed state on the balloon catheter, to facilitate winding its way through arteries to the point where it is to be deployed by pressurization of the balloon catheter. During the expansion from a compressed to an extended state, the struts of the mesh-type stent may be partially reduced in cross sectional area due to plastic strain that results from having surpassed the elastic limit of the alloy. After deployment, because of reduced thickness, the struts may exhibit even greater indications of less-than-ideal fluoroscopic radiopacity. To enhance the fluorescent radiopacity of these stainless steel stents, strut thicknesses can be increased, but this will be at the expense of overall flexibility and expandability.

Alternatives to use of UNS S31673 alloys have been sought due to the less-than-ideal radiopacities exhibited by deployed coronary stents made of these alloys. In their stent handbook, Serruys and Rensing [1] compare most coronary stents that are available today in terms of their mechanism for deployment and other features such as radiopacity and flexibility. They noted that the following approaches have been used: tantalum, platinum wire (as a core inside a cobalt alloy tube), and gold electroplating. Other means of applying radiopaque coatings are a topic of current research interest [2]; these include coatings of iridium, platinum and gold. These alternatives to UNS S31673 alloys have used external means to enhance radiopacity or replaced it with more radiopaque material.

Background and Initial Approach

Boston Scientific Corporation/Interventional Technologies (BSC/IVT) developed a balloon-expandable coronary stent (LP Stent™[8]) that is made from stainless steel foil. The foil is formed into tubing and the stent is then fabricated by a photo-etch process.

To better understand the structural and functional embodiments of its LP Stent design, IVT conducted an internal study [3] of available coronary stents at its corporate research and development laboratories. The results of this study correlated well with IVT's initial design study, which indicated UNS S31673 alloys represented the most universal solution to the design and manufacturing features that were to be incorporated into the LP Stent. However, all stainless steel stents that compared well to the flexibility of BSC/IVT's LP Stent were considered insufficiently radiopaque.

Since the photo-etch process chosen to fabricate the intricate LP Stent design was specific to iron-base alloys, substituting tantalum would not only invalidate the work that went into developing and refining this unique process and require an alternate process to be developed, but it would potentially make the stent design too radiopaque. A platinum and cobalt alloy wire design could not be applied to the LP Stent design or fabrication process. With the electropolished finish, coatings would not adhere well to the LP Stent and may be brittle, which could compromise the flexible design.

Having considered the above, it was decided to establish a research program to study the addition of an additional element, tantalum, unspecified in F139, to the UNS S31673 alloy, thus maintaining adherence to this specification while increasing its radiopacity.

In the United States and elsewhere, government regulatory bodies monitor evolution and implementation of all new stent designs, their materials of construction, and analyze risks associated with *in vivo* and *in vitro* testing. Since radiopacity is a functional rather than a structural requirement, F138 and F139 alloys have not been subjected to regulation in the past. ASTM Committee F04 (Medical and Surgical Materials and Devices) has recently addressed this issue and a document is in draft. ASTM Test Methods for Radiopacity of Plastics for Medical Use, F649m discusses radiopacity and provides several comparative approaches based on use of film radiography. F640 refers to the attenuation law (Beer-Lambert), citing ASTM Terminology Relating to Metallography, E7, where transmissivity [4], T, the ratio of transmitted X-ray intensity I_t to incident intensity I_e is

$$I_t / I_e = exp [- (\mu) X] = T \qquad (2)$$

where μ is the linear attenuation coefficient and X the thickness of the absorbing material.

The above applies for an idealized case [5] of a narrow-beam X-ray photon of incident intensity I_e penetrating a layer of material of thickness X (where μX is dimensionless). The remaining photons emerge from the attenuator with transmitted intensity I_t according to the Beer-Lambert law, Eq. 2. Published data are often listed as the mass attenuation coefficient, μ/ρ, where ρ in g/cm^3, is the density of the element. Values of densities and of linear and mass absorption coefficients, at 80 keV and at 100 keV, are in Table 1 for the elements Cr, Fe, Ni, Mo, Ta, and Pt. As shown in Eq. 3, the ratio of incident X-ray intensities to transmitted intensities is the radiopacity [4], R, of the attenuating material

$$I_e / I_t = exp [(\mu) X] = R \qquad (3)$$

---

[8] Trademark applied for: Boston Scientific Corporation/Interventional Technologies, San Diego, CA.

Table 1 – *Linear and Mass Absorption Coefficients and Densities [4]*

	Cr	Fe	Ni	Mo	Ta	Pt
ρ	7.180	7.874	8.902	10.220	16.650	21.450
μ/ρ 80 keV	0.491	0.595	0.731	1.962	7.587	8.731
μ 80 keV	3.522	4.687	6.504	20.052	126.324	187.28
μ/ρ 100 keV	0.317	0.372	0.444	1.096	4.302	4.993
μ 100 keV	2.273	2.927	3.952	11.201	71.628	107.10

Eq. 3 shows that as either the linear absorption coefficient or the thickness of the material is changed, so does radiopacity. For film radiography, we have these same relationships, where the optical transmission density of the radiographic film, D, is as shown below [5]

$$D = log \, I_e / I_t. \tag{4}$$

Here I_e is incident light from the optical densitometer on the radiographic film (absorber), I_t is the light transmitted through the absorber, and I_e / I_t is the opacity of the absorber.

From the above, with stent wall thickness $X = 12.7 \times 10^{-3}$ cm, we calculate T and R for Ta and Pt and for primary elements of an alloy similar to UNS S31673, Table 2.

Table 2 – *Radiopacities & Transmissivities for Ta, Pt, and Primary Elements of 316L*

	Ta	Pt	Cr	Fe	Ni	Mo
$R_{80 \, keV}$	4.974	10.788	1.046	1.061	1.086	1.290
$T_{80 \, keV}$	0.201	0.093	0.956	0.942	0.921	0.775
$R_{100 \, keV}$	2.484	3.897	1.029	1.038	1.051	1.153
$T_{100 \, keV}$	0.403	0.257	0.972	0.964	0.951	0.867

Table 3 shows the Table 2 values for Ta and Pt, while Table 4 shows calculated values, using appropriate weight percentages, for primary elements of a 316L type stainless steel. Low transmission of both Ta and Pt contrasts with extremely high transmission of 316L.

Table 3 – *Calculated Radiopacities & Transmissivities for Tantalum and Platinum*

	Ta	Pt	$R_{80 \, keV}$	$T_{80 \, keV}$	$R_{100 \, keV}$	$T_{100 \, keV}$
w	100	-	4.974	0.201	2.484	0.403
w	-	100	10.788	0.093	3.897	0.257

Table 4 – *Calculated Radiopacities & Transmissivities for Primary Elements of 316L*

	Cr	Fe	Ni	Mo	$R_{80 \, keV}$	$T_{80 \, keV}$	$R_{100 \, keV}$	$T_{100 \, keV}$
w	18	65.5	14	2.5	1.066	0.938	1.040	0.961

As can be seen from Tables 5 and 6, when stainless steel with either tantalum or platinum is compared to the native 316L-type alloy, a decrease in transmissivity is obtained based on the enhanced radiopacity of the resulting alloy.

Table 5 – *Calculated Transmissivities for a Stainless Steel Containing 5 w Ta or 5 w Pt*

	Cr	Fe	Ni	Mo	Ta	Pt	$T_{80 keV}$	$T_{100 keV}$
w	18	61.5	13	2.5	5	-	0.901	0.940
w	18	61.5	13	2.5	-	5	0.893	0.934

Table 6 – *Calculated Radiopacities for a Stainless Steel Containing 5 w Ta or 5 w Pt*

	Cr	Fe	Ni	Mo	Ta	Pt	$R_{80 keV}$	$R_{100 keV}$
w	18	61.5	13	2.5	5	-	1.110	1.064
w	18	61.5	13	2.5	-	5	1.120	1.070

Initially, the argument was in favor of adding tantalum since it is not a noble metal and thus would be much more economical as an alloying element. It is a carbide former, used in austenitic steels such as AISI 347 and AISI 348 in amounts up to 0.9 w to decrease the alloy susceptibility to intergranular corrosion [6]. While determining the solubility of tantalum in UNS S31673 alloys is usually considered too difficult, a quaternary stainless steel can be devised from binary data [7], comprised of 18 w Cr, 14 w Ni; added fourth (high-density) element, M, balance Fe. For such an alloy, it was estimated that roughly 2.9 w Ta would be soluble.

An experiment was devised in which industrial radiographs were taken of a stainless steel base partially covered with a foil step-wedge made of tantalum; the thicknesses were approximately 2.5 %, 4.0 %, and 5.0 % of the stainless steel base. This allowed the use of an optical film densitometer to compare the resulting film densities. Based on these results, it was determined that between 1 and 5 w tantalum would be required to slightly enhance radiopacity of coronary stents made of the resulting alloy over the X-ray energy range used in a catheterization laboratory (~65 keV to ~120 keV).

Tantalum was added to a commercial UNS S31673 alloy meeting F138 specifications, BioDur[9] 316LS and cast in 100 g ingots. Five ingots containing nominally 1.0 w to 5.0 w Ta in the stainless steel matrix were cast. Compositions of the alloys are in Table 7.

Table 7 – *Compositions of Remelted BioDur 316LS containing Ta*

	IVT # 18	IVT # 19	IVT # 20	IVT # 21	IVT # 22
Nominal w	1.00	2.00	3.00	4.00	5.00
Actual w	0.84	1.87	2.58	3.56	4.40

The production of the alloys and their subsequent rolling was accomplished at the U. S. Department of Energy's Albany Research Center (ARC). These ingots were made in an arc furnace, using a triple-melt procedure and one-third atmosphere argon; the ingot

---

[9] Registered trademark of Carpenter Technology Corporation, Reading, PA.

(button) was contained on a water-cooled copper hearth and the components were melted using a thoriated W tip to establish and control the arc, much as a welding rod might be used. The buttons were heated slowly to 870°C, then heated rapidly to 1150-1260°C; they were then hot-rolled from an average thickness of 8.5 mm to 3.0 mm in 15 % reductions, with five minutes for reheats between passes, annealed at 1040°C and water-quenched. The resulting shape was then milled to the thickness (2.54 mm) of the stainless steel base that had been radiographed along with the tantalum step wedge so the radiographic results could be compared. The film density measurements, D, compared well with those from the plate-stepwedge.

X-ray diffraction results of the five cast and rolled specimens indicated the presence of an eta phase, Fe_2Ta, which is a Laves-type topologically close-packed (TCP) structure [6] that began to appear with the 1.91 w Ta specimen. This indicated that the solubility of tantalum in the BioDur 316LS alloy was less than initially predicted. The solubility for tungsten can be similarly predicted to be about 13.6 w. Tungsten is attractive from the point of view that, like tantalum, it is a dense element that would promote radiopacity if added to the stainless steel matrix. The possibility of using tungsten was pursued as a companion experiment to the use of tantalum; five 100 g buttons were cast as previously described, containing from 1.0 to 5.0 w W. These were rolled into plate, machined, and radiographed, confirming radiopacity expectations. However, at 4.0 w W and above, X-ray diffraction clearly indicated the presence of ferrite.

Analysis

From the above experiments, it was obvious that sufficient amounts of tantalum or tungsten would not be soluble in the 316LS matrix to achieve the objectives of enhancing a functional requirement, radiopacity, while maintaining or improving upon structural requirements. Analysis of these experiments entailed looking more closely at the problem to be solved and determining how to proceed in order to succeed with another alloying element since the functional (enhanced radiopacity) experiments were considered to be successful.

In AISI 347 and AISI 348 austenitic stainless steels, tantalum and niobium are added because they are carbide formers and may be used [4] singly or together, in amounts of up to ten times the carbon content in these alloys, to stabilize the grade against chromium carbide formation. This decreases the susceptibility to chromium depletion, which would lead to intergranular corrosion in harsh environments. In the UNS S31673 matrix, there is no excess carbon, thus in the case of tantalum additions, there is a Laves-type TCP-structure, the Fe_2Ta eta phase, and at higher tantalum contents, some indications of the formation of ferrite. The tungsten additions clearly formed ferrite, along with an unidentified phase, especially at higher contents. Tantalum and tungsten are known ferrite-formers [6], so the presence of ferrite in these alloys it to be expected.

Approach

The precious metals, iridium, platinum and gold can be considered as potential alloying elements. Biocompatibility would thus not be a first-order issue if one of these were to be selected as an unspecified additional element in UNS S31673 alloys.

Solubility of these elements in the simple quaternary described above (18 w Cr, 14 w Ni, M, balance Fe) is excellent; we find, at 900°C, iridium and platinum are completely soluble in this quaternary and gold can be dissolved up to 37 w. The maximum amounts of noble elements envisioned to enhance radiopacity of coronary stents made by adding such unspecified additional elements to UNS S31673 are well below these solubility levels. When considering the use of iridium, platinum and gold as alloying elements, platinum was selected, in spite of its high price, since iridium was even more expensive and gold does not act as an austenite stabilizer [8].

UNS S31673 alloys must meet ASTM requirements for ferrite content and inclusion content. The presence of topologically close packed phases (TCP) in such alloys is unacceptable because of their effect on alloy ductility

The approach applied by DuPont [9] and described recently by its originators Morinaga et al [10] is used to predict the onset of TCPs; New PHACOMP was developed for and is principally used in the development of Ni-base superalloys. The original PHACOMP, which New PHACOMP would replace, emerged during the 1960s in response to TCP (sigma phase) problems with superalloys in high-temperature service and is attributable to Boesch and Slaney [11]. An overview of the state of the art of the original PHACOMP technology, circa 1987, is given by Sims [12]. Barrows and Newkirk [13] provide a model that describes the gamma phase-sigma phase boundary (solvus) more closely than earlier works, in terms of concentration and temperature. The methodology of [10] was developed in the early 1980s to address problems encountered in using Ni_3Al (gamma-prime) arising from the use of aluminum in nickel-base superalloys. The so-called cluster model surrounding nickel aluminide, with its formula $MNi_{12}Al_6$, led Morinaga et al to obtain the effect of a transition metal M on the electronic structure of the nickel aluminide in terms of energy levels (eigenvalues), which are expressed in electron volts (eV) relative to the Ni_3Al Fermi level; this level is arbitrarily set to zero for both Ni and Ni_3Al. These eigenvalues, due to the d-orbitals of the transition metals, are referred to as Md levels, or parameters, expressed in eV. In [10], a list of elements typically used in superalloys and steels is provided, along with their respective Md parameters. The New PHACOMP approach defines the average Md, which is the compositional value for an alloy, as

$$Md(avg) = \sum [x_i (Md)_i] \qquad (5)$$

where x_i is the atomic fraction of component element i and $(Md)_i$ is the value of Md for each element i constituting the alloy. It was shown by Morinaga et al that the values of Md(avg) roughly approximate the single phase gamma boundaries in a large number of ternary alloys. Further, as an example, it was shown that when Md(avg) was greater than 0.925 eV at 1200°C, the TCP phases were precipitated out of the gamma phase.

It was decided to use New PHACOMP to determine whether TCPs would form on adding certain unspecified additional elements to a UNS S31673 matrix. At the time, the Md parameters for the three noble metals under consideration (Ir, Pt, Au) had not been published and assumed values were utilized, based on the Md parameters available. The

Md for Ir was subsequently published in [10]; Morinaga has also provided[10] the Md parameters for Pt (0.764 eV), Au (0.627 eV), Pd (0.779 eV), and Ag (0.659 eV), along with corresponding bond orders (Bo) of these elements, as in [10], with Bo parameters of 0.920 eV (Pt), 0.528 eV (Au), 0.751 eV (Pd), and 0.391 eV (Ag).

Using appropriate Md parameters from the above discussion for the hypothetical quaternary alloy discussed above, we find the average Md parameters are greater for Ta and W but approximately equal for Ir, Pt, and Au

Table 8 – *Md(avg) for Hypothetical Quaternary with 0 w and 5 w Ta, W, Ir, Pt, Au*

5 *wt%* Ta	5 *wt%* W	5 *wt%* Ir	quaternary	5 *wt%* Pt	5 *wt%* Au
Md(avg) = 0.918 eV	Md(avg) = 0.909 eV	Md(avg) = 0.897 eV	Md(avg) = 0.895 eV	Md(avg) = 0.895 eV	Md(avg) = 0.893 eV

Using appropriate Md parameters in TCP-free F138 alloy (Carpenter BioDur 316LS), average Md parameters increase with the BCC elements but remain stable with Ir, Pt, Au

Table 9 – *Md(avg) for BioDur 316LS with 0 w and 5 w Ta, W, Ir, Pt, Au*

5 *wt%* Ta + 316LS	5 *wt%* W + 316LS	5 *wt%* Ir + 316LS	BioDur 316LS	5 *wt%* Pt + 316LS	5 *wt%* Au + 316LS
Md(avg) = 0.936 eV	Md(avg) = 0.927 eV	Md(avg) = 0.915 eV	Md(avg) = 0.915 eV	Md(avg) = 0.913 eV	Md(avg) = 0.911 eV

For Ir only in a 316LS base, we have the following average Md parameters

Table 10 – *Md(avg) for BioDur 316LS with 0 w to 60 w Ir*

BioDur 316LS	7.5 *w* Ir + 316LS	15 *w* Ir + 316LS	30 *w* Ir + 316LS	45 *w* Ir + 316LS	60 *w* Ir + 316LS
Md(avg) = 0.915 eV	Md(avg) = 0.915 eV	Md(avg) = 0.915 eV	Md(avg) = 0.914 eV	Md(avg) = 0.914 eV	Md(avg) = 0.913 eV

These 100 g ingots of platinum containing alloys were cast, rolled, annealed, and machined to shape. X-ray diffraction was used to determine the presence of either TCP phases or ferrite. Whereas tantalum, with an Md of 2.224 eV, resulted in an alloy containing a TCP (eta phase), and tungsten, with an Md of 1.655 eV, resulted in an alloy containing ferrite, the diffraction results showed an absence of ferrite or TCPs in the BioDur 316LS containing platinum. Radiopacity measurements, as with tantalum and tungsten, were as expected; sufficient enhancement in radiopacity of the resulting coronary stents would be provided by approximately 5.0 *w* Pt. Thus it was decided to cast a 50 kg ingot in order to try all applicable manufacturing processes. Later, a further series

---

[10] Morinaga, M., Nagoya University, Nagoya, JP, personal communication with Charles Craig, Interventional Technologies, Inc., San Diego, CA, October 2001.

of small ingots, with platinum contents up to 10 w, was cast. These were then processed as before and subjected to the same analysis; no indications of TCPs were found and radiopacity results compared well with expectations. Tubes were then manufactured from the 5 w Pt foil. These tubes were examined by optical and transmission electron microscopy (TEM). No indications were found of any of these tubes containing TCPs.

Although enhancing the radiopacity of the UNS S31673 alloys by intentionally adding platinum as unspecified additional elements appears to be new, alloying stainless steels with platinum group metals for other purposes is not new, dating back to 1911 [13]. More modern efforts to use such materials appear to be based on extensive, corrosion-related research conducted in the former Soviet Union beginning in the late 1940s, which first reached a large audience outside that community in a translated textbook [14] during the late 1960s. McGill [15, 16] has reviewed the effects of platinum group metals on the corrosion and mechanical properties of stainless steels.

Approximately 14 kg of the first 50 kg ingot containing 5 w platinum in 316LS was rolled into sheet and then into foil and tubing suitable for prototype fabrication of a next-generation LP Stent. This was examined for pitting resistance and susceptibility to corrosion in accordance with F138 and F139 and is reported by Covino *et al* [17], where it is shown that this alloy fully complies with the pitting and corrosion requirements of F138 and F139.

Summary and Conclusions

The addition of platinum to a commercially-available alloy complying to F138, BioDur 316LS, has provided enhancement in the radiopacity of the resulting stainless steel, referred to here as PERSS. PERSS may not qualify under F138 or F139 due to the intentional addition of dense elements, but the criteria of those specifications is used for reference purposes. For this new alloy to be useful for coronary stents the modified alloy must still be capable of being processed and to survive *in vivo*. Corrosion behavior (intergranular corrosion susceptibility; pitting resistance), as well as metallurgical and mechanical properties, to include freedom from formation of delta ferrite and low microinclusion content, must be similar to BioDur 316LS, as specified by F138 and F139. These aims are achieved by BioDur 316LS stainless steels alloyed with platinum.

References

[1]   Serruys, P. W. and Rensing, B., Eds., *Handbook of Coronary Stents, 4th edition*, Martin Dunitz, Ltd., London, 2001.

[2]   Sahagian, R. "Critical Insight: Marking Devices with Radiopaque Coatings," *Medical Device & Diagnostic Industry*, Vol. 21, No. 5, 1999, pp. 160-166.

[3]   Radisch, H. "Comparisons of the LP Stent with Other Stent Designs – 2nd edition," internal report, Interventional Technologies, Inc., San Diego, CA, 1999.

[4]   Hubbell, J. H. and Seltzer, S. M. *Tables of X-ray Mass Attenuation Coefficients*

and Mass Energy-Absorption Coefficients (Version 1.03), National Institute of Standards and Technology (NIST), 1997 [Online]. Available: http://physics.nist.gov/xaamdi [2002, February 17], NIST, Gaithersburg, MD.

[5]   ASM International, *ASM Handbook®, Volume 17: Nondestructive Evaluation and Quality Control*, ASM International, Materials Park, OH, 1989, p. 323.

[6]   Beddoes, J., and Parr, J. G. *Introduction to Stainless Steels, 3rd edition*, ASM International, Materials Park, OH, 1999, pp. 137-138.

[7]   Okamoto, H. *Desk Handbook: Phase Diagrams for Binary Alloys*, ASM International, Materials Park, OH, 2000.

[8]   Moema, J., and Paton, R., "The Influence of Gold and Ruthenium on the Austenitic Stability of Type 316L Stainless Steels," internal report by Mintek (Randburg, SA), for Interventional Technologies, Inc., San Diego, CA, 2001.

[9]   DuPont, J. N., "A Combined Solubility Product/New PHACOMP Approach for Estimating Temperatures of Secondary Solidification Reactions in Superalloy Weld Metals," *Metallurgical and Material Transactions*, Vol. 29A, 1998, pp. 1449-1456.

[10]   Morinaga, M., Murata, Y., and Yukawa, H., "Recent Progress in the New PHACOMP Approach," *Materials Design Approaches and Experiences (Proceedings of Symposium sponsored by the High Temperature Alloys Committee of the Structural Alloys Division (SMD) of TMS (The Minerals, Metals & Materials Society)*, Zhao, J. -C., Fahrmann, M., and Pollock, T. M., Eds., TMS, Warrendale, PA, 2001, pp. 15-28.

[11]   Boesch, W. J., and Slaney, J. S., "Preventing Sigma Phase Embrittlement in Nickel Base Superalloys," *Metal Progress*, July 1964, pp. 109-111.

[12]   Sims, C. T., "Prediction of Phase Composition," *Superalloys II*, Sims, C. T., Stoloff, N. S., and Hagel, W. C., Eds., Wiley, New York, 1987, pp. 217-239.

[13]   Monnarz, P., "Contribution to the Study of Ferrochrome Alloys, with Special Consideration Given to Acid Resistance," *Metallurgie*, Vol. 8, No. 7, 1911, pp. 160-176.

[14]   Tomashov, N. D., and Chernova, G. P., *Passivity and Protection of Metals Against Corrosion*, Plenum Press, New York, 1967.

[15]   McGill, I. R., "Platinum Metals in Stainless Steels: A Review of Corrosion and Mechanical Properties," *Platinum Metals Review*, Vol. 34, No. 2, 1990, pp. 85-97.

[16]   McGill, I. R. "Platinum Metals in Stainless Steels: Part II: Further Corrosion and Mechanical Properties," *Platinum Metals Review*, 34, No. 3, 1990, pp. 144-154.

[17]   Covino, B. S., Jr., Craig, C. H., Cramer, S. D., Bullard, S. J., Ziomek-Moroz, M., Jablonski, P. D., Turner, P. C., Radisch, H. R., Jr., Gokcen, N. A., Friend, C. M., and Edwards, M. R., "Corrosion Behavior of Platinum-Enhanced Radiopaque Stainless Steel (PERSS®) for Dilation-Balloon Expandable Coronary Stents," *Stainless Steels for Medical and Surgical Applications, ASTM STP 1438*, G. L. Winters and M. J. Nutt, Eds., ASTM International, West Conshohocken, PA, 2003.

Markus Windler,[1] and Rainer Steger[1]

Mechanical and Corrosion Properties of Forged Hip Stems made of High-Nitrogen Stainless Steel

Reference: Windler, M., and Steger, R., "**Mechanical and Corrosion Properties of Forged Hip Stems made of High-Nitrogen Stainless Steel,**" *Stainless Steels for Medical and Surgical Applications, ASTM STP 1438*, G. L. Winters and M. J. Nutt, Eds., ASTM International, West Conshohocken, PA, 2003.

Abstract: The purpose of the study was to determine the mechanical and corrosion properties of forged, commercially available, femoral hip stems. Two different stem designs were selected (the MS-30, sizes 6 and 16, and the MUELLER straight stem, sizes 7.5 and 15.0). They were made of high-nitrogen stainless steel according to ISO 5832-9 and ASTM F1586. The samples for determining the mechanical properties were taken from the proximal part of the prostheses. The metallurgical and the potentio-dynamic corrosion behaviours were investigated in three different transverse cross-sectional planes. The mechanical properties in the forged condition were as follows: Yield strength 1051 – 1172 MPa, tensile strength 1138 – 1238 MPa and elongation 15 – 19%. Vickers hardness values of between 354 and 393 HV were measured. The breakdown potential fell from +1000 $mV_{(SCE)}$ (wrought bar) to +600 to +950 $mV_{(SCE)}$ (forged hip stems) for pH 4 and 37°C. The rotational bending fatigue value for 10 million cycles was 587 MPa.

Keywords: high-nitrogen stainless steel, corrosion properties, mechanical properties, microstructure

Nomenclature

Breakdown potential – The least noble potential where pitting or crevice corrosion, or both, will initiate and propagate [ASTM Standard Terminology Relating to Corrosion Testing (G15)].

---

[1]Director, Materials Research, and Research Scientist, respectively, Material Research Department, Sulzer Orthopedics Ltd., P.O. Box 65, 8404 Winterthur, Switzerland

Introduction

Stainless steel has been employed as surgical implant material for many years. The quality of the steel in the pioneering days was poor, and numerous deficiencies such as fatigue failures and severe corrosion were reported [1]. The breakthrough of stainless steel as an implant material came with the development of the material with the designation AISI 316L. This type of steel is still used today, primarily for the products of osteosynthesis like plates, nails and screws [2,3]. Endoprostheses made of this type of steel since the 1960s, e.g., the Charnley hip stem, have been implanted and retained successfully in the body for many years [4-6]. Reports of corrosion phenomena and fatigue failures of this steel in-vivo have been made in the literature [2,4,7]. A new type of steel was introduced in the field of orthopedic surgery in the mid-1980s [4]. The chromium and manganese contents of the alloy were raised and up to 0.5% nitrogen was also introduced to improve the corrosion resistance and increase the strength [8]. This material was standardized under the designation "Wrought High Nitrogen Stainless Steel" 1992: ISO 5832-9 and ASTM F1586 – 95. The application for this highly alloyed stainless steel in the field of orthopedic surgery have been modular, cemented hip prostheses and femoral heads, which articulate against polyethylene. In this study, we analysed the mechanical, metallurgical and corrosion properties of forged hip stems.

Material

The smallest and the largest size of the "MS-30" hip stem design, as well as the smallest and third largest size of the "MUELLER straight stem" design were investigated (Table 1). All femoral stem components were taken from the regular production of Sulzer Orthopedics Ltd., Switzerland, and were made from the highly alloyed stainless steel "high-nitrogen stainless steel," tradename Protasul™-S30. As far as the chemical composition and the mechanical properties are concerned, the material fulfilled the requirements of ISO 5832-9 and ASTM Standard Specification for Wrought Nitrogen Strengthened –21Chromium – 10Nickel –3Manganese –2.5Molybdenum Stainless Steel Bar for Surgical Implants (F1586). The stainless steel bars with a diameter of 22 mm were mill annealed and formed into hip prostheses by means of the "drop-forging process." The transverse cross-section (anterior-posterior) of the MS-30 hip stem becomes larger as the size increases, whereas the cross-section (anterior-posterior) of the MUELLER straight stem remains the same even though the size increases (Figure 1).

Table 1 – *Investigated Hip Stem Design, Size and Number of used Specimen*

Hip stem design	Size	No. of Specimen
MS-30	6 (smallest)	10
MS-30	16 (largest)	10
MUELLER straight stem	7.5 (smallest)	10
MUELLER straight stem	15.0	25

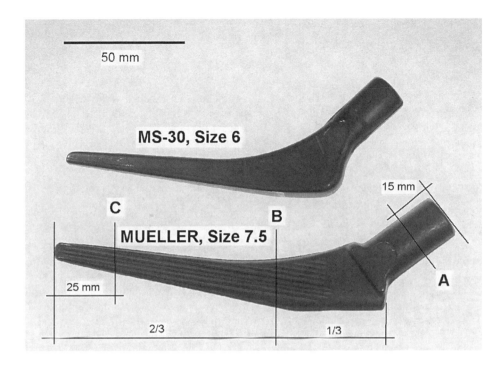

Figure 1 – *MS-30 hip stem, size 6 (top) and MUELLER straight stem, size 7.5 (bottom). Microstructure analysis and corrosion tests were done at planes A, B and C*

Methods

Tensile Properties

The test specimen for the tensile properties were machined from the proximal prosthetic stem of forged blanks. The gauge diameter of each tensile specimen was 6 mm, except for those samples made from MUELLER stems, size 7.5. The throat diameter of these stems was 4 mm. Six tests were performed for each stem type in accordance to European Standard, Metallic Materials; Tensile testing; Part 1: Method of testing (10 002). The elongations were determined for 5D gauge lengths. The mechanical values were statistically analysed with the Student t-test ($p < 0.05$).

Microstructure Analysis

The microstructure analysis and also the corrosion tests were made on three transverse planes of the hip stems (A – C). Plane A was located 15 mm below the face of the taper; plane B was two-thirds in length between distal tip and proximal shoulder of the prosthesis; and plane C was 25 mm from distal tip of the stem (Figure 1). The metallographical sections were etched and examined with 500-times magnification under a high power light microscope (Leica DMRX, Wetzlar, Germany).

Hardness Measurement

The Vickers hardness (HV10) was determined at the two ends of the tensile specimen. The measurements were made in accordance to ISO, Metallic materials – Vickers hardness test – Part 1: Test methode (6507-1). All hardness measurements were made 3 times and averaged.

In addition, the Vickers hardness was measured on all three metallographical planes of the MS-30 stem, size 16, and the MUELLER straight stem, size 15.0. The measuring positions were located anterior, posterior, lateral, medial and in the center.

Potentio-dynamic Corrosion Test

Potentio-dynamic polarization curves of the hip stems were determined per ASTM Standard Reference Test Method for Making Potentiostatic and Potentiodynamic Anodic Polarization Measurements (G5) using an EG&G (VersaSat II) Potentiostat, EG&G (SoftCorr III) Software and an EG&G K46 corrosion cell (EG&G Instruments, Princeton, USA). The measurements were made in the cross-section planes A, B and C (Figure 1). The coupon surfaces were ground to 1200 grit and masked with a self-dried polymer (Erne Galvanotechnik, Dättlikon, Switzerland, Product: Abdecklack No. 1). The test surfaces were measured in size and immersed in 1 litre of sodium chloride solution (0.9%) at 40°C, pH 4 (adjusted with HCl) and with nitrogen bubbling during the whole process. A cathodic pre-polarization (2 minutes at 100 $\mu A/cm^2$) was made 250 mV negative to the rest potential to clean the immersed surface. After waiting 30 minutes to allow the system to come to equilibrium, the test was started with a scan rate of 10 mV/min. Saturated calomel electrodes (SCE) were used for reference purposes. All the tests were made twice, reusing the old sample after refinishing.

Rotating Beam Fatigue

A high cycle rotating beam fatigue test were used to determine the fatigue properties with constant force mode. The test conditions were: 100 Hz for 10 million cycles in air at room temperature and stress ratio R = –1. All specimens had a diameter of 4 mm and were grit blasted (Ra 1 – 2 μm). Sixteen (16) specimens were machined from the proximal part of the MUELLER stems, size 15.0. Probit analysis was used to calculate the fatigue strength at 50, 90, 95 and 99% survival.

Results

Tensile Properties
The tensile properties are summarized in Table 2 and Figures 2, 3. With the MS-30 stem, the tensile strength reduces significantly, namely to the extent of 8.1% (p<0.001), from size 6 to size 16, and 10.5% in the case of the yield strength (p<0.001). The Vicker hardness also declines by 9.8% (p<0.001), but there is no recognizable difference in the elongation (p=0.75). In contrast to this, no statistical difference could be established between the investigated MUELLER straight stems size 7.5 and 15.0. This also applies for the yield strengths values (p>0.3), the hardnesses (p>0.3) and the elongations (p>0.7).

The relations of hardness and tensile properties is shown in Figure 4. The yield strength and tensile strength rise linearly with increasing hardness.

Table 2 – *Tensile Properties of Forged Hip Stems, Design MS-30 Size 6 and 16 and MUELLER Straigth Stem Size 7.5 and 15.0*

Design	MS-30	MS-30	MUELLER	MUELLER
Size	6	16	7.5	15.0
Yield Strength [MPa]	1172 ± 19	1051 ± 16	1115 ± 25	1105 ± 14
Tensile Strength [MPa]	1238 ± 16	1138 ± 11	1197 ± 24	1186 ± 9
Elongation [%]	15 ± 3	16 + 2	19 ± 3	18 ± 3
Reduction of Area [%]	59.0 ± 1.5	62.0 ± 1.5	66.7 ± 1.0	60.0 ± 0.6
Vicker Hardness	393 ± 11	354 ± 5	370 ± 5	373 ± 4

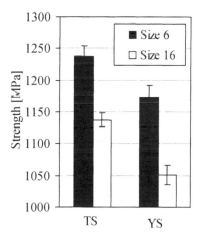

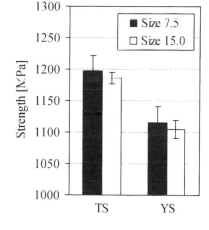

Figure 2 – *Mechanical strength of forged MS-30 hip stems, size 6 and 16*

Figure 3 – *Mechanical strength of forged MUELLER hip stems, size 7.5 and 15.0*

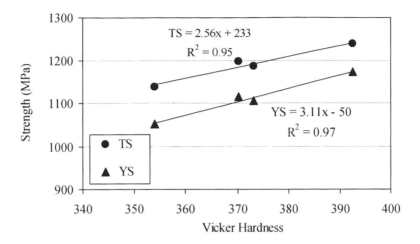

Figure 4 – *Relation between mechanical strength and Vicker hardness.*
NOTE: TS = Tensile Strength, YS = Yield Strength

Microstructure Analysis

All the metallographical sections of the "high-nitrogen stainless steels" had an austenitic matrix. No delta ferrite could be observed up to 100x magnification. As a result of the forging process, the structure is deformed badly in the vicinity of the flash. Two types of inclusions were observed in all the transverse cross-sections of the prostheses. Type 1 are fine, homogeneously distributed [Cr, Mo]-carbide with a diameter of less than 1 μm. Type 2 are larger inclusions with a diameter of up to 10 μm and identified as [Cr, Nb]-nitrides. No inclusions could be observed at the grain boundary. The microstructure in the necks of all of the stems (plane A) was recrystallized in the anterior and posterior regions of the taper (Figure 5) and was elongated near the flash in the medial and lateral regions (Figure 6).

Vicker Hardness

The average hardnesses measured on the tensile specimens were between 354 HV for the MS-30 size 16 and 393 HV for the MS-30 size 6 (Table 1). The values for the MUELLER hip stems were 370 HV (size 7.5) and 373 HV (size 15.0).

The hardness values measured in different areas in the three cross-section planes are shown in Table 3. The highest values were always measured near the flash (medial and lateral) and in the center of the femoral stems. Compared with the tensile specimen the Vicker hardness measured in plane B was between 7 and 10% higher.

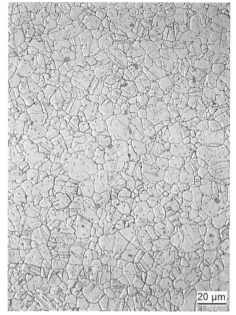

Figure 5 – *Microstructure in plane A (neck region) which is fully recrystallized*

Figure 6 – *Microstructure in plane A (neck region) with elongated grains near the flash*

Table 3 – *Vicker Hardness Values Measured at Three Sectional Planes A – C and Different Locations. Hardness Values from the Tensile Specimen were at the Bottom*

Plane	Position	MS-30, size 16	MUELLER, size 15.0
A	anterior / posterior	356	327
A	medial / lateral	433	403
A	center	408	418
B	anterior / posterior	361	398
B	medial / lateral	385	407
B	center	393	402
C	anterior / posterior	346	406
C	medial / lateral	405	449
C	center	418	424
	tensile specimen	354 + 5	373 + 4

Corrosion Test

The breakdown potentials ranging from +800 to +980 mV$_{(SCE)}$ was measured on the investigated planes A – C of the hip prosthesis designs (Figure 7). No differences could be established with respect to the corrosion-resistance as a function of the prosthesis size and/or location. The current density in the passive range between 0.1 to 1 µA/cm^2.

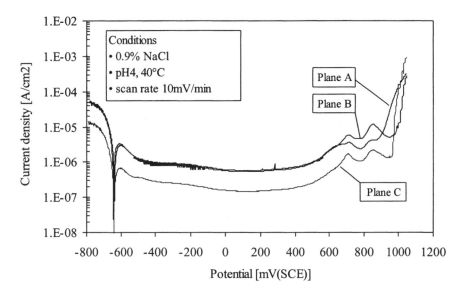

Figure 7 – *Potentio-dynamic corrosion with forged MUELLER hip stem, size 7.5. The breakdown potential in the cross-sectional plans A to C ranging between +840 and +980 mV$_{(SCE)}$*

Rotation Beam Fatigue

The plot of all fatigue specimens are in Figure 8. At 10^7 cycles, the fatigue strength of forged high-nitrogen stainless steel were calculated as follows:

50% survive – 692 MPa
90% survive – 634 MPa
95% survive – 618 MPa
99% survive – 587 MPa.

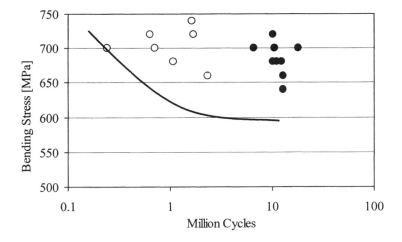

Figure 8 – *Rotation banding fatigue curve in air at room temperature. Black spots represent non fractured samples and white spots fractured samples*

Discussion

The minimum mechanical properties for the investigated, highly alloyed nitrogen stainless steel in the forged state are:

- Tensile Strength   TS   min.   1100 MPa
- Yield Strength   YS   min.   1000 MPa
- Elongation   E   min.   10%
- Fatigue Strength   (10^7 cycles)   587 MPa

The mechanical properties of forged hip prostheses can be determined easily in tensile and fatigue tests. On a daily basis, hip stem components are mechanically loaded in every single step over many years in the patient. Consequently, it is important to be conversant with the fatigue limit of the final product. However, the documentation of the endurance fatigue limit of the device was not the objective of this investigation and has not been measured in this study. It is possible that this alloy may exhibit greater reduction in its fatigue strength under such conditions compared to CoCrMo alloys.

Smethurst [9] investigated the properties of cold-worked high-nitrogen stainless steel (Ortron 90). The tensile properties were a bit lower (yield strength 810 MPa, tensile strength 1150 MPa, elongation 15%) and similar values for Vicker hardness (HV 413) and fatigue strength (583 MPa at 10^7 cycles) than this study.

A literature comparison with other metallic materials, which are employed for endoprostheses, shows that CoCrMo cast alloy has the lowest mechanical strength of them all. This applies, first and foremost, to the fatigue behaviour. The reasons for this are the coarse as-cast structure and sporadic microporosities. With the aid of the isostatic process (HIP), however, it is possible to reduce the number and size of the pores. As far as the mechanical properties are concerned, high-nitrogen stainless steel" is comparable with those of the wrought CoCrMo alloys [10]. This applies to both high-carbon and low-carbon CoCrMo alloy.

Alpha/beta and beta titanium alloys, which are employed primarily for cementless applications, exhibit lower tensile strength but similar fatigue strength [10]. In addition, the fatigue behaviour of this titanium alloy is notch-sensitive [11].

Truman [8] did potentio-dynamic corrosion tests with various steels in sodium chloride solution at 25°C. The pitting potential with the high-nitrogen stainless steel were highest with +950 mV$_{(SCE)}$ as compared with 317S16 (+320 mV) and 316S16 (+140 mV). Those results were confirmed by Smethurst [9], who investigated this material in the cold-worked state (Ortron 90). In this study the breakdown potential of the forged "high-nitrogen stainless steel" is slightly lower than in the initial soft-annealed state. Incoming inspections of the raw material are absolutely essential to maintain the high quality of the forged components. The breakdown-potential of the investigated products is comparable with that of the CoCrMo alloys.

CONCLUSIONS

Hip prostheses made from the material "high-nitrogen stainless steel," which are manufactured according to a forging process, have high mechanical properties in combination with high ductile characteristics.

The more this highly alloyed steel is formed, the higher its mechanical properties and hardness. The structure is badly deformed in the vicinity of the flash. There are no segregations on the grain boundaries.

The corrosion-resistance of this steel is good. Nevertheless, only bar material with high breakdown potential should be used as raw material for forged products. The corrosion resistance declines as a result of the forging process. As a result, the forging process should be optimzed with a view to combining the mechanical properties with high corrosion resistance.

High-nitrogen stainless steel has also been employed for cemented hip prostheses in Europe for more than 15 years. Up to now, there have been no reports of any negative results such as fractured stems or corrosive surface changes, which could be associated with this material.

References

[1]   Frank, E. and Zitter, H., *Metallische Implantate in der Knochenchirurgie*, Springer Verlag, 1971.

[2]   Cook, S.D., Renz, E.A., Barrack, R.L., Thomas, K.A., Harding, A.F., Haddad, R.J., Jr., and Milicic, M., "Clinical and Metallurgical Analysis of Retrieved

Internal Fixation Device," *Clinical Orthopaedics and Related Research*, No. 194, 1985, pp. 236 – 247.

[3]   Disegi, J.A. and Eschbach L., "Stainless Steel in Bone Surgery," *Injury*, Vol. 31, 2000, Supplement 4, pp. D2-D6.

[4]   Wroblewski, B.M., *Revision Surgery in Total Hip Arthroplasty*, Springer Verlag, 1990.

[5]   Sochart, D.H., Porter, M.L., and Lancashire, W., "The Long-Term Results of Charnley Low-Friction Arthroplasty in Young Patients Who Have Congenital Dislocation, Degenerative Osteoarthritis or Rheumatoid Arthritis," *Journal of Bone and Joint Surgery*, Vol. 79-A, 1997, pp. 1599 – 1617.

[6]   Callaghan J.J., Forest E.E., Olejniczak, J.P., Goetz, D.D., and Johnston, R.C., "Charnley Total Hip Arthroplasty in Patients Less Than Fifty Years Old," *Journal of Bone and Joint Surgery*, Vol. 80-A, 1988, pp. 704 – 714.

[7]   Wright, T.M., Burstein, A.H., and Bartel, D.L., "Retrieval Analysis of Total Joint Replacement Components: A Six-Year Experience," *Corrosion and Degradation of Implant Materials*, ASTM STP 859, A.C. Fraker and C.D. Griffin, Eds., American Society for Testing Materials, Philadelphia, 1985, pp. 415 – 428.

[8]   Truman, J.E., "An Austenitic Stainless Steel of Imporved Strength and Corrosion Resistance," *Stainless Steel Industry*, Vol. 6, No. 23, 1978, pp. 21 – 23.

[9]   Smethurst, E., "A New Stainless Steel Alloy for Surgical Implants Compared to 316S12," *Biomaterials*, 1981, Vol. 2, pp. 116 – 119.

[10]   Brehme, J., and Biehl, V., "Metallic Biomaterials," *Handbook of Biomaterial Properties*, J. Black and G. Hastings, Eds., Chapman & Hall, 1998, pp. 135 – 214.

[11]   Grover, H.J., "Metal Fatigue in Some Orthopedic Implants," *Journal of Materials*, Vol. 1, No.2, 1966, pp. 413 – 420.

John A. Disegi[1] and Lyle D. Zardiackas[2]

Metallurgical and Mechanical Evaluation of 316L Stainless Steel Orthopaedic Cable

---

Reference: Disegi, J. A. and Zardiackas, L. D., **"Metallurgical and Mechanical Evaluation of 316L Stainless Steel Orthopaedic Cable,"** *Stainless Steels for Medical and Surgical Applications, ASTM STP 1438*, G. L. Winters and M. J. Nutt, Eds., ASTM International, West Conshohocken, PA, 2003.

Abstract: Stainless steel cable systems have been designed for a multitude of orthopaedic implant applications. Various implant fixation, cerclage, and tension banding techniques may be used with cable constructs to stabilize a variety of simple and complex bone fractures. Multifilament cable products, however, can pose special challenges regarding metallurgical evaluation and mechanical property testing. The present project investigated the metallurgical and mechanical properties of a new 316L stainless steel cable system designed for general trauma surgery. Important cable attributes such as strand configuration, cable construction, and finishing options are discussed. The advantages of inductively coupled plasma spectroscopy analysis are presented for the compositional verification of solid cable specimens. Metallographic methods for the examination of nonmetallic inclusion limits and grain size are described for a cable construct composed of 75 fine wires. The microstructure associated with laser remelted cable ends is documented via light microscopy. Unique tension test methods are described for the determination of failure load and elongation of 1.1 and 1.7 mm diameter cable sizes. Test results are compared with generalized requirements compiled in ASTM F 2180 Standard Specification for Metallic Implantable Strands and Cables.

Keywords: metal (for surgical implants), wire, strand, cable, stainless steel, surgical implants

Stainless steel cable systems are designed for a multitude of orthopaedic implant applications. Typical clinical indications for cable [1] include fracture fixation stabilization of olecranon, patella, femur, humerus, pelvic, acetabular, and ankle fractures. Additional clinical uses include acromioclavicular dislocations, prophylactic banding during total joint procedures, and temporary reduction during open reduction procedures.

---

[1]Materials Development Manager, Synthes (USA) Technical Center, 1301 Goshen Parkway, West Chester, PA, 19380.

[2]Professor and Coordinator of Biomaterials and Professor of Orthopaedic Surgery, University of Mississippi Medical Center, 2500 North State Street, Jackson, MS, 39216.

The implants and instruments utilized with cable systems for orthopaedic trauma represent sophisticated designs since the clinical techniques are very specialized. Orthopaedic cable typically displays improved tensile failure load [2], enhanced fatigue endurance limit [3], and better handling characteristics when compared to monofilament wire of the same diameter. Intraoperative advantages for the surgeon include the absence of sheared monofilament wire ends that can cut through surgical gloves and cause potential disease transmission problems during surgery. Cable products, however, can pose special challenges regarding metallurgical evaluation and mechanical property testing. The present project investigated the metallurgical and mechanical properties of a new 316L stainless steel cable system designed for general trauma surgery.

Materials and Methods

Cable Construction

The starting coil material used for the manufacture of the cable product examined in this study met the prevailing requirements specified in ASTM Specification for Wrought 18 Chromium-14 Nickel-2.5 Molybdenum Stainless Steel Bar and Wire for Surgical Implants (F 138).

Proper terminology related to stranding and cabling configurations is essential in order to discuss construction and design requirements for orthopaedic cable. Round wire is the individual product form that is utilized to produce a strand. Strand is a group of wires helically twisted together while cable is a group of strands helically twisted together. The construction designation for strands and cables is known as MxN, where M represents the number of strands in the cable and N represents the number of wires in each strand. Some examples of strand construction are 1x7 and 1x3 while some common cable constructions are 7x7 and 7x19. The lay or twist is the helical form taken by the wires and by the strands in a cable. The lay may be right or left depending whether the orientation is in the same or opposite direction as the thread on a right-hand screw. Pitch is the distance parallel to the axis of the strand or cable in which the wire or strand makes one complete turn about the axis. A 1x7 strand is comprised of 1 wire surrounded by 6 wires with a left-hand lay and a uniform pitch of 8 to 16 times the nominal strand diameter. A 1x19 strand is characterized by an inner 1x7 strand with a right-hand lay and a uniform pitch of 8 to 12 times the nominal strand diameter. The outer 12 wires have a left-hand lay with a uniform pitch of 9 to 11 times the nominal strand diameter. Other types of specialized strand configurations may be used depending on design criteria and intended applications. Cabling configurations refer to the manner in which the strands are constructed to achieve a final cable diameter. Some common cable configurations include 7x7 and 7x19 construction. The 7x7 cable consists of an inner 1x7 strand with a right-hand lay and a uniform pitch of 12 to16 times the nominal strand diameter. The outer 1x7 strands have a left-hand lay with a uniform pitch of 8 to 16 times the nominal strand diameter. Overall, the 7x7 cable has a right-hand lay with a uniform pitch of 7 to10 times the nominal cable diameter. The strand, pitch, and lay configuration for a 7x19 cable is fairly complex and beyond the scope of this presentation. Various other cable constructions may be used, including hybrid designs that represent non-standard configurations. The present study evaluated a cable comprised of a uniquely designed 1x19 inner core surrounded by eight 1x7 outer strands. The fine wire size was varied to provide either a 1.1 mm or 1.7 mm cable diameter. A cross-sectional illustration of the cable containing 75 wires is shown in Figure 1.

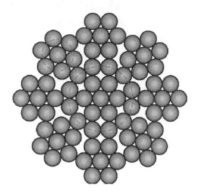

Figure 1 – *Cross-sectional schematic of 1.7 mm cable containing 75 wires (30X).*

Cable manufacturing operations include laser or tungsten inert gas (TIG) thermal treatments to secure the ends of the cable while hollow crimp blocks are used to provide a means for threading, tensioning, and crimping the cable. Auxiliary implants may include cerclage positioning pins and cerclage buttons. Cerclage pins maintain proper cable position when threaded through a bone plate hole while cerclage buttons help to augment screw purchase, especially for unicortical screw fixation around a prosthesis. An orthopaedic cable system will also include specialized surgical instruments such as a cable passer, calibrated tensioner, crimper, and cutter. An example of a stainless steel cable system with cerclage positioning pins and a cerclage button to stabilize a stainless bone plate is shown in Figure 2.

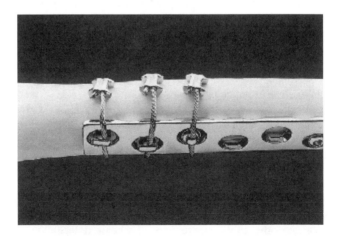

Figure 2 – *Stainless cable system with bone plate (1X).*

Metallurgical Evaluation

Laser treated cable ends were cut, cold mounted in epoxy resin, polished with a series of polishing suspensions to a final metallographic finish using 0.05 micron aluminum oxide (Al_2O_3), and etched in a solution of ferric chloride ($FeCl_3$) saturated hydrochloric acid (HCl) with a small amount of nitric acid (HNO_3). The microstructure in the vicinity of the remelted cable end was examined by light microscopy. Composition was determined by cutting a 40 mm long cable length, folding the cable length in two, and inserting the folded cable length into a special fixture. Five samples from each cable lot were analyzed. Manganese (Mn), silicon (Si), nickel (Ni), chromium (Cr), and molybdenum (Mo) content were analyzed using a Spectro inductively coupled plasma (ICP) spectroscopy with a spark stand attachment, which allows direct sampling of solids rather than acid dissolution. Prior to analysis, the ICP equipment was calibrated with primary standards used for the routine analysis of implant quality 316L stainless steel. Mean and standard deviation values were calculated for each element analyzed in the product analysis study. A 15 mm long specimen was cut, cold mounted, polished, and rated for inclusion content in the unetched condition per ASTM Test Methods for Determining the Inclusion Content of Steel (E 45). Five samples per lot (n = 5) were rated for nonmetallic inclusion content. Five 15 mm long samples per lot were obtained for transverse grain size measurements, etched with $FeCl_3$ saturated HCl plus a small amount of HNO_3, and rated according to ASTM Test Methods for Determining Average Grain Size (E 112).

Tension Testing

Either 1.1 mm or 1.7 mm diameter cable test samples about 100 mm in length were provided for uniaxial tension testing in a vertical plane according to ASTM Test Methods for Tension Testing of Metallic Materials (E 8). The cable ends were laser welded to prevent untwisting during the tension test. A 254 mm gage length was tested at a 2.00 mm/sec stroke rate to failure. A plot of load versus deflection was obtained during the tension test. The 0.2% yield strength and reduction of area were not determined. A minimum of five samples (n = 5) representing various implant cable lots were tested. Failure load and % elongation were recorded. The mean and standard deviation values were calculated for each cable lot. Tension testing was performed with a Model 810 MTS servohydraulic test machine equipped with load cells calibrated with standards traceable to the National Institute of Standards and Technology (NIST).

Results and Discussion

Metallographic examination of the laser processed cable ends indicated that a relatively uniform dendritic microstructure was present. The dendritic microstructure appeared similar to recast austenitic stainless structures that are produced by fast melting followed by a high rate of solidification. Voids and thermal oxidation were not observed in the remelted regions. Inert gas shrouding during the laser remelting process produced a homogeneous microstructure that was free of significant oxidation. Laser thermal treatment has the added advantage of providing highly localized remelting with a small

heat affected zone (HAZ). A light microscopic image of the laser processed 316L stainless
steel microstructure is shown in Figure 3.

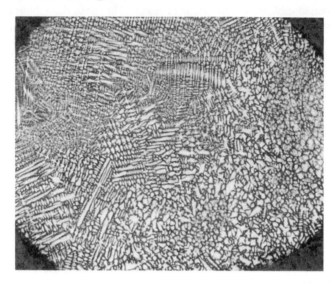

Figure 3 - *Remelted structure of 1.7 mm diameter laser treated cable end (100X).*

ICP compositional results were straightforward and no unusual problems were
experienced. The check analysis values for Mn, Si, Ni, Cr and Mo were within the
product analysis tolerance limits specified in F 138. Product analysis tolerances cover
variations between laboratories in the measurement of chemical content. ICP results for
three cable lots are compared to the certified heat analysis of the starting coil stock in
Table 1.

Table 1 - *ICP Product Analysis Results for 1.1 mm Cable*

| | Weight % | | | | | |
| | Lot A | | Lot B | | Lot C | |
Element	Heat (n = 2)	Product (n = 5)	Heat (n = 2)	Product (n = 5)	Heat (n = 2)	Product (n = 5)
Mn	1.77	1.85 ± 0.03	1.77	1.84 ± 0.06	1.76	1.88 ± 0.00
Si	0.50	0.44 ± 0.02	0.46	0.35 ± 0.03	0.46	0.39 ± 0.01
Ni	14.76	14.54 ± 0.30	14.73	14.33 ± 0.12	14.72	14.71 ± 0.16
Cr	17.46	18.32 ± 0.70	17.50	17.28 ± 0.12	17.44	17.60 ± 0.19
Mo	2.82	2.52 ± 0.07	2.80	2.61 ± 0.06	2.79	2.61 ± 0.07

The alloy suppliers usually report the heat composition values in duplicate on the primary certificate of tests so standard deviations were not calculated for the mean values. Product analysis test results (n = 5) for Mn, Si, Ni, Cr, and Mo indicated that excellent standard deviations were obtained. The use of the ICP spark system is considered an advantage because analysis time is significantly reduced and errors that may be introduced during classical wet chemical analysis are avoided. Standardization with solid primary standards also provides better control of interelement effects when compared to the use of individual elemental standards. Also, improved detection limits are generally observed with ICP when compared to X-ray fluorescence (XRF) procedures.

Transverse metallographic mounts were used to examine the inclusion content of the stranded fine wires. During the polishing operation about 20-25% of the fine wires became repositioned in the longitudinal plane and this orientation was used to evaluate the nonmetallic inclusion content. Nonmetallic inclusion ratings in the unetched condition were within the limits specified in F 138. Only thin and heavy Type D oxides were observed when a series of eighteen lots of 1.1 mm diameter and sixteen lots of 1.7 mm diameter cable were rated for nonmetallic inclusions. The repetitive fine wire die drawing operations tend to deform and disperse Type A, Type B, and Type C inclusions whereas the Type D oxides tend to resist deformation during manufacturing.

Grain size in the transverse plane was difficult to rate at 100X magnification due to the combination of cold work and small wire diameter. The nominal wire diameter was either 0.10 mm or 0.15 mm depending on the cable size that was examined. E 112, Section 10, Comparison Procedure, defines the maximum value (finest grain size) as ASTM 8 for a twinned austenitic structure and ASTM 10 for an untwinned austenitic structure. Grain size was rated finer than ASTM 10 for the majority of the cable lots that were examined. The stainless cable met the F 138 grain size requirement of ASTM 5 or finer that is specified for bar and wire product. However, the measurement of grain size was not straightforward and testing limitations were identified for orthopaedic cable composed of small diameter wire.

Preliminary tension test results (n = 5) indicated that failure load and elongation values were not reproducible and unacceptable standard deviations were obtained for both the 1.1 mm and 1.7 mm diameter cable sizes. The early tests were performed with 400 mm long cable specimens and conventional wire tension grips. Examination of the load versus deflection curves indicated that cable slippage was occurring in the wire grips. Initial discussions with a cable producer, Pioneer Cable Technology, Marquette, MI, suggested that longer test specimens and specialized cable grips with roller assemblies would be required to provide reproducible tension testing results. Special cable grips were constructed and 1450 mm long tension test specimens with laser welded ends were utilized in order to establish a standardized tension test procedure. A long cable specimen was needed so that both ends of the cable could be threaded around the 25 mm diameter roller and locking assemblies that are attached to each cable grip. The modified tension test arrangement eliminated slippage problems and provided excellent data reproducibility. It was also noted that careful specimen alignment was critical to ensure uniform cable elongation within the gage section. Elongation was determined by monitoring the amount of crosshead separation during tension testing to failure (not peak load) because it was not possible to measure accurately the cable length change after failure. Figure 4 shows a cable specimen inserted into the specially fabricated tension test grips.

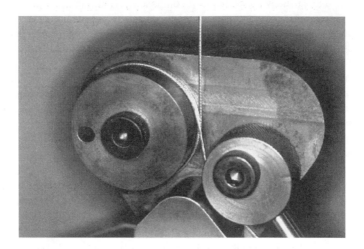

Figure 4 - *Roller grip assembly used for cable tension testing (2X).*

Mean failure loads, mean % elongation, and standard deviations for random production lots of 1.1 mm and 1.7 mm diameter cables are compiled in Table 2.

Table 2 – *Cable Failure Load and Elongation Results (n = 5)*

Cable Diameter (mm)	Lot	Mean Failure Load, N	Mean Elongation, %
1.1	A	1195 ± 2.9	3.9 ± 0.13
	B	1215 ± 12.1	4.2 ± 0.08
	C	1212 ± 5.6	4.2 ± 0.14
	D	1193 ± 1.2	4.4 ± 0.13
1.7	E	2774 ± 13.5	5.1 ± 0.18
	F	2751 ± 18.4	5.1 ± 0.16
	G	2770 ± 33.4	4.2 ± 0.17
	H	2801 ± 7.4	4.6 ± 0.09

The magnitude of the cable failure load and elongation are highly dependent on whether the fine wire filaments are manufactured in the strand annealed or cold drawn condition. Strand annealing parameters and the amount of cold work introduced into the fine wire during the last wire drawing operation will have a significant effect on the finish mechanical properties attained for cable. Engineering specifications for the implant 316L stainless cable sizes under investigation define minimum failure loads that must be met on a consistent basis. Minimum ultimate tensile strength (UTS) is not specified because of errors that may be introduced in calculating the true cross-sectional area of the cable. The option of using swaging operations to size the cable during manufacture and the tightness of the strand are factors that can influence the accuracy of the cross-sectional area measurements. Theoretical formulas for various strand configurations are included in the F 2180 standard but cable designs may not always meet idealized cross-sectional area calculations. The desire to standardize UTS limits for cable must be balanced against the improved accuracy that is obtained when area measurement errors are eliminated.

Conclusions

A metallurgical and mechanical property evaluation of 1.1 and 1.7 mm diameter 316L stainless steel cable intended for surgical implants revealed the following

1. Inert gas shrouded laser remelting is a satisfactory method for captivating the ends of multifilament cable and this high temperature process provided a homogeneous dendritic structure that was free of thermal oxidation.

2. Standard metallographic techniques are satisfactory for the examination of nonmetallic inclusions although only type D globular oxides were identified. A grain size rating finer than ASTM 10 was generally observed but the combination of cold work and small wire diameter contributed to grain size measurement difficulties.

3. ICP spectroscopy analysis yielded reproducible Mn, Si, Cr, Ni, and Mo compositional values that were within ASTM F 138 product analysis tolerance limits.

4. Special roller grip assemblies, extra long cable specimens, and careful alignment techniques are required to provide reproducible tension test results.

References

[1]   Synthes (USA), "The Orthopaedic Cable System Technique Guide," Brochure GP1369-A, 1999, pp. 2-20.
[2]   Dall, D.M., "Reconstruction of the Femur in Total Hip Replacement Using Multifilament Cerclage Cables Fastened with Crimp Sleeves," In: *Bone Implant Grafting*, J. Older, Ed., Springer-Verlag, New York, 1992, pp. 135-155.
[3]   Lie, A., O'Connor, D.O., and Harris, W.H., "Comparison of Cerclage Techniques Using a Hose Clamp Versus Monofilament Cerclage Wire or Cable," *Journal of Arthoplasty*, Vol. No. 12, 7, 1997, pp. 772-776.

Processing, Quality Assurance Concerns, and MRI Testing

J. Zachary Dennis,[1] Charles H. Craig,[1] Herbert R. Radisch, Jr.,[1] Edward J. Pannek, Jr.,[1] Paul C. Turner,[2] Albert G. Hicks,[3] Matthew Jenusaitis,[1] Nev A. Gokcen,[4] Clifford M. Friend,[5] and Michael R. Edwards[5]

Processing Platinum Enhanced Radiopaque Stainless Steel (PERSS®[6]) for Use as Balloon-Expandable Coronary Stents

---

Reference: Dennis, J. Z., Craig, C. H., Radisch, H. R., Jr., Pannek, E. J., Jr., Turner, P. C., Hicks, A. G., Jenusaitis, M., Gokcen, N. A., Friend, C. M., and Edwards, M. R., "**Processing Platinum Enhanced Radiopaque Stainless Steel (PERSS®) for Use as Balloon-Expandable Coronary Stents,**" *Stainless Steels for Medical and Surgical Applications, ASTM STP 1438*, G. L. Winters and M. J. Nutt, Eds., ASTM International, West Conshohocken, PA, 2003.

Abstract: A platinum-enhanced variant of UNS S31673 stainless steel has been developed for use in fabricating balloon-expandable coronary stents. PERSS® is sufficiently radiopaque to be detected by current radiographic methods and maintains compliance with ASTM requirements. Boston Scientific Corporation/Interventional Technologies (BSC/IVT) has implemented a pilot program for the development of PERSS with the intent of achieving vertical integration of the manufacturing process. PERSS ingots containing 5 wt% platinum were cast by vacuum induction melting, refined by vacuum arc remelting, upset in a forge, then hot and cold-rolled into sheet and foil. The sheet was cold-rolled on a 20-high cluster mill to a foil thickness of less than 0.25 mm (0.01 inches). While the final product otherwise meets the ASTM specification for UNS S31673 alloys, intentional addition of unspecified additional elements precludes its compliance with same.

Keywords: coronary stent, stainless steel, platinum, vacuum induction melting, vacuum arc remelting, Sendzimir mill, PERSS

---

[1] Manufacturing Engineer, Research & Development Engineer, Vice President (R&D), Vice President (Process Development), and General Manager, respectively, Boston Scientific Corporation/Interventional Technologies, 3574 Ruffin Road, San Diego, CA, 92123.

[2] Associate Director for Thermal Treatment Technologies, Albany Research Center, U.S. Department of Energy, 1450 Queen Ave., Albany, OR, 97321.

[3] Technical Manager, Rolled Products Division, The Arnold Engineering Co., 300 N. W. Street, Marengo, IL, 60152.

[4] Consultant, 385 Palos Verdes Dr. W, Palos Verdes Estates, CA, 90274.

[5] Professor and Head, and Senior Lecturer, respectively, Department of Materials and Medical Sciences, Cranfield Postgraduate Medical School, Shrivenham, Swindon SN6 8LA, United Kingdom.

[6] Registered trademark: Boston Scientific Corporation/Interventional Technologies, San Diego, CA.

Introduction

Balloon-expandable coronary stents are typically made from thin-walled tubes of surgical grade stainless steel made in accordance with ASTM Specification for Wrought 18 Chromium-14 Nickel-2.5 Molybdenum Stainless Steel Sheet and Strip for Surgical Implants (UNS S31673), F139. This material has sufficiently low carbon content to ensure freedom from intergranular corrosion susceptibility, while pitting resistance is obtained by maintaining a specific weight percentage of chromium and molybdenum. Stents made from commercially available variants of UNS S31673 stainless steel that is made to F139 such as BioDur®[7] 316LS are quite suitable in terms of their structural properties and their biocompatibility, but may not be suitable in terms of fluoroscopic radiopacity, a functional property that determines whether the stents are visible radiographically once they have been deployed inside the coronary artery. The PERSS alloy was developed to provide a solution to this problem by an unspecified additional element, platinum, which addresses the functional property without compromising the structural or biocompatibility properties. Development of the PERSS alloy is described by Craig et al [1].

Processing of the PERSS alloy is strongly influenced by design-mandated concerns over dimensional control of the final thickness of the foil and over maintaining its final grain size. BSC/IVT uses welded tubes made from this alloy to fabricate stents, which are made by rolling foil into a tube, laser-welding the seam, then drawing it to the required diameter of the stent. BSC/IVT fabricates stents by a chemical etching process, which requires tubes of an extremely consistent wall thickness and grain size in order to produce implant grade medical products. Grain size significantly affects the strength and ductility of the stent and is controlled for cold-worked and annealed structures principally by the amount of cold working [2]. The effect of the annealing temperature is much less, especially when the amount of prior cold work is large. Thus, in order to produce a specific grain size after annealing, as is required to produce the appropriate mechanical properties for stents, careful control of the cold working before annealing is essential. These material conditions must be met before the tube is chemically etched.

Based on constraints of thickness and grain size, processing requirements for manufacturing the foil were determined and are addressed here. Figure 1 shows the processing steps for PERSS alloys prior to tube production and stent fabrication. The alloy is formed by Vacuum Induction Melting (VIM) a commercially available stainless steel, BioDur 316LS, in rod form, along with the chosen unspecified additional element, platinum, and any additional specified elements such as chromium and molybdenum required to maintain PERSS within the compositional specifications of F139. The alloy is refined through Vacuum Arc Remelting (VAR) and molded into an ingot. The ingot is taken through a forging process where it is formed into a billet. The billet is formed into a sheet by hot-rolling in a 2-high rolling mill and cold-rolling in a 4-high rolling mill. The foil is then formed from the sheet by a 40% final reduction in thickness by a 20-high Sendzimir cluster rolling mill (Z-mill).

---

[7] Registered trademark Carpenter Technology Corporation, Reading, PA.

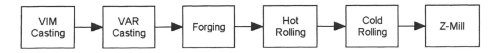

Figure 1 - *Block diagram of the stent material production process prior to tube forming*

Background

VIM of the stainless steel was chosen in order to reduce the level of nonmetallic inclusions in the alloy, which can tend to promote unwanted corrosion. VIM is a metallurgical process that uses an induction furnace inside a vacuum chamber to melt and cast steel (as well as other alloys). VIM consists of heating the alloy components together in a crucible that is surrounded by a water-cooled copper coil. High frequency current passes through the coil and melts the materials within the crucible as well as causing a powerful electromagnetic stirring action. The use of a vacuum helps to minimize the amount of impurities present in the alloy by keeping oxides and other nonmetallic products from forming.

A second melting of the VIM-produced alloy may be accomplished by VAR in order to reduce the chemical segregation in the ingot, as well as producing further reductions in the level of nonmetallic inclusions. VAR consists of maintaining a high current DC arc between the electrode made from the VIM-produced PERSS alloy and a molten metal pool of the alloy that is contained in a water-cooled copper crucible. The VAR process, as with the VIM process, is kept under vacuum to maintain alloy cleanliness and eliminate impurities. The remelting process produces an ingot with good internal structure and excellent chemical homogeneity.

The reduction of the ingot to plate was carried out by initially hot upsetting the ingot and then hot rolling. Forging the molded ingot into a billet is performed by compressing the ingot between two flat dies, or "upsetting". The forging process changes the microstructure of the workpiece from a cast to a wrought structure, i.e., from a chemically homogenous ingot with non-uniform grains to a wrought billet with uniform grains. Hot rolling is performed above the recrystallization temperature of the alloy. A billet is heated and drawn through a pair of hardened steel rollers that reduces the thickness of the material over several passes to produce a plate form. The grains initially elongate and subsequently recrystallize into smaller, more uniform grains, providing greater strength and ductility than is provided by the metallurgical structure of the billet.

For the reduction of the plate to thin sheet, it was necessary to cold roll the alloy at room temperature, because this gave better dimensional tolerances and a superior surface finish. Cold rolling is performed to reduce plate thickness without allowing the grains to recrystallize.

The final cold rolling of the PERSS sheet into foil requires a 40% reduction in thickness with the foil thickness required to be very consistent both along the width and the length of the foil. Normal rolling mills are affected by roll deflection, defined as a tendency for the rolls to bend outward in response to the roll forces. This causes a crown to be formed on the rolled material; the center is observed to be thicker than the outer edges. This effect can be countered by using a larger roll and giving it a barrel shape (camber) to offset the effects of roll deflection. Larger rolls, however, are more susceptible to roll flattening, where the rolls bulge into an oblong shape in response to the roll forces. Roll flattening can cause defects in the final material and limits the amount that the material can be reduced.

The Z-mill is of a class of rolling mills known as "cluster" mills (see Figure 2). Two small-diameter rolls that contact the metal are supported by a group of larger rolls. The smaller diameter rolls enable the mill to perform the 40% reduction of the material without suffering the effects of roll flattening. The smaller diameter rolls also reduce the roll force and power requirements, and help prevent horizontal spreading of the material. The larger supporting rolls prevent the working rolls from deflecting, so a consistent foil thickness can be maintained. These rolls are particularly useful in rolling thin sections and materials that are hard. Since stainless steels have high work-hardening coefficients, these mills have often been applied in the rolling of fine gages of stainless steels. Further details of Sendzimir mills may be found in [3].

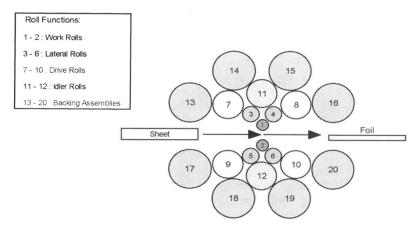

Figure 2 - *20-high Z-Mill roll configuration*

Foil Production

The initial processing of the alloy was performed at the U. S. Department of Energy's Albany Research Center (ARC) located in Albany, Oregon. It consisted of the melting, forging and rolling of the alloy to sheet approximately 0.060 in thick. The alloy was then rolled to product size, 0.006 in thick, by The Arnold Engineering Company, located in Marango, IL. BioDur 316LS stainless steel rod, chromium, molybdenum, and platinum were melted together in a VIM furnace. The VIM system used in the development program is shown in Figure 3, and the ingot produced from the VIM process is shown in Figure 4. The ingot has approximate dimensions of 15 cm diameter by 20 cm long. The composition of the platinum enhanced stainless steel ingot was determined and is presented in comparison to the typical composition of BioDur 316LS in Table 1 below.

Table 1 – *Compositions of UNS S31673, BioDur 316LS, and PERSS alloys*

Element	Symbol	ASTM F139	BioDur 316 LS	PERSS ingot #50
Carbon	C	0.030 wt% max.	0.024 wt%	0.023 wt%
Manganese	Mn	2.0 wt% max.	1.80 wt%	1.54 wt%
Silicon	Si	0.75 wt% max.	0.44 wt%	0.45 wt%
Chromium	Cr	17.0 – 19.0 wt%	17.66 wt%	18.67 wt%
Nickel	Ni	13.0 – 15.0 wt%	14.66 wt%	13.25 wt%
Molybdenum	Mo	2.25 – 3.0 wt%	2.78 wt%	2.94 wt%
Platinum	Pt	-	-	5.32 wt%

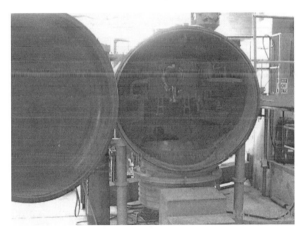

Figure 3 – *Vacuum induction melting furnace at Albany Research Center*[8]

---

[8] Figure 3 – 8 courtesy Albany Research Center.

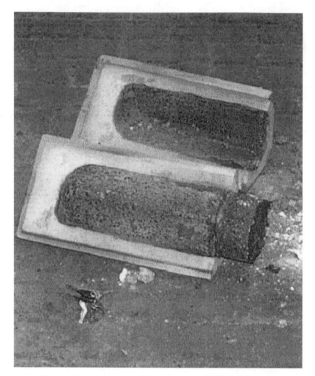

Figure 4 - *Vacuum induction melt PERSS ingot*

To further refine the material and improve its quality the VIM ingot was subjected to the VAR process. The ingot was quartered and welded together to form a consumable electrode and then secured in an evacuated chamber. The amount of current passing through the bars was gradually increased from 1500 A at 26 V to a maximum of 4800 A at 32 V. After VAR, the re-solidified ingot had an approximate diameter of 15 cm and an approximate length of 20 cm.

To prepare the material for the hot-rolling process, the ingot was forged into a rectangular block (billet). The ingot was heated to 1230°C for a soak time of five hours and transferred to the forge shown in Figure 5. The material was upset through a series of compressions, reheating the material between actions of the forge to produce a billet approximately 9.5 cm x 17 cm x 22 cm.

The process of hot and cold- rolling the billet into plate form in a 2-high rolling mill took place in several stages, with a typical reduction of 10% per pass. The billet was rolled into a slab at an initial temperature of 1230°C and reheated between the subsequent passes to maintain the elevated temperature. The slab was rolled into a plate with a final thickness of 1.33 cm (0.522") and was of sufficient consistency that it was not necessary to re-flatten the material on the forge. The 2-high rolling mill used in the development program is shown in Figure 6, while Figure 7 shows the hot plate emerging from the mill. Figure 8 shows the sheet of material obtained after cold-rolling on the 2-high rolling mill. The material was annealed at 1040°C for 14 minutes before fan-assisted cooling to room temperature. The plate was transferred to a 4-high rolling mill and cold-rolled by an extensive series of 5% reductions with occasional fifteen-minute anneals at 1040 °C. The 4-high rolling mill is shown in Figure 9. The sheet that was obtained through the first part of the cold-rolling process had a thickness of 1.63 mm (0.064"). The cold-rolled sheet was coiled and secured for a vacuum batch anneal at 950°C. The strip was cleaned and trimmed and the thickness further reduced by cold-rolling to a thickness of 0.69 mm (0.027") on the 4-high mill.

Prior to the final reduction in the Z-mill, the strip of PERSS material was trimmed to a width of 15.88 cm (6.25") and strip annealed at 1065°C at approximately 2 m per minute (6 feet per minute) in a horizontal furnace. The material was then loaded onto the Z-mill and reduced to a final thickness of 0.15 mm (0.0063"). A final anneal was performed at 1050°C at approximately 1 m per minute (3 feet per minute) in the horizontal furnace. Figure 10 shows a Z-mill such as that used for the process development described above.

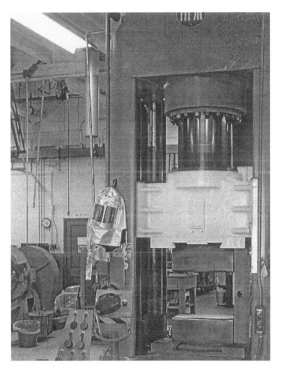

Figure 5 – *Forging press at Albany Research Center*

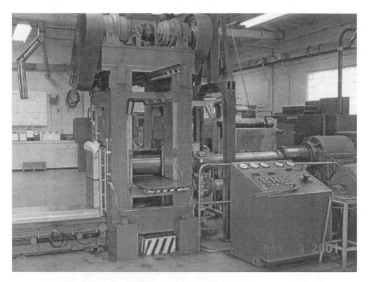

Figure 6 – *2/4-high rolling mill at Albany Research Center*

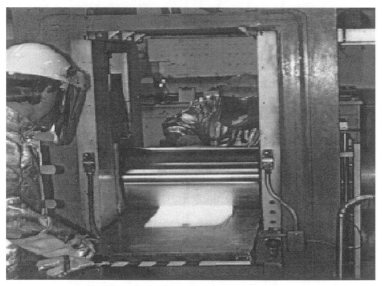

Figure 7 – *Hot-rolled PERSS plate emerging from 2-high mill at Albany Research Center*

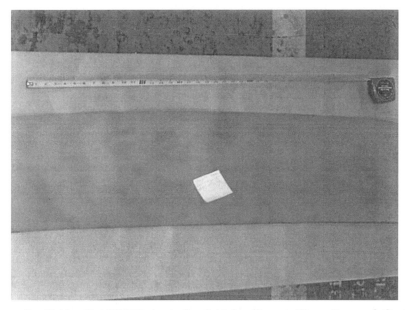

Figure 8 – *Cold-rolled PERSS sheet after 2-high rolling at Albany Research Center*

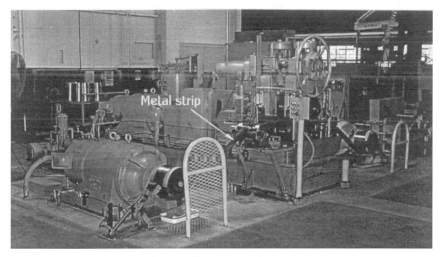

Figure 9 – *4-high rolling mill at Arnold Engineering*

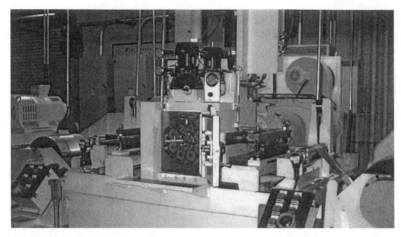

Figure 10 – *20-high cluster mill at Boston Scientific/Interventional Technologies*

Summary and Conclusions

A platinum-enhanced variant of UNS S31673 stainless steel has been developed by BSC/IVT. PERSS has an enhanced radiopacity compared to UNS S31673 stainless steels without additional unspecified elements, which makes it ideal for coronary stent applications. Procedures described in this paper discuss the process of taking the initial PERSS ingot and converting it into a form that can be used with BSC/IVT's chemical etching process to produce stents.

BSC/IVT has developed a pilot program for internal production of its new PERSS alloy. The Z-mill was shown to be capable of providing the precise reduction in thickness necessary for the foil to be used in the stent manufacturing process.

Acknowledgments

The authors would like to express their gratitude to the U.S. Department of Energy's Albany Research (Portland, OR), The Arnold Engineering Company (Marengo, IL), and Intergrated (*sic*) Industrial Systems (Yalesville, CT) for assistance in the processing of this material. Without their contributions, the timely completion of this research would have been much more difficult.

References

[1]   Craig, C. H., Radisch, H. R., Jr., Trozera, T. A., Turner, P. C., Govier, R. D., Vesely, E.J., Jr., Gokcen, N. A., Friend, C. M., and Edwards, M. R., "Development of a Platinum Enhanced Radiopaque Stainless Steel (PERSS®)," *Stainless Steels for Medical and Surgical Applications, ASTM STP 1438*, G. L. Winters and M. J. Nutt, Eds., ASTM International, West Conshohocken, PA, 2003.

[2]   Humphreys, F. J., and Hatherly, M., *Recrystallization and Related Annealing Phenomena*, Pergamon, Oxford, 1996, pp. 205-206.

[3]   Lahoti, G. D., and Semiatin, S. L., in *Metals Handbook, 9th Edition, Volume 14, Forming and Forging*, ASM International, Materials Park, OH, 1988, pp. 343-360.

Markus Windler,[1] Rainer Steger,[1] and Gary L. Winters[2]

Quality Aspects of High-Nitrogen Stainless Steel for Surgical Implants

Reference: Windler, M., Steger, R., and Winters, G. L., "Quality Aspects of High-Nitrogen Stainless Steel for Surgical Implants," *Stainless Steels for Medical and Surgical Applications, ASTM STP 1438*, G. L. Winters and M. J. Nutt, Eds., ASTM International, West Conshohocken, PA, 2003.

Abstract: High-nitrogen stainless steel has been used in orthopedic implants because of its high strength, good corrosion resistance and biocompatibility. In this study six annealed wrought high-nitrogen stainless steel sample bars from five different manufacturers were characterized in terms of chemical composition, mechanical properties, hardness, metallurgical structure and corrosion resistance. The metallurgical investigation, which determined the microstructure, grain size and inclusion content, was made with a light microscope, image analysis and SEM with EDX. The potentio-dynamic corrosion behaviour in the cross-sectional plane was measured at pH 4 and 40°C. No major differences were found in the chemical compositions, mechanical properties, hardness or metallurgies of the six sample materials. The only difference between the materials was established in the corrosion test, where the breakdown potential varied between -150 and $+900$ mV$_{(SCE)}$. However, no correlation could be established between the corrosion results and chemical composition, microstructure, or type / number of the inclusions. Additional heat treatment improved the material with low breakdown potential. It is recommended that minimum requirements should be established for the breakdown potential and incorporated in the current material standards.

Keywords: high nitrogen stainless steel, corrosion properties, mechanical properties, microstructure, inclusions

[1]Director, Materials Research, and Research Scientist, respectively, Material Research Department, Sulzer Orthopedics Ltd., P.O. Box 65, 8404 Winterthur, Switzerland.
[2]Materials Engineer, Material Research Department, Sulzer Orthopedics Inc., Spectrum Drive 9900, Austin, TX, 78717, U.S.A.

Introduction

Stainless steel has been employed as surgical implant material for many years. The quality of the steel in the pioneering days was poor and numerous deficiencies such as fatigue failures and severe corrosion were reported [1]. The breakthrough of stainless steel as an implant material came with the development of the material with the designation AISI 316L. This type of stainless steel is still used today, primarily for the products of osteosynthesis like plates, nails and screws [2,3]. Endoprostheses made of this type of steel since the 1960s, e.g. the Charnley hip stem, have been implanted and retained successfully in the body for many years [4-6]. Reports of corrosion phenomena and fatigue failures of this stainless steel in-vivo have been made in the literature [2,4,7]. A new type of stainless steel was introduced in the field of orthopedic surgery in the mid 1980s [4]. The chromium and manganese contents of the alloy were raised and up to 0.5% nitrogen was also introduced to improve the corrosion resistance and increase the strength [8]. This material was standardized under the designation "Wrought High Nitrogen Stainless Steel" 1992: ISO 5832-9 and ASTM F1586 – 95. This highly alloyed stainless steel is employed primarily for cemented hip prostheses and is well established in Europe. As a result of the increasing demand for material in the mid-1990s, more and more steelworks began to manufacture this stainless steel.

This study was made to document the variation in quality of this high alloyed stainless steel, which is produced by various manufacturers. In addition to a quantitative microstructural analysis, the corrosion resistance was studied in the potentio-dynamic test. The biocompatibility of a metal is influenced decisively by the corrosion resistance. Reports have been made of the negative biological effects of corrosion products by various metals [1,9,10].

Material

Six wrought high-nitrogen stainless steel sample bars (A, B-1, B-2, C, D, and E) from five different manufacturers ("A" – "E") were compared in this evaluation. The commercially manufactured bars, which had diameters of 22 to 33 mm and were annealed (1050°C, 1 h, quenched with water), met the requirements of ISO 5832-9 and ASTM Standard Specification for Wrought Nitrogen Strengthened –21Chromium – 10Nickel – 3Manganese –2.5Molybdenum Stainless Steel Bar for Surgical Implants (F1586) for chemical composition and mechanical properties (Table 1). The values in Table 1 were taken from the manufacturer's material certificates. This material will be used for femoral hip stems which underwent afterwards a forging process.

Methods

Microstructure Analysis

Metallographic sections of all the bars were prepared in the longitudinal and transverse directions and etched and studied with high powered optical microscope (Leica DMRX, Wetzlar, Germany). Typical structural pictures with a magnification of 500x were made of all materials in the scanning electronic microscope (JSM-IC 848 A, Joel, J-Tokio). With the aid of image analysis software (Soft Imaging System, Analysis 3.0, Münster, Germany), the inclusions in the steel were determined according to type, number and size. The chemical elements of the inclusions were determined by means of EDX Analysis (Energy Dispersive Analysis) (TRACOR Analysator TN 5421, Noran Instruments Ltd., Middleton, WI, USA). A structural analysis consisted of 5 images, each with a size of 200 μm x 150 μm.

An X-ray diffraction analysis was made on the transverse section of Material "E" to identify the inclusions (Goniometer, Cu K_α rays with $\lambda = 0.15418$ nm).

Table 1 - *Chemical Composition and Mechanical Properties of Studied Materials*

	"A"	"B-1"	"B-2"	"C"	"D"	"E"	ISO 5832-9
Diameter	ø22mm	ø33mm	ø33mm	ø22mm	ø22mm	ø33 mm	n.s.
Carbon [%]	0.034	0.02	0.032	0.043	0.03	0.034	0.08 max.
Chromium [%]	20.9	20.2	21.25	21.27	20.5	20.71	19.5 to 22
Nickel [%]	9.55	10.15	10.55	9.15	9.8	9.82	9 to 11
Manganese [%]	4.12	3.65	4.05	3.51	3.99	3.81	2 to 4.25
Molybdenum [%]	2.15	2.4	2.28	2.36	2.1	2.17	2 to 3
Nitrogen [%]	0.39	0.55	0.43	0.41	0.37	0.39	0.25 to 0.5
Niobium [%]	0.31	0.38	0.27	0.36	n.m.	0.27	0.25 to 0.8
Phosphorus [%]	0.021	0.023	0.025	0.011	0.018	0.016	0.025 max.
Sulphur [%]	<0.002	0.0001	0.001	0.001	0.001	0.001	0.01 max.
Copper [%]	0.013	0.08	0.23	0.06	0.1	0.06	0.25 max.
Silicon [%]	0.34	0.73	0.19	0.14	0.25	0.15	075 max.
Iron [%]	Balance	Balance	Balance	Balance	Balance	Balance	Balance
Properties							
TS [MPa]	880	1017	902	900	869	868	740 min.
YS (0.2%) [MPa]	506	600	565	539	621	482	430 min.
Elongation [%]	39	35	41	36	35	46	35 min.
Brinell Hardness	241	276	252	254	251	229	n.s.
Grain Size No.	10	8	7 - 8	10	5 – 10	8	> 5

NOTES: TS = tensile strength, YS = yield strength, n.s. = not specified, n.m. = not measured by the vender. The Brinell Hardness values were measured in our lab and were not from the vendors' certificates.

Hardness Measurement

The Brinell hardness survey was made in the center of each metallographic transverse section. The Brinell hardness (2.5/187.5) was determined according to ISO Metallic materials – Brinell hardness test – Part 1: Test method (ISO 6506-1), using an EMCO Tester, M4A-025, Hallein, Austria. Each survey consisted of three measurements.

Potentio-dynamic Corrosion Test

A potentio-dynamic polarization curve of each sample were determined per ASTM Standard Reference Test Method for Making Potentiostatic and Potentiodynamic Anodic Polarization Measurements (G5) using an EG&G (VersaSat II) Potentiostat, EG&G (SoftCorr III) Software and an EG&G K46 corrosion cell (EG&G Instruments, Princeton, USA). The samples were prepared so that the measurement surface of each sample were transverse planes of the original bar. The sample surfaces were ground to 1200 grit. A surface area of 1 cm^2 was immersed in 1 litre of sodium chloride solution (0.9%) at 40°C, pH 4 (adjusted with hydrochlorid acid) and with nitrogen bubbling during the whole process. A cathodic pre-polarization (2 minutes at 100 $\mu A/cm^2$) was made 250 mV negative to the rest potential to clean the immersed surface. After waiting 30 minutes to allow the system to come to equilibrium, the test was started with a scan rate of 10 mV/min. Saturated calomel electrodes (SCE) were used for reference purposes. All the tests were made twice reusing the old sample after refinishing.

Corrosion Test after Heat Treatment

Four specimens each with a length of 20 mm were separated from the material produced by manufacturer "E" (ø22 mm). These specimen were subjected to different heat treatments at temperatures of 850°C, 900°C, 950°C, 1000°C, 1050°C and 1100°C in a High-Therm VMK 1400 air furnace (Linn, Hirschbach, Germany). After a holding time of 1h, the specimens were quenched in air. Electrochemical tests were performed on the transverse section of each sample. Two tests were performed for each heat treatment reusing the old sample after refinishing. Transversal cross sections were made after heat treatment to check grain growth, as well as qualification of inclusion content by light microscope.

Results

Microstructure Analysis

All metallographic sections of the high-nitrogen stainless steels had an austentic matrix with a grain size of between 7 and 10. No delta ferrite could be observed with a magnification of up to 100x. The structure of the transverse sections was isotropic and the structure of the longitudinal sections was elongated in the rolling direction. Three forms of inclusions were observed in the longitudinal and transverse cross sections. Type 1 inclusions were fine and homogeneously-distributed with a diameter of less than 1 μm. They were identified as [Cr, Mo]-carbides after qualitative EDX analysis detected the presence of the elements Cr and Mo in these features. Type 2 inclusions were larger, more elongated in the rolling direction, had a diameter of up to 10 μm and consisted of Cr, Nb and N (Figure 1). On the basis of the X-ray diffraction analysis, these inclusions were tetragonal [Cr, Nb]-nitrides; Card Number No. 25-0240 according to JCPDS [11]. Type 3 inclusions were black, non-metallics up to 15 μm in diameter and had a composition of aluminum (Figure 2). These inclusions were alumina-slag and resulted from the deoxidation process. The number of Type 2 and Type 3 inclusions are shown in Figures 3 and 4.

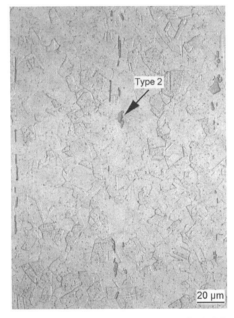 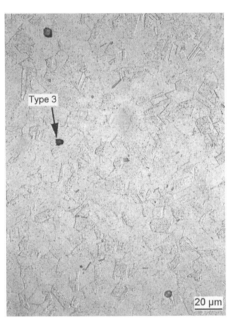

Figure 1 - *Microstructure, Material "B-2" in the longitudinal cross-section. Type 2 inclusion consisted of [Cr, Nb]-nitride*

Figure 2 - *Microstructure, Material "B-2" in the transverse cros-section. Type 3 inclusion consisted of alumina-slag*

Potentio-dynamic Corrosion Test

Typical potentio-dynamic plots are shown in Figure 5. The rest potential (or open circuit potential) varied between –700 mV and –400 mV for all the tests, and a corrosion rate of about 1 μA/cm^2 was observed in the passive range. The breakdown potential for the different bars was noticeably different (Table 2). The breakdown potential varied over a range of –150mV and +900mV. The plot of material "C", had severe transients above

−100 mV and the breakdown potential could only be determined in these cases with difficulty.

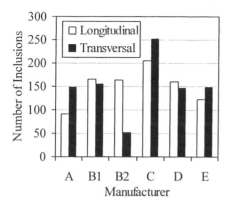

Figure 3 - *Number of Type 2 inclusions [Cr, Nb]-nitride in the longitudinal and transverse cross sections*

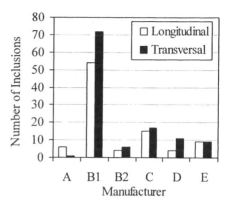

Figure 4 - *Number of Type 3 inclusions (slag) in the longitudinal and transverse cross sections*

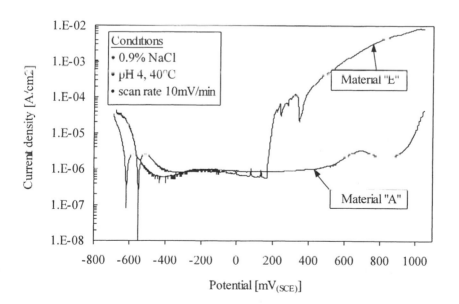

Figure 5 - *Potentio-dynamic corrosion test of high-nitrogen stainless steel. Breakdown potential for Material "A" = +910 mV$_{(SCE)}$ and Material "E" = +200 mV$_{(SCE)}$*

Corrosion Test after Heat Treatment

The breakdown potentials of the heat-treated specimens are listed in Table 2. The heat treatments up to 900°C did not have any influence on the breakdown potential. An improvement could only be realized from 950°C upwards, but with numerous transients in the passive range. The potentio-dynamic corrosions curves had no transients after heat treatments of ≥1000°C, with breakdown potentials in the range of +850 to +920 mV$_{(SCE)}$ (Figure 6). A small grain growth was recognized after the heat treatment ≥1050°C and about 50% of the type 2 inclusions (Cr,Nb-nitrides) had been dissolved into the matrix.

Table 2 - *Breakdown Potential for Different Qualities of High-Nitrogen Stainless Steel*

Material	Breakdown Potential [mV$_{(SCE)}$]	Remarks
"A"	+910 / +800	pitting corrosion
"B-1"	+520 / +380	crevice corrosion
"B-2"	+890 / +820	pitting corrosion
"C"	approx. +640 / approx. +810	transients above −100 mV
"D"	+230 / −150	crevice corrosion
"E"	+160 / +200	crevice corrosion
"E" 850°C / 900°C	+180 to +220	crevice corrosion
"E" 950°C	approx. +600	transients above +100 mV
"E" 1000°C – 1100°C	+850 to +920	pitting corrosion

Discussion

With high-nitrogen stainless steel, the substantial difference in the breakdown potential of various material lots and manufacturers cannot be explained on the basis of the microstructural analysis. The material is not easy to manufacture – a statement, which is substantiated by the following facts. The material lots "C" and "D" were the first times that the respective manufactures had attempted to make this material. In all probability, the material qualities, i.e., corrosion resistance, fluctuated markedly because the fabrication operations were not optimal. In view of the quality problems, Manufacturer "E" does not market this material any more.

Inclusions in the stainless steel can have a marked effect on the corrosion resistance. In our opinion, the larger [Cr, Nb]-nitrides have a greater influence on the corrosion resistance than the very small chromium-molybdenum carbides. As a result of the additional heat treatment ≥1000°C, the [Cr, Nb, N]-inclusions may have been dissolved into the matrix, with a positive effect on the corrosion resistance. In general, inhomogeneities in the material can be reduced by means of heat treatment.

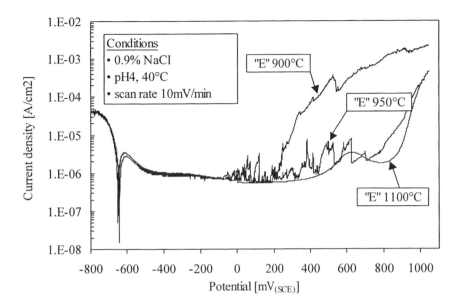

Figure 6 - *Potentio-dynamic corrosion test of Material "E" after heat treatments at 900°C, 950°C and 1100°C*

The corrosion resistance in the stainless steels could be affected by the presence of sigma-phase (σ) and / or delta-ferrite (δ) [12]. σ-phase can occurs if the material were held for some time between about 700 and 810°C. The crystal structure is tetragonal, hard and brittle. δ-ferrite can form directly from austenite during the cold working process. If the rolling/heating operations, which the mill used to balance grain size, mechanical properties and the requirements to be annealed were not adequate, then stainless steels may form small amounts of σ-phase and δ-ferrite. Both phases usually cannot be found in the optical microstructure, but they can be removed by annealing.

With good material lots, the corrosion resistance of high-nitrogen stainless steel is distinctly higher than those of the conventional stainless steels, type ISO 5832-1 or AISI 316L. The breakdown potential for AISI 316L was measured in the range of +100mV to +350mV(SCE) by various authors depending on pH and temperature [13,14]. In the main, the differences are attributable to the different structural and deformation conditions. In comparison with the stainless steel alloys, the breakdown potential by CoCrMo alloys ranges from +400 to +600mV(SCE) [15,16]. These values are valid for CoCrMo cast alloy [ASTM Standard Specification for Cobalt –28Chromium –6Molybdenum Casting Alloy and Cast Products for Surgical Implants (F75)] as well as for wrought or forged CoCrMo alloys [ASTM Standard Specification for Wrought Cobalt – 28Chromium –

6Molybdenum Alloy for Surgical Implants (F1537) or ASTM Standard Specification for Cobalt –28Chromium –6Molybdenum Alloy Forgings for Surgical Implants (F799)].

The majority of the potentio-dynamic corrosion tests described in the literature were made in sodium chlorid solutions or Ringer's solution at 37°C and pH 7 (near physiological conditions). Corrosion phenomena, which are mainly attributable to crevice corrosion, have been found by the analysis of implants [17]. Fontana [18] developed the basic model for crevice corrosion. According to this theory, metal consumes oxygen in a cathodic reaction and oxygen cannot be replaced in a crevice because the small dimensions of the crevice impeds the diffusion of oxygen into the crevice. At the final stage the pH of the crevice drops to a lower value and the unprotected metal dissolves. The tests in this study were therefore conducted at pH 4 to simulate the acidic condition of the crevice.

Conclusions

As far as the chemical composition and the mechanical properties were concerned, all six bar materials of the high-nitrogen stainless steel specimen fulfilled the requirements of the standards ISO 5832-9 and ASTM F1586.

A critical difference was found for the corrosion resistance, whereby the best material lot had a breakdown potential of about +900 mV and, in contrast, the poorest material lot exhibited a breakdown by a potential of –150 mV.

The breakdown potential can be improved considerably by means of a subsequent heat treatment at ≥1000°C. The reason for this, however, was not indicated in this work. Nevertheless, it is interesting to find that an additional heat treatment had a positive effect on bars that have already been mill annealed.

From the point of view of corrosion resistance, it is possible to differentiate between "Good Material Lots" and "Poor Material Lots" with the aid of a simple potentio-dynamic corrosion test. This corrosion test, together with minimum requirements, should be incorporated in the ISO and ASTM standards for the material "High-Nitrogen Stainless Steel" in future.

References

[1]   Frank, E., and Zitter, H., *Metallische Implantate in der Knochenchirurgie*, Springer Verlag, 1971.

[2]   Cook, S.D., Renz, E.A., Barrack, R.L., Thomas, K. A., Harding, A.F., Haddad, R.J., Jr., and Milicic, M., "Clinical and Metallurgical Analysis of Retrieved Internal Fixation Device," *Clinical Orthopaedics and Related Res*earch, No. 194, 1985, pp. 236 – 247.

[3]   Disegi, J.A., and Eschbach, L., "Stainless Steel in Bone Surgery," *Injury*, Vol. 31, 2000, Supplement 4, pp. D2-D6.

[4]   Wroblewski, B.M., *Revision Surgery in Total Hip Arthroplasty*, Springer Verlag, 1990.

[5]   Sochart, D.H., Porter, M.L., and Lancashire, W., "The Long-Term Results of Charnley Low-Friction Arthroplasty in Young Patients Who Have Congenital Dislocation, Degenerative Osteoarthritis or Rheumatoid Arthritis," *J. Bone and Joint Surgery*, Vol. 79-A, 1997, pp. 1599 – 1617.

[6]   Callaghan, J.J., Forest, E.E., Olejniczak, J.P., Goetz, D.D., and Johnston, R.C., "Charnley Total Hip Arthroplasty in Patients Less Than Fifty Years Old," *J. Bone and Joint Surgery*, Vol. 80-A, 1988, pp. 704 – 714.

[7]   Wright, T.M., Burstein, A.H., and Bartel, D.L., "Retrieval Analysis of Total Joint Replacement Components: A Six-Year Experience," *Corrosion and Degradation of Implant Materials*, ASTM STP 859, A.C. Fraker and C.D. Griffin, Eds., American Society for Testing Materials, Philadelphia, 1985, pp. 415 – 428.

[8]   Brehme, J., and Biehl, V., "Metallic Biomaterials," *Handbook of Biomaterial Properties*, J. Black and G. Hastings, Eds., Chapman & Hall, 1998, pp. 135 – 214.

[9]   Merritt, K., and Brown, S.A.; "Biological Effects of Corrosion Products from Metals," *Corrosion and Degradation of Implant Materials*, ASTM STP 859, A.C. Fraker and C.D. Griffin, Eds., American Society for Testing Materials, Philadelphia, 1985, pp. 195 – 207.

[10] Black, J., *Biological Performance of Materials: Fundamentals of Biocompatibility*, Marcel Dekker, Inc., 1999.

[11] *Mineral Powder Diffraction File*, JCPDS International Centre for Diffraction Data, Swarthmore, U.S.A., 1986.

[12] "Atmospheric and Aqueous Corrosion," *Stainless Steels, ASM Specialty Handbook*, J.R. Davis, Ed., ASM International, Materials Park, Ohio, U.S.A., 1994, pp. 133 – 180.

[13] Sheety, R.H., Gilbertson, L.N., and Jacobs, C.H., "The New Surface Finish – A Method of Improving the Properties of 316L Stainless Steel," [abstract], *Transaction of the Society of Biomaterials*, New York, 1987, p. 233.

[14] Ogundele, G.I., and White, W.E., "Polarization Studies on Surgical-Grade Stainless Steels in Hanks' Physiological Solution," *Corrosion and Degradation of Implant Materials*, ASTM STP 859, A.C. Fraker and C.D. Griffin, Eds., American Society for Testing Materials, Philadelphia, 1985, pp. 117 – 135.

[15] Kuhn, A.T., "Corrosion of Co-Cr Alloys in Aqueous Environments," *Biomaterials*, Vol. 2, 1981, pp. 68 – 77.

[16] Devine, T.M., and Wulff, J., "The Comparative Crevice Corrosion Resistance of Co-Cr Base Surgical Implant Alloys," *J. Electrochem. Soc.: Electrochemical Science and Technology*, Vol. 123, 1976, pp. 1433 – 1437.

[17] Willert, H.-G., Broback, L.-G., Buchhorn, G.H., Jensen, P.H., Köster, G., Lang, I., Ochsner, P., and Schenk, R., "Crevice Corrosion of Cemented Titanium Alloy Stems in Total Hip Replacements," *Clinical Orthopaedics and Related Research*, No. 333, 1996, pp. 51 – 75.

[18] Fontana, M.G., and Greene, N.D., *Corrosion Engineering*, 3rd Edition, McGraw-Hill, New York, 1986.

Terry O. Woods[1]

MRI Safety and Compatibility of Implants and Medical Devices

Reference: Woods, T. O., "**MRI Safety and Compatibility of Implants and Medical Devices**," *Stainless Steels for Medical and Surgical Applications, ASTM STP 1438,* G. L. Winters and M. J. Nutt, Eds., ASTM International, West Conshohocken, PA, 2003.

Abstract: Since MRI (magnetic resonance imaging) scanners became available in the 1980's, they have rapidly become one of the most common clinical imaging tools. The MR environment produces unique safety and compatibility issues for materials used in implants and medical devices. The principal issues for MR safety and compatibility are magnetically induced displacement force and torque, radio frequency (RF) heating, and image artifact. This paper defines and discusses the potential hazards produced by implants and devices in the MR environment, with an emphasis on stainless steels. It also describes MR safety and compatibility test methods developed by ASTM and summarizes ongoing MR standards development work.

Keywords: MRI, MRI safety, MRI compatibility, implants, medical devices

Introduction

MRI (magnetic resonance imaging) scanners became commercially available in the mid 1980s. The high quality of the diagnostic information provided has led to their adoption as one of the most common clinical imaging tools. Demand for greater image resolution and faster scan times has driven the evolution of scanner technology over the last 15 years with several-fold increases in field strength and temporal and spatial gradient fields over those present in early scanners. Interventional MR (magnetic resonance) procedures, performed inside or near the scanner, are the newest facet of MR technology to place increased demands for safety and compatibility on stainless steel surgical instruments and other intraoperative devices like patient monitors and anaesthesia equipment. It is likely that everyone in the developed world will be exposed to an MRI scan at some time in his or her life, so the issues of MR safety and compatibility of implants and medical devices are ones that directly impact millions of patients.

The MR environment produces unique safety and compatibility issues for materials used in implants and medical devices. The FDA proposed definitions for MR safety and compatibility in "A Primer on Medical Device Interactions with Magnetic Resonance Imaging Systems," which was released for comment in February 1997 [1]. These definitions were published in the ASTM Standard Test Method for Evaluation of MR

[1]Mechanical Engineer, Food and Drug Administration, Center for Devices and Radiological Health, 9200 Corporate Boulevard, HFZ-150, Rockville, MD, 20850.

Artifacts from Passive Implants (F2119). A device is considered MR safe if it presents no hazards to the patient or other individuals. An MR compatible device is MR safe and in addition does not significantly affect the diagnostic information nor have its operations affected by the MR scanner. For both definitions, the MR conditions in which the device was tested must be specified because a device that is found to be safe or compatible under one set of conditions may not be found to be so under more extreme MR conditions. This is a particularly important warning currently because most devices that are claimed to be MR safe or compatible have been tested in 1.5 tesla scanners. Recently, 3 tesla scanners with much harsher MR environments have been introduced and it is likely that some devices that were safe or compatible in a 1.5 tesla system will no longer be safe or compatible in a 3 tesla scanner.

Just a few years ago, a needle biopsy was the most complicated interventional MR procedure. Today however, MR guided neurosurgery is commonly performed in some centers because the MR gives a unique capability to identify tumor boundaries intraoperatively. The rapid and widespread development and increasing complexity of procedures performed in the MR suite is exponentially increasing the demand for MR safe and compatible devices. Development of these interventional and intraoperative MR capabilities requires a fully configured MR safe operating room, one which potentially contains many stainless steel components. The types of applications where stainless steels might be found in a device in the MR environment include passive implants (stents, aneurysm clips, sutures), active implants (neurostimulators), external passive devices (patient positioning devices, electrical leads, surgical hand tools, iv poles, equipment carts, gas bottles), and external electrically active devices (patient monitors, anaesthesia equipment, defibrillators). These medical devices range in complexity from the bearings in a castor on a cart to a life-sustaining implant like an endovascular stent-graft, and yet in the wrong circumstances, both could potentially interact with an MRI scanner to cause serious problems for the patient.

The principal issues for MR safety and compatibility are magnetically induced displacement force and torque, radio frequency (RF) heating, and image artifact. Gradient field induced voltages are also a potential problem for implants. Adverse events ranging from deaths caused by magnetically induced displacement force and torque to third degree burns and images containing large void areas due to the presence of magnetic materials have happened in the past and continue to happen. Specific examples are presented below. Fortunately, serious accidents are not common, though they do continue to happen every year. A number of organizations including the FDA, the Radiological Society of North America, the American College of Radiologists, the National Electrical Manufacturers Association (NEMA) MR Technical Committee, and ECRI (formerly the Emergency Care Research Institute) are working to increase MR safety awareness through publications, courses, web sites and standards development activities [2-4].

Standards Development Efforts

ASTM Standard Specification for the Requirements and Disclosure of Self-Closing Aneurysm Clips (F1542-94), was the first standard to outline a test method for determining MR safety, though it addresses only the magnetically induced displacement force. In 1998, ASTM Committee F04 on Medical and Surgical Materials and Devices, Subcommittee 15, Materials Test Methods, formed a task group to develop standards addressing MR safety and compatibility of implants and medical devices. The group has completed the ASTM Standard Test Method for Measurement of Magnetically Induced Displacement Force on Passive Implants in the Magnetic Resonance Environment (F2052), the ASTM Standard Test Method for Measurement of Radio Frequency Induced Heating near Passive Implants During Magnetic Resonance Imaging (F2182), and F2119 for determining image artifact. The group is also working on a test method for measuring magnetically induced torque on passive implants. These standards are the first general test methods addressing MR safety and compatibility of medical devices. Their scope is currently limited to passive implanted devices, but the test methods are also appropriate for a range of active implants as well as passive and active devices that are not implants. ISO 9713 Neurosurgical implants – Self-closing intracranial aneurysm clips, requires MR testing to determine magnetically induced forces and torques and image artifacts, but gives no test methods. IEC 60601-2-33, Particular Requirements for the Safety of Magnetic Resonance Equipment for Medical Diagnosis, defines operating limits for MR scanners. In particular, it defines safety limits for specific absorption rate (SAR) in the head, whole body and local tissue [5]. These limits help to define the allowable amount of RF induced heating.

MRI Effects on Materials and Devices

All materials are either ferromagnetic, paramagnetic, or diamagnetic. As defined in ASTM F2052, a ferromagnetic material has ordered and parallel magnetic moments that produce magnetization in one direction; a paramagnetic material has a relative permeability which is slightly greater than unity, and which is practically independent of the magnetizing force; and a diamagnetic material has a relative permeability less than unity. The most common ferromagnetic materials are iron, cobalt, and nickel [6]. Magnetic susceptibilities for even the most weakly magnetic ferromagnetic materials are orders of magnitude greater than the magnetic susceptibilities of paramagnetic and diamagnetic materials [7]. Common examples of paramagnetic materials are titanium, aluminum, and platinum [6, 8, 9]. Many metals, copper, for instance, and most nonmetals are diamagnetic [6].

Martensitic and ferritic stainless steels are ferromagnetic. Ferromagnetic stainless steels, like the 400 series Class 4 martensitic stainless steel and the Class 6 ferritic stainless steel in the ASTM Standard Specification for Stainless Steel Billet, Bar, and Wire for Surgical Instruments (F899), are not MR safe. Austenitic stainless steels are paramagnetic at room temperature [8]. They include the austenitic stainless steels in the ASTM Standard Specification for Wrought 18 Chromium-14 Nickel-2.5 Molybdenum Stainless Steel Bar and Wire for Surgical Implants (UNS S31673) (F138), the ASTM Standard Specification for Wrought 18 Chromium-14 Nickel-2.5 Molybdenum Stainless Sheet and Strip for Surgical Implants (UNS S31673) (F139), the ASTM Standard Specification for Wrought Nitrogen Strengthened 22 Chromium-12.5 Nickel-5 Manganese-2.5 Molybdenum Stainless Steel Bar and Wire for Surgical Implants (F1314), the ASTM Standard Specification for Wrought 18 Chromium-14 Nickel-2.5 Molybdenum Stainless Steel Surgical Fixation Wire (UNS S31673) (F1350), the ASTM

Standard Specification for Wrought Nitrogen Strengthened-21 Chromium-10 Nickel-3 Manganese-2.5 Molybdenum Stainless Steel Bar for Surgical Implants (F1586), and the Class 3 austenitic stainless steel specified in ASTM F899.

These austenitic stainless steels are safe for some MR applications, though cold work [10-12] and heat treatments [6, 13] during manufacturing may produce regions of magnetic martensite or ferrite that can render a device unsafe in the MR environment. For instance, it has been shown that martensite transformation produced during heavy cold working of 316 stainless steel can increase the susceptibility from 0.003 to 9 [8], transforming a paramagnetic and potentially MR safe material into an unsafe ferromagnetic material. Because processing can change the magnetic properties of the material, it is important that the MR safety and compatibility testing for any device be performed on a finished device. It is also important to consider possible lot to lot variations in magnetic properties of starting materials and possible effects of processing changes on the magnetic properties of a finished device when determining the frequency and sample size needed for MR safety and compatibility testing. In spite of these caveats, there are many applications for which the appropriate austenitic stainless steel is an acceptable material for a device or device component in the MR environment.

Magnetically Induced Displacement Force

A magnetic displacement force is produced when a magnetic object is exposed to a spatial gradient in a magnetic field. This force is responsible for the "projectile effect" familiar to anyone who has held a small magnet near a paper clip or other small magnetic object. Even though this magnetic field effect is well-known to virtually everyone, accidents caused when magnetic objects become projectiles in the large magnetic fields around MR scanners continue to happen. This is in part due to the fact that the field strength and gradient fields in MR scanners are many times greater than the magnetic fields to which most people are accustomed. The field strength in a 3 tesla MR scanner, the largest currently available clinical system, is more than 50,000 times the earth's magnetic field strength

Objects ranging from scissors and IV poles to forklift tines and "sandbags" containing steel shot have been pulled into the bores of MR scanners, sometimes causing serious injuries [1]. An iron filing in a patient's eye was displaced by a scanner's magnetic field, causing the patient to lose vision in that eye permanently [14]. Numerous accidents have occurred when gas cylinders were pulled into MR scanners. In July 2001, a child undergoing an MR scan was killed when he was struck in the head by an oxygen bottle that was pulled into the scanner [15]. This accident occurred the same month an article was published presenting five projectile cylinder accidents which had taken place in two institutions, four of which had occurred in the previous three years [16]. The authors suggested that in spite of MR safety education, projectile cylinder accidents may be increasing because more patients are being scanned while they are on life support systems [16]. Ironically, even an object as seemingly innocuous as a pillow can become a projectile in a magnetic field. A pillow containing coil springs that were not detected during pre-scan screening by a hand-held magnet was attracted into an MR scanner, fortunately without causing any injuries [17]. Later measurements showed that 16% of the mass of the pillow consisted of metal. Experiments were performed to determine velocities developed by objects moving from the creep point (the point furthest from the magnet at which the object would accelerate within 30 s of being placed there) into the bore of the 1.5 tesla scanner. The 1 kg pillow reached a maximum velocity of 33.7 km/h after undergoing a maximum acceleration of 9.9 g, while a 91 g metal glasses case reached a maximum velocity of 77.8 km/h [17].

Large magnetic fields can also affect the operation of devices. At least one patient with an implanted cardiac pacemaker died when the MR system interrupted the functioning of the pacemaker, and an implanted insulin infusion pump was found to be non-functional after being exposed to an MR scanner [1]. Recent work in our laboratory has shown that the flow rate produced by some portable oxygen regulators is altered at the entrance to the bore of a 2 tesla MR scanner [18].

The magnetically induced displacement force, $\mathbf{F}$, is a function of the magnitude of the magnetic field gradient and the magnetic moment of the object (which is in turn a function of the object's magnetization and volume). Or, $\mathbf{F} = \nabla(\mathbf{m} \bullet \mathbf{B})$, where $\mathbf{m}$ is the dipole moment and $\mathbf{B}$ is the magnetic field strength [19]. Since the magnetization, $\mathbf{M}$, is proportional to $\mathbf{m}$, it is also true that $\mathbf{F} \propto \nabla(\mathbf{M} \bullet \mathbf{B})$. For diamagnetic and paramagnetic materials and for ferromagnetic materials below their magnetic saturation point, the force is proportional to the product of the magnetic field strength and the gradient of the magnetic field strength, $(|\mathbf{B}| \, |\nabla \mathbf{B}|)$ [9]. For ferromagnetic materials that have reached saturation, the force is proportional to the gradient of the magnetic field strength, $\nabla \mathbf{B}$ [9].

The displacement force must be measured at the location of the maximum spatial gradient or the location of the maximum product of the spatial gradient and the field strength so it is necessary to determine that location. Magnet system designers often incorporate shielding, which contains the field within a smaller volume around the magnet. This shielding can produce greater gradients in the magnetic field, which will produce greater displacement forces on magnetic objects. Shielding can also complicate the spatial distribution of the field and its gradient. For a scanner with a horizontal static field, B_o, along the long axis (Z axis) of the magnet, the maximum spatial gradient should occur in the Z direction near or inside the entrance to the magnet bore. This is due to the fact that the field lines run along the Z axis until they reach the portal of the magnet and then begin to bend around in the X and Y directions.

The magnetically induced deflection force may be measured using the method described in ASTM F2052. In general, a device can be considered to experience an acceptable level of magnetically induced deflection force if the measured force is less than the weight of the device.

Magnetically Induced Torque

A torque is produced as an object attempts to align itself with the magnetic field produced by the imaging magnet, just as a compass needle aligns itself with the earth's magnetic field. This effect has also caused the death of at least one MR patient. Magnetically induced torque rotated an intracranial aneurysm clip in a patient who had entered the MR scan room, but who had not entered the scanner and so had not entered the most extreme field conditions. The aneurysm clip tore adjacent blood vessels and the patient hemorrhaged and died [20].

The torque is a function of the strength of the magnetic field and the characteristics, both material and geometric, of the magnetically active object. It is related to the geometry, composition, distribution of mass, and magnetic properties of the object and the strength of the magnetic field. The torque may be written as:

$$\mathbf{T} = \mathbf{m} \times \mathbf{B}, \tag{1}$$

where $\mathbf{m}$ is the dipole moment and $\mathbf{B}$ is the magnetic field strength [19].

So, for an object with a given dipole moment, the maximum magnetic torque produced on an object will occur when the object is in the region of the highest magnetic field strength, that is, in the imaging volume.

For an MRI scanner with a horizontal magnetic field:

$$\mathbf{B} = B_o \hat{z} \tag{2}$$

and

$$\mathbf{m} = (m_x \hat{x} + m_y \hat{y} + m_z \hat{z}) \tag{3}$$

so,

$$\mathbf{T} = (m_x \hat{x} + m_y \hat{y} + m_z \hat{z}) \times B_o \hat{z} = B_o m_y \hat{x} - B_o m_x \hat{y} \tag{4}$$

or

$$\mathbf{T} = T_x \hat{x} + T_y \hat{y} \tag{5}$$

Therefore, for a scanner with a horizontal magnetic field, the torque may have components in the x and y directions. It is very important to note that while the direction of $\mathbf{B}$ is always in the z direction, the direction of $\mathbf{m}$ varies as the orientation of the device varies with respect to the scanner. So, as the orientation of an object changes with respect to the scanner, the magnitude of the torque (and the magnitudes of the components of the torque in the x and y directions) will change.

If an object has a spherical symmetry, it will have no "main axis," and there will be no preferred orientation with the magnetic field and no torque experienced, even if the object has substantial (but uniform) magnetic susceptibility. However, a spherically symmetric object would still experience a magnetically induced displacement force.

A number of methods have been used to measure the magnetically induced torque. There is currently no published standard test method, however one method is the subject of an F04.15 draft standard test method. In all of these test methods, the maximum magnetically induced torque is compared to the maximum torque on the device produced by gravitational forces. In addition to the other MR safety constraints, the maximum magnetically induced torque acting on a device must be less than or equal to the gravitational torque for a device to be determined to be safe in the MR environment.

RF Heating

RF heating is heating of the body produced by currents induced by the pulsed RF imaging gradients applied during scanning. The potential for this problem is greatly increased by the presence of metallic implants or other medical devices, particularly ones with the shape of a long wire, for instance in an electrode for a nerve or cardiac stimulator [21]. Patients have been burned severely when they were positioned improperly within an MR scanner so that conductive loops were formed, for instance when clasping their hands together, or when lying so that there was a small point contact between a patient's calves. Many burns have been reported involving leads that were coiled to produce loops and then were allowed to touch the patient inside the scanner, including burns severe enough to require skin grafts [1, 22]. There also have been many incidents with pulse oximeters, some requiring skin grafts, and some severe enough to require amputation of portions of fingers or toes [23, 24].

As with torque testing, a number of methods have been used to determine RF heating. ASTM F2182, a test method for measuring RF induced heating of passive implants was published in 2002. This method is the only published standard test method for determining RF induced heating of medical devices. The FDA follows the IEC60601-2-33 guidelines for acceptable levels of RF heating during clinical scanning.

Image Artifact

In MR images, artifacts may appear as void regions where no signal is seen or as geometric distortions of the true image [8]. There are three primary mechanisms for production of an MR imaging artifact by an implant [25, 26]. A ferromagnetic material may produce a static field in addition to the uniform magnetic field produced by the magnet. This will perturb the relationship between position and frequency that is essential for accurate image reconstruction [26]. Magnetic objects may produce appreciable distortion if they have a magnetic susceptibility sufficiently different than that for tissue. The presence of such objects can lead to macroscopic imperfections of the magnetic field that lead to nonparallel flux lines [25]. The extent of the artifact depends upon the magnetic susceptibility, mass, shape, orientation, and position of the object, as well as the method used for image processing. Finally, an implant may exhibit an induced eddy current due to the incident RF magnetic field. This will alter the RF field near the implant, thereby creating distortion. The extent of this artifact depends upon the factors listed above as well as the conductivity of the implant.

The image artifact does not generally affect the MR safety of a device, though there has been at least one report of surgery that was performed on a patient based on an artifact that was present in an MR image [1]. The amount and location of the artifact with respect to the location of the region the clinician wishes to image does impact the MR compatibility of a device. It is also important to note that a complete absence of artifact is not always desirable. Manufacturers have gone to considerable effort to design MR safe biopsy needles that have a small enough artifact to allow the region of interest to be visible but enough artifact to allow the needle to be visualized as it is inserted so that it may be precisely positioned in the tissue that is to be sampled. ASTM F2119 identifies a protocol for determining image artifact using standardized pulse sequences.

Discussion and Conclusions

With the advent and rapid proliferation of MR scanning technology, medical devices have been faced with new safety issues. The principal issues affecting MR safety and compatibility are magnetically induced displacement force and torque, RF induced heating and image artifacts. This paper identifies test methods that can be used to determine the safety and compatibility of a device in the MR environment. The current ASTM test methods, which are the only existing published standard test methods addressing MR safety and compatibility of medical devices, are written for passive implanted devices. There is a great need for continued work to expand the scope of these test methods and to develop additional test methods for electrically active implants and devices that are not implants.

Stainless steels have been and will continue to be widely used in medical devices. If properly chosen and fabricated, devices composed of or containing austenitic stainless steel can be safe in the MR environment. However, because of potential hazards caused by the presence of medical devices in and near MR scanners, manufacturers and users must take extreme care to ensure that any device composed of or containing stainless steel is MR safe and that "identical" devices from different lots of raw material or · different production runs are also MR safe.

References

[1]   Center for Devices and Radiological Health, "A Primer on Medical Device Interactions with Magnetic Resonance Imaging Systems," http://www.fda.gov/cdrh/ode/primerf6.html, February 7, 1997.

[2]   Center for Devices and Radiological Health, http://www.fda.gov/cdrh/safety/mrisafety.html, "MRI Safety Web Site."

[3]   ECRI, "The Safe Use of Equipment in the Magnetic Resonance Environment," *Health Devices*, Vol. 30, 2001, pp. 421-444.

[4]   E. Kanal, *Special Cross-Specialty Categorical Course in Diagnostic Radiology: Practical MR Safety Considerations for Physicians, Physicists, and Technologists 2001*. RSNA, Oak Brook, IL, 2001.

[5]   L. A. Zaremba, "Regulatory Issues in MR Safety," in *Special Cross-Specialty Categorical Course in Diagnostic Radiology: Practical MR Safety Considerations for Physicians, Physicists, and Technologists 2001*, E. Kanal, Ed. RSNA, Oak Brook, IL, 2001, pp. 103-110.

[6]   R. M. Bozorth, *Ferromagnetism*. IEEE, Inc., New York, NY, 1978.

[7]   L. H. Van Vlack, *Materials Science for Engineers*. Addison-Wesley, Reading, MA, 1970.

[8]   J. F. Schenck, "The Role of Magnetic Susceptibility in Magnetic Resonance Imaging: MRI Magnetic Compatibility of the First and Second Kinds," *Medical Physics*, Vol. 23, 1996, pp. 815-850.

[9]   E. M. Purcell, *Electricity and Magnetism, Berkeley Physics Course, Volume 2*. McGraw-Hill, New York, 1985.

[10]   J. T. McFadden, "Metallurgical Principles in Neurosurgery," *Journal of Neurosurgery*, Vol. 31, 1969, pp. 373-385.

[11]   M. Dujovny, N. Kossovsky, R. Kossowsky, R. Valdivia, J. S. Suk, F. G. Diaz, K. Berman, and W. Cleary, "Aneurysm Clip Motion during Magnetic Resonance Imaging: In Vivo Experimental Study with Metallurgical Factor Analysis," *Neurosurgery*, Vol. 17, 1985, pp. 543-548.

[12]   M. Dujovny, N. Kossovsky, R. Kossowsky, F. G. Diaz, and J. I. Ausman, "Magnetic Aneurysm Clips: Correlation with Martensite Content and

Implications for Nuclear Magnetic Resonance Examination," *Surgical Forum*, Vol. 34, 1983, pp. 525-527.

[13]   R. M. Brick, A. W. Pense, and R. B. Gordon, *Structure and Properties of Engineering Materials*, 4th ed., McGraw Hill, New York, 1977.

[14]   CDRH, MDR-R100222, http://www.fda.gov/cdrh/maude.html, 1/8/85.

[15]   D. W. Chen, "Boy, 6, dies of skull injury during M.R.I.," *New York Times*. New York, July 31, 2001, pp. B1, B5.

[16]   G. Chaljub, L. A. Karmer, R. F. Johnson III, J. R. F. Johnson, H. Singh, and W. Crow, "Projectile Cylinder Accidents Resulting from the Presence of Ferromagnetic Nitrous Oxide or Oxygen Tanks in the MR Suite," *American Journal of Roentgenology*, Vol. 177, 2001, pp. 27-30.

[17]   B. Condon, D. M. Hadley, and R. Hodgson, "The ferromagnetic pillow: a potential MR hazard not detectable by a hand-held magnet," *The British Journal of Radiology*, Vol. 74, 2001, pp. 847-851.

[18]   T. O. Woods, L. W. Grossman, A. A. Graham, and J. N. Johannessen, "The Effect of a 2T Magnetic Field on Flow Delivered by Oxygen Regulators," 2002 FDA Science Forum - FDA: Building a Multidisciplinary Foundation, Washington, DC, 2002.

[19]   R. J. Thome and J. M. Tarrh, *MHD and Fusion Magnetics, Field and Force Design Concepts,* John Wiley & Sons, New York 1982.

[20]   R. P. Klucznik, D. A. Carrier, R. Pyka, and R. W. Haid, "Placement of a Ferromagnetic Intracerebral Aneurysm Clip in a Magnetic Field with a Fatal Outcome," *Radiology*, Vol. 187, 1993, pp. 855-856.

[21]   J. A. Nyenhuis, J. D. Bourland, and A. V. Kildishev, "Safety Considerations of Rapidly Switched Gradients in MR Environments," in *Special Cross-Specialty Categorical Course in Diagnostic Radiology: Practical MR Safety Considerations for Physicians, Physicists, and Technologists 2001*, E. Kanal, Ed. RSNA, Oak Brook, IL, 2001, pp. 103-110.

[22]   CDRH, MDR-M709484, http://www.fda.gov/cdrh/maude.html, 5/1/95.

[23]   CDRH, MDR-M297255, http://www.fda.gov/cdrh/maude.html, 6/26/92.

[24]   CDRH, MDR-M729534, http://www.fda.gov/cdrh/maude.html, 9/22/95.

[25]   E. M. Bellon, et. al, "MR Artifacts: A Review," *American Journal of Roentgenology*, Vol. 147, 1986, pp. 1271-1281.

[26]   F. G. Shellock, "Biological Effects and Safety Aspects of Magnetic Resonance Imaging," *Magnetic Resonance Quarterly*, Vol. 5, 1989, pp. 243-261.

Corrosion

Lukas Eschbach, Gianni Bigolin, Werner Hirsiger, and Beat Gasser[1]

Fatigue of Small Bone Fragment Fixation Plates Made from Low-Nickel Steel

Reference: Eschbach, L., Bigolin, G., Hirsiger, W., and Gasser B., "**Fatigue of Small Bone Fragment Fixation Plates Made from Low-Nickel Steel,**" *Stainless Steels for Medical and Surgical Applications, ASTM STP 1438*, G. L. Winters and M. J. Nutt, Eds., ASTM International, West Conshohocken, PA, 2003.

Abstract: Today's implant quality stainless steels contain up to 16 wt% nickel although nickel ions are the most widespread skin contact allergens. Previously sensitized persons may develop allergic reactions when nickel is released from stainless steel medical implants. New low-nickel stainless steels combine the benefits of excellent mechanical properties with virtual absence of nickel.

Miniature bone plates and corresponding 2.0 mm screws for the fixation of small bone fragments were produced of a low-nickel stainless steel. The implants were tested in a static reverse-bending setup and under dynamic conditions, and compared to commercially pure (CP) titanium and standard 316L implant steel counterparts. The low-nickel plate could withstand over 200 cycles of bending, whereas the titanium plate broke at 26 cycles. This confirms the higher tolerance of the low-nickel plate to multiple contouring during surgery.

Nevertheless, high cycle fatigue tests under physiologic conditions showed that the low-nickel steel plates exhibit lower resistance to cyclic loads than titanium and 316L plates. SEM investigations of the fatigue fractures confirmed that the cracks preferentially propagate along grain boundaries leading to intergranular fracture of the low-nickel steel. It is suggested that the intergranular crack initiation facilitates the early failure under high cycle fatigue conditions, whereas plastic bending properties are not affected. The tendency to intergranular crack initiation in the low-nickel steel could stem from surface deformation (work hardening) introduced during machining and related embrittlement in the surface zone.

Keywords: Low-nickel steel, fatigue resistance, bending properties, bone plate, bone screw.

---

[1] Scientific co-worker, technical co-worker, technical co-worker, and head of basic research, Dr Robert Mathys Foundation, Bischmattstrasse 12, CH-2544 Bettlach, Switzerland.

Introduction and General Overview of Low-Nickel Steels

High Nitrogen Stainless Steels

Today's implant quality stainless steels contain 9 to 16 wt% nickel although nickel ions are the most widespread skin contact allergens, and more than 20% of the European female population suffers from nickel allergy [1]. Previously sensitized persons may develop allergic reactions and significantly more aseptic or septic complications when nickel is released from stainless steel medical implants [2]. Therefore, titanium implants are used in patients with known nickel allergies. Titanium and titanium alloys have better biocompatibility and corrosion resistance than stainless steel, but titanium disadvantages include lower mechanical strength, reduced toughness, and higher price.

High nitrogen stainless steels were developed during the 1980s after the successful introduction of the pressurized electro-slag-remelting process. They were first thought to increase the performance of petrol, offshore and power generation facilities, because of the positive effect of nitrogen on strength and corrosion resistance. However, nitrogen as an alloying element in steel has the additional benefit of stabilizing the austenitic phase. In fact, nitrogen has been found to be 18 times more efficient than nickel in stabilizing the gamma phase [3]. It is therefore possible to replace nickel by nitrogen in austenitic stainless steels. The resulting virtually nickel-free steels have attracted the attention of producers of medical implants as well as watch case manufacturers, as possible problems with nickel allergies can be omitted.

Some low-nickel stainless steel compositions have been developed for medical or implant applications during the last years (Table 1). All compositions have a high manganese content, which is necessary for increased nitrogen solubility. In alloys with highest manganese contents, nitrogen is even brought into solution without pressure. For the production of the lower manganese composition, remelting under pressurized nitrogen is needed to bring enough nitrogen into the melt. Nitrogen replaces nickel in advanced low-nickel stainless steels, is a powerful austenite stabilizing element, and therefore prevents the formation of secondary magnetic phases.

Table 1 – *Typical composition (wt%) of known low-Ni steels for medical applications. Balance: Fe*

Low-Ni steel	Cr	Mn	Mo	Ni	Nb	C	N
Carpenter BioDur ™ 108 [2]	21	23	1	< 0.05		≤ 0.08	> 0.90
Boehler P558 [3]	17	11	3	< 0.2		0.2	0.5
VSG P2000 [4]	18	14	3	-	≤ 0.25	≤ 0.15	0.75-1.00
Aubert & Duval Nonic M1 [5]	18	22	3	< 0.05		≤ 0.08	0.60-0.90

---

[2] Carpenter Technology Corporation, Reading, PA.
[3] Boehler Edelstahl GMBH, Kapfenberg, Austria.
[4] VSG Energie- und Schmiedetechnik, Essen, Germany.
[5] AUBERT & DUVAL, Neuilly-sur-Seine, France.

Mechanical Properties

Nitrogen strengthened low-nickel stainless steels typically show excellent static mechanical properties, which are clearly better than today's standard implant stainless steels [1,4,5]. In the annealed (soft) condition, the strength is much higher than in the conventional 316L implant stainless steel, whereas elongation values lie in the same range (Table 2) [1]. It is well known that the strength of austenitic stainless steels can be increased by cold deformation, whereas the elongation properties are reduced. This is usually done with implant raw material when higher strength is required. Low-nickel stainless steels exhibit a stronger potential for work hardening than conventional stainless steels (Figure 1). Earlier studies have shown that the strengthening effect of cold deformation increases with increasing nitrogen content [6]. This opens new possibilities for high-strength implant applications or for the dimensional reduction (miniaturizing) of implant systems where anatomically limited space is an issue.

Table 2 – *Typical mechanical properties of standard and low-nickel stainless implant steel (17% Cr, 12% Mn, 3% Mo, and 0.9% N) in the annealed condition [1].*

	316L Implant steel (ISO 5832-1)	Low Ni steel
Tensile yield strength, TYS	220 - 260 MPa	610 - 720 MPa
Ultimate tensile strength, UTS	500 - 540 MPa	980 - 1120 MPa
Elongation at break	55 - 65 %	55 - 65 %

Not much is known about the fatigue properties of low-nickel steels. Although the static mechanical properties of these steels are very promising, there are some indications that fatigue strength is below that of 316L implant material. In one study, this fact was related to a manufacturing process that was not optimal [7].

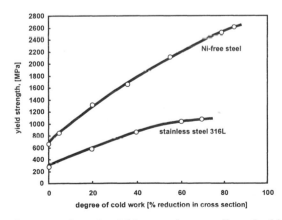

Figure 1 – *Increase of tensile yield strength as an effect of cold work [1].*

Corrosion Resistance and Biocompatibility

The low-nickel steels are very corrosion resistant because of their high chromium, molybdenum, and nitrogen content [8]. The pitting resistance equivalent (PRE) is an empirical formula to quantify the effect of different alloying elements on localized corrosion resistance. It can, for example, be derived from measurements of the critical crevice corrosion temperature. For standard nickel containing stainless steel the PRE is defined as %Cr + 3.3 x %Mo. This sum shall be at least 26 for implantable compositions, according to ASTM F 138 and ISO 5832-1, where this formula is stated as compositional requirement. For the high-nitrogen steel BioDur 108, the PRE has been defined as %Cr + 3.2 x %Mo + 8 x %N [9]. For compositions similar to the Boehler P558 or the VSG P2000, the PRE has been found to be %Cr + 3.3 x %Mo + 20 x %C + 20 x %N [1]. This results in PRE values between 30 and 45 for the nitrogen containing steels. Regardless of the formula used to calculate the PRE, it is clear that nitrogen provides significantly increased corrosion resistance. The improved corrosion resistance has been confirmed in laboratory tests and represents a reduction of metallic ions and corrosion products available to interact with the biological environment. In anodic polarization measurements, the pitting potential of BioDur 108 was found to be higher than that of 316L implant steel but lower than in commercially pure titanium [10]. The repassivation potential on the other hand was lower than in 316L, which could indicate some limitations if the passive layer is destroyed.

Wear corrosion resistance of Boehler P558 was compared to standard implant steels in a recent study [11]. P558 performed much better than implant quality 316L (ISO 5832-1, ASTM F 138) and Rex734 (ISO 5832-9, ASTM F 1586) in slurry wear tests, pin-on-disk, and crevice corrosion temperature measurements. The resistance against pitting corrosion was found to be equivalent to that of Rex734.

Although low-nickel stainless steels are still under evaluation with regard to surgical implant applications, the biocompatibility appears to be satisfactory. Investigations on cell toxicity have been made, and no adverse reactions were detected [12 - 14]. Furthermore, an animal study focused on the different effects of implant quality stainless steel, pure titanium, and low-nickel steel on blood circulation [15]. Using the hamster dorsal skinfold chamber model and intravital microscopy, it was demonstrated that reducing the nickel content in stainless steel implants has a positive effect on local microvascular parameters.

Further Considerations

Unfortunately, the high strength and toughness of low-nickel stainless steels are responsible for poor machinability. The ability to optimize machining parameters and the use of near net shapes represent future challenges for implant manufacturers. Trials of forging and Metal Injection Molding [16] of low-nickel steels have successfully been carried out.

Introducing new materials for implants always asks the question of adverse reactions provoked by direct contact of implants of different materials (galvanic coupling). Implant quality 316L and low-nickel stainless steel plate and screw samples were investigated in pure and mixed fretting corrosion combinations [17]. The mixed combinations showed even less fretting than both pure combinations. Based on this result, it was concluded that no additional problems of fretting corrosion are to be expected using this low-nickel stainless steel in combination with conventional implant quality stainless steel.

Low-nickel stainless steels typically contain a residual nickel content of $\leq 0.1\%$. Although this content is very low compared to all stainless implant steels, the biological effect of this residual nickel content on a strongly sensitized patient is unknown. Additionally, there are occasional cases of chromium allergy. For these patients, low-nickel steels will not be a reasonable alternative to titanium implants.

The price (low-nickel steels are expected to cost about twice the price of 316L implant steel raw material [18]), availability, and machinability of these new low-nickel implant steels will be influential in determining the widespread use in bone surgery.

However, the scope of this study was to evaluate the feasibility of producing an implant system from new low-nickel steel and to compare the relevant mechanical properties to standard implant materials.

Low-Nickel Steel as a Candidate Material for Small Bone Plates

Synthes® Compact Lock Plates[6] are small implants for the fixation of midface and mandible fractures as well as for osteotomies and reconstructions (Figure 2). These plates have an overall length of about 40 mm. Corresponding bone screws have an outer diameter of 2.0 mm, are self-drilling and self-tapping due to their special tip design, and have a threaded conical head that locks in the plate hole, providing angular stability. Today, this fixation system is made of CP titanium (plates) and titanium alloy Ti-6Al-7Nb (screws). Known disadvantages of the titanium system include limited formability of the plate (multiple contouring is not possible, the titanium plate risks to break), low cutting performance of the self-drilling screws in hard bone because of the limited hardness of Ti-6Al-7Nb, possible tendon irritations, and too high an amount of tissue ingrowth on the titanium surface, resulting in difficulties at explantation of temporary implants.

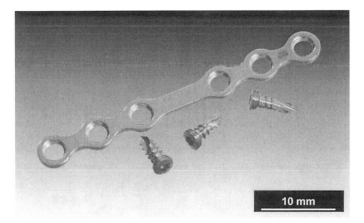

Figure 2 – *Compact Lock Plate and 2.0 mm screw prototypes.*

[6] Synthes AG, Chur, Switzerland.

The purpose of this study was to produce the implants of the Compact Lock 2.0 system with low-nickel stainless steel to overcome all the mentioned disadvantages without causing new allergic problems. The prototype system was then to be compared with the current titanium system and prototype plates made of implant quality 316L stainless steel. Reverse bending tests were proposed to confirm the superior intraoperative contourability (multiple bending treatment) and high cycle fatigue tests to ensure the long-term durability of the new material during service.

Materials and Test Methods

Compact Lock Plate Prototypes

Compact 6-hole plates and corresponding 2.0 mm screws (Figure 2) for the fixation of small bone fragments were made of Carpenter BioDur 108 low-nickel stainless steel (tensile properties of the raw material see Table 3, transverse micrographs see Figure 3) using conventional machining techniques. The plates were compared to identical plates made of CP titanium and standard 316L implant steel (Table 3).

Table 3 – *Mechanical properties of raw material, according to supplier's test certificates (BioDur 108) and internal recertification results (other materials).*

	Tensile yield strength	Ultimate tensile strength	Elongation at break
BioDur 108 round bar (screws)	938 MPa	1227 MPa	31 %
BioDur 108 strip (plates)	642 MPa	1001 MPa	46 %
316L implant steel strip (plates)	not measured	837 MPa	17.5 %
CP titanium sheet (plates)	553 MPa	680 MPa	23.9 %

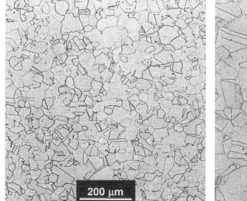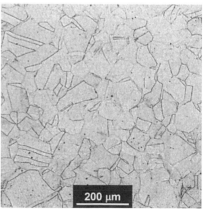

Figure 3 – *Transverse micrograph of the BioDur 108 raw material used for production of plates and screws; (a) 1.5 mm strip raw material, (b) 4 mm diameter round bar.*

Test Setup

In a first setup, the bone plates were tested for tolerance against multiple reverse bending procedures. The plates were fixed on one side and plastically bent up and down in a range of ± 10 mm by a motor-driven actuator at a cantilever of 22 mm (Figure 4). The velocity of the bending device was 200 mm/min (5 cycles/min) and deformation was continued until plate rupture. The fractures were always placed through the middle of the central hole where the highest bending moment occurs.

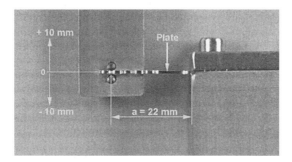

Figure 4 – *Test set-up for reverse bending testing.*

The high cycle fatigue properties of all three plate types were compared in a combined compression-flexion setup (Figure 5). The plates were fixed with 6 screws (0.3 Nm fixation torque) onto cylinders of polyoxymethylene (POM). A gap of 6 mm between the POM parts simulated the situation of load bearing through the plate without bony support. Dynamic compression load at a minimum to maximum load ration of R = 0.1 was applied vertically on the POM cylinders with a frequency of 6 Hz. The complete setup was placed in a container with 1% NaCl-solution and kept at 37°C to simulate a physiologic situation. Tests were performed at different maximum loads, using new specimen for every test, and were conducted until failure of the plate or 2.5 mio cycles, respectively.

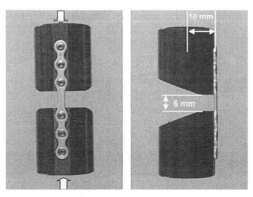

Figure 5 – *Test set-up for dynamic bending testing, frontal and lateral view.*

Results

Reverse Bending and Fatigue Tests

The results of the reverse bending test are summarized in Figure 6. CP titanium plates broke after 26 ± 7 cycles (3 samples, failure after 24, 25, and 29 cycles), whereas BioDur 108 plates could withstand a mean number of 226 ± 46 cycles (208, 226, and 245 cycles). Plates of 316L stainless steel were not investigated in this setup. The results confirm the significantly ($p = 0.001$) higher tolerance against multiple plastic deformation of stainless steel compared to CP titanium. The higher damage tolerance of steel plates prevents from possible fractures during contouring operations.

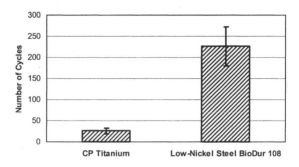

Figure 6 – *Number of cycles to failure in reverse bending test.*

The results of the fatigue tests are summarized in the Woehler diagram (Figure 7). Differences in fatigue resistance are mainly found at the highest loads: At 20 N maximum load, the first BioDur 108 plate broke at about 5 000 cycles, whereas the best 316L plate withstood 676 000 cycles. At this load, the titanium plates showed intermediate fatigue resistance with failures between 60 000 and 85 000 cycles.

At lower maximum loads, CP titanium and 316L plates showed comparable fatigue resistance, but BioDur 108 plates were still inferior.

Scanning Electron Microscopy

The fracture surfaces of the BioDur 108 plates were analyzed by scanning electron microscope (SEM) and compared to 316L stainless steel plates to find out more about possible reasons for early fatigue failures. For this SEM investigation, plates were used that had been tested at highest fatigue loads (20 N maximum load, 2 N minimum load). The BioDur 108 plate was the one that broke after 4978 cycles already, the 316L plate was the best one that broke after 676 584 cycles.

All fatigue fractures occurred at one of the central holes, where the cross section of the plate is reduced because of the hole, and multidirectional loads are found as a consequence of the tight fixation by screws (Figure 8).

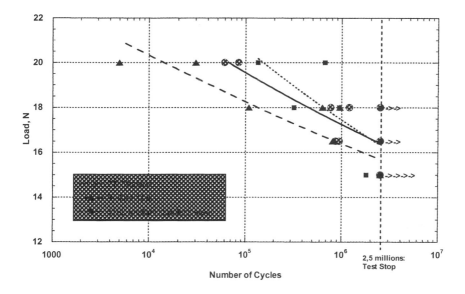

Figure 7 – *Woehler-diagram: Highest fatigue resistance at high loads is found in 316L plates, followed by CP titanium plates and BioDur 108 plates. At lower loads, differences in fatigue resistance are smaller.*

Figure 9 a provides an overview of the fracture surface of the BioDur 108 plate. Crack initiations were found on both sides of the plate. The cracks propagated from the upper and lower side to the center of the plate, where the remaining overload fracture surface is located. A second crack zone was usually found on the opposite side of the fatigue failure. The examination of the crack initiation site (Figure 9 b) of these secondary cracks at the plate surface was very helpful in characterizing the type of fracture. It was found, that the fatigue cracks in BioDur 108 have a great percentage of intercrystalline propagation (Figure 10 a). It seems that the grain boundaries are a site of preferred fatigue crack propagation in the BioDur 108 stainless steel. In addition, a spreading of the fractures along parallel gliding planes can be observed (Figure 10 b).

The secondary, incomplete crack in the 316L stainless steel plate is shown in an upper (Figure 11a) and a lower plate side view (11 b). The fatigue cracking results in a strong deformation of the thread in the plate hole. The crack initiation zone is characterized by multiple small crack sites. The image of the same zone at stronger magnification (Figure 12 a) makes clear that cracking is not intercrystalline such as in the BioDur 108 alloy, but much more transcrystalline. Nevertheless, the fracture characteristic of the 316L plate seems similar in terms of spreading of cracks along parallel gliding planes (Figure 12 b).

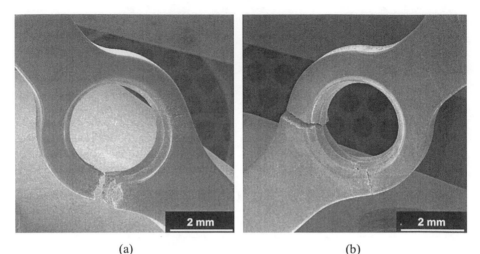

(a)   (b)

Figure 8 – *Upper side view of the fatigue-tested BioDur 108 plate (a) and 316L stainless steel plate (b).*

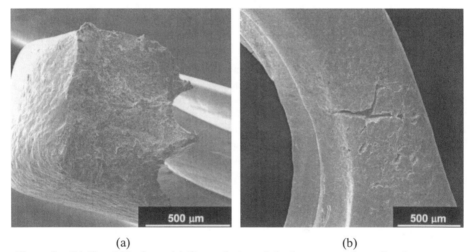

(a)   (b)

Figure 9 – *BioDur 108 plate: (a) General view of the fracture surface. Crack initiation was at the top and the bottom of the plate and the cracks propagated from both sides to the center of the plate. (b) Crack initiation zone on the upper plate side.*

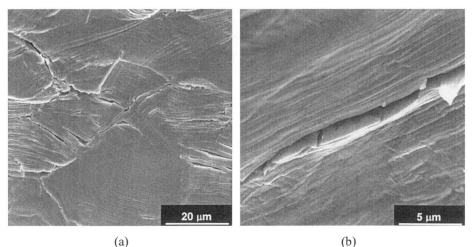

(a)   (b)

Figure 10 – *Surface of BioDur 108 specimen near the initiation site of fatigue cracks:*
(a) Intercrystalline fatigue crack propagation;
(b) Spreading of cracks along gliding planes.

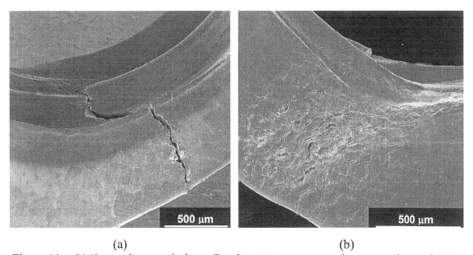

(a)   (b)

Figure 11 – *316L stainless steel plate: Crack initiation zone on the upper plate side (a)*
and on the lower plate side (b).

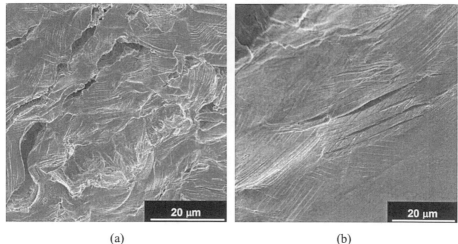

(a)   (b)

Figure 12 – *Surface of 316L specimen near the initiation site of fatigue cracks:*
(a) Transcrystalline fatigue crack propagation;
(b) Spreading of cracks along gliding planes.

Since it could be observed that the fatigue cracks in BioDur 108 show a much greater percentage of intergranular fracture, the metallographic specimens were analyzed by SEM too. Especially the grain boundaries were checked for possible foreign phases or precipitation particles. But it was impossible to find any reason for the weakness of grain boundaries.

Discussion and Conclusions

Miniature bone plates were produced of new BioDur 108 low-nickel stainless steel to overcome known disadvantages of titanium, such as poor ductility and formability. Reverse bending tests confirmed that the low-nickel steel plates are significantly more tolerant to multiple bending procedures than titanium plates.

Nevertheless, high cycle fatigue tests under physiologic conditions showed that the low-nickel steel plates exhibit lower resistance to cyclic loads than titanium and 316L plates of identical size and design. Although the static tensile strength of low-nickel steel is clearly superior to both pure titanium and implant quality 316L stainless steel, this new steel showed lowest performance under dynamic conditions, especially at high loads. SEM investigations of the fatigue fractures confirmed that a different fracture mode is characteristic for the BioDur 108 plates: a great percentage of the cracks propagate along grain boundaries leading to intergranular fracture.

It was thought that the high nitrogen content of over 0.90 % could lead to the precipitation of nitrides on the grain boundaries, and hence facilitate intergranular fracture. But it was not possible to detect foreign phases at the grain boundaries by SEM investigation of the fracture surfaces and the metallographic specimens.

Low-nickel steels with high nitrogen content seem to be prone to reduced high cycle fatigue resistance due to preferred intergranular fracture. This is in accordance with previous reports confirming the inferior fatigue resistance compared to other implant materials [7].

Crack initiation is a critical step under high cycle fatigue conditions, much more critical than under plastic bending conditions. It is likely that the intergranular crack initiation facilitates the early failure under high cycle fatigue conditions, whereas plastic bending properties are not affected. This would explain the different outcome of the BioDur 108 plates in the two tests presented here. The tendency to intergranular crack initiation could come from surface deformation (work hardening) introduced during machining and related embrittlement in the surface zone. Further development in the processing and machining of low-nickel steel products could help to improve the microstructure of these materials and overcome the possible problem of reduced high cycle fatigue resistance documented in this study.

References

[1]   Speidel, M. O., and Uggowitzer, P. J., "Biocompatible Nickel-Free Stainless Steels to Avoid Nickel Allergy," *Materials in Medicine, Proceedings of Materials Day 1998*, ETH Zürich, Department of Materials, pp. 191-208.

[2]   Hierholzer, S. and Hierholzer, G., "Internal Fixation and Metal Allergy – Clinical Investigations, Immunology and Histology of the Implant Tissue Interface," *Thieme Medical Publishers*, New York, 1992.

[3]   Speidel, M. O., "Stickstofflegierte Stähle – eine Übersicht," *Ergebnisse der Werkstoff-Forschung* Band 4, Thubal-Kain, Zürich, 1991, pp. 1-17.

[4]   Uggowitzer, P. J., Magdowski, R., and Speidel, M. O., "Nickel Free High Nitrogen Austenitic Steels," *ISIJ International*, The Iron and Steel Institute of Japan, Vol. 36, No. 7, 1996, pp. 901-908.

[5]   Stein, G. and Hucklenbroich, I., "Biokompatible stickstofflegierte Austenite für Anwendungen am und im menschlichen Körper," *Werkstoffwoche '98, Band IV, Symposium 4, Werkstoffe für die Medizintechnik*, H. Planck and H. Stallforth, Eds., Wiley VCH, Weinheim, 1999, pp. 3-9.

[6]   Menzel, J., Kirschner, W., and Stein, G., "High Nitrogen Containing Ni-Free Austenitic Steels for Medical Applications," *ISIJ International*, The Iron and Steel Institute of Japan, Vol. 36, No. 7, 1996, pp. 893-900.

[7]   Fink, U., Weik, T., and Gümpel, P., "Nickel-Free Austenitic Steels as a Future Implant Material," *13th Europ. Conf. on Biomaterials, Göteborg, Sweden, Sept. 4-7*, 1997, p. 140.

[8]   Cigada, A., Rondelli, G., Vicentini, B., Brunella, F., and Dallaspezia, G., "Corrosion Behaviour of High Nitrogen Stainless Steels for Biomedical Applications," *Compatability of Biomedical Implants, San Francisco, California, USA, 23-25 May*, 1994, pp.185-195.

[9]   Brown, R. S. and Gebeau, R. C., "Strength and Corrosion Resistance of BioDur 108 Alloy," *Proceedings of the Sixth World Biomaterials Congress*, Kamuela, Hawaii, May 15-20, 2000, p. 828.

[10]   Disegi, J. A., Zardiackas, L. D., and Mitchell, D. W., "Anodic Polarization Evaluation of Nickel-Free Implant Quality Stainless Steel," *Proceedings of the Sixth World Biomaterials Congress*, Kamuela, Hawaii, May 15-20, 2000, p. 816.

[11]   Thomann, U. I. and Uggowitzer, P. J., "Wear-Corrosion Behavior of Biocompatible Austenitic Stainless Steels," *Wear*, Vol. 239, 2000, pp. 48-58.

[12]   Carpenter Technology Corporation Alloy Data, BioDur^{TM} 108 Alloy, Carpenter Technology corp., Reading, PA, 1999.

[13]   Internal Report on Cytotoxicity of Low-Nickel Steels, Robert Mathys Foundation, Bettlach, Switzerland, 1998.

[14]   Hochörtler, G., Bernauer, J., and Kriszt, K., "Corrosion Behaviour and Nickel Release of Alloys with Various Nickel Contents," *Materials for Medical Engineering, Proceedings of Euromat 99*, Vol. 2, H. Stallforth and P. Revell, Eds., Wiley-VCH, Weinheim, 2000, pp. 204-209.

[15]   Kraft, C. N., Burian, B., Perlick, L., Wimmer, M. A., Wallny, T., Schmitt, O., and Diedrich, O., "Impact of a Nickel-Reduced Stainless Steel Implant on Striated Muscle Microcirculation, A Comparative In Vivo Study," *Journal of Biomedical Materials Research*, Vol. 57, 2001, pp. 404-412.

[16]   Uggowitzer, P. J., Speidel, M. O., and Wohlfromm, H., "PANACEA Provides the Answer to Ni Allergy," *MPR (Metal Powder Report)*, Sept. 1998, pp. 48-52.

[17]   Eschbach, L., Marti, A., and Gasser, B., "Fretting Corrosion Testing of Internal Fixation Plates and Screws," *Materials for Medical Engineering, Proceedings of Euromat 99*, Vol. 2, H. Stallforth and P. Revell, Eds., Wiley-VCH, Weinheim, 2000, pp. 193-198.

[18]   Kramer, K.-H., "Implants for Surgery – A Survey on Metallic Materials," *Materials for Medical Engineering, Proceedings of Euromat 99*, Vol. 2, H. Stallforth and P. Revell, Eds., Wiley-VCH, Weinheim, 2000, pp. 9-29.

Lyle D. Zardiackas[1], Scott Williamson[1], Michael Roach[1], and Jay-Anthony Bogan[1]

Comparison of Anodic Polarization and Galvanic Corrosion of a Low-Nickel Stainless Steel to 316LS and 22Cr-13Ni-5Mn Stainless Steels

Reference: Zardiackas, L. D., Williamson, S., Roach, M., and Bogan, J. A., **"Comparison of Anodic Polarization and Galvanic Corrosion of a Low-Nickel Stainless Steel to 316L S and 22Cr-13Ni-5Mn Stainless Steels,"** *Stainless Steels for Medical and Surgical Applications, ASTM STP 1438*, G. L. Winters and M. J. Nutt, Eds., ASTM International, West Conshohocken, PA 2003.

Abstract: Over the years, numerous biomedical implants have been produced from austenitic stainless steels due to their exceptional mechanical and corrosion properties. High nickel content has been used to stabilize the austenitic microstructure, but the presence of these nickel concentrations has been implicated as a cause of metal sensitivity reactions in a minor portion of the population. In a partial response to the possibility of hypersensitivity reactions, low-nickel stainless steels with a high nitrogen content to stabilize the austenitic microstructure have been developed. In this study, the anodic polarization and galvanic corrosion behavior of one such low-nickel alloy (BioDur[®2] 108 Carpenter Technology) was compared to BioDur[®] 316LS and BioDur[®] 22Cr-13Ni-5Mn. For anodic polarization, duplicate samples with a surface ground to 600 grit and duplicate samples with a metallographic polish were tested in accordance with ASTM G5 at a sweep rate of 0.6 V/hr, initiated 200 mV below the rest potential. Samples for galvanic testing were metallographically polished, the rest potentials were recorded prior to test initiation, and duplicate coupled tests were run for a period of 48 hours for each alloy combination. The galvanic current and couple potential were recorded in accordance with ASTM G71. Anodic polarization results revealed BioDur[®] 108 to have a pitting potential similar to BioDur[®] 22Cr-13Ni-5Mn and significantly higher than that of BioDur[®] 316LS. In addition, substantially higher pitting levels on BioDur[®] 316LS were also noted during post-anodic metallographic examination. None of the alloy combinations revealed substantial galvanic coupled currents indicating little susceptibility to galvanic corrosion. No evidence of pitting or crevice corrosion was found on any of the galvanically coupled surfaces.

Keywords: corrosion, galvanic, stainless steel, low-nickel

[1]Professor and Coordinator of Biomaterials and Professor of Orthopaedic Surgery, senior materials engineer, materials engineer and senior materials engineer, respectively, University of Mississippi Medical Center, SOD / Biomaterials, 2500 North State Street, Jackson, MS, 39216.
[2]Carpenter Technology Corporation, Reading, PA, USA.

Introduction

Austenitic stainless steels are widely used in the production of biomedical implants. They provide high strength, good corrosion resistance, and are cost effective [1]. However, up to this time medical grade stainless steels have used a significant amount of nickel to maintain their austenitic microstructure. Nickel is reported to account for as much as 90% of the clinically observed sensitivity to metals and may lead to other complications when released from stainless steel implants [1,2]. Fretting and wear, in addition to other forms of corrosion, of stainless steel devices may lead to metallic ion release into the tissues surrounding the implants. Histological analyses of these tissues have shown a nickel concentration as high as 2% [3]. Carpenter Specialty Alloys has developed a low-nickel austenitic stainless steel (BioDur® 108) in partial response to concerns over the possibility of nickel induced sensitivity reactions. A nitrogen concentration of at least 0.85% is used to maintain the austenitic microstructure of this low-nickel alloy. In addition, this high nitrogen content is also reported to contribute to the high strength and good corrosion resistance of the material [4,5].

In physiological solutions, several studies have documented greater pitting corrosion susceptibility of implant quality 316L stainless steel compared to other austenitic stainless steels used for implant devices [4,5,6]. Potentiodynamic studies on 316L steel in salt solutions reveal a small passive range, a low breakdown potential, and a large hysteresis loop between the forward and reverse scans which is indicative of a material susceptible to pitting corrosion [6,7]. Implant retrieval studies have shown that localized corrosion is generally not sufficient to result in the mechanical failure of 316L devices. However, the release of corrosion products over the term of implantation may lead to tissue inflamation, primarily due to nickel ion release, and possible device loosening contributing to the need for implant removal [8]. Nevertheless, the corrosion resistance for implant quality 316L remains generally acceptable for many implant applications [9]. High manganese austenitic stainless steels, such as 22Cr-13Ni-5Mn, benefit from a combination of molybdenum and elevated nitrogen levels as well as chromium to raise their pitting potential [10]. Cyclic polarization studies in Ringer's solution reveal 22Cr-13Ni-5Mn to exhibit a much larger passive region, higher pitting potentials, and a very small hysteresis compared to 316L, indicating superior pitting resistance [4,6,11]. Initial studies on the corrosion properties of BioDur® 108 stainless steel suggest excellent pitting and crevice corrosion resistance with similar oxide breakdown potential to those of 22Cr-13Ni-5Mn stainless steel [4,5].

The direct contact or electrical couple of two different metals leads to the formation of a galvanic couple [10,12]. Differences in composition and processing of implant quality austenitic stainless steels may lead to galvanic corrosion effects if dissimilar metals are in contact. Initial studies of mixed metal combinations of BioDur® 108 and implant stainless steels have shown good results in fretting tests [1]. However, previous studies have shown that even mixing implant plates and screws of the same material from different manufacturers may lead to galvanic effects [13].

The purpose of this study was to characterize the anodic polarization and galvanic corrosion of BioDur® 108 (alloy A), as compared to both BioDur® 316LS (alloy B) and BioDur® 22 Cr-13 Ni-5 Mn (alloy C) due to their long and successful history as implants.

Materials and Methods

Samples were prepared from a single lot of 8 mm centerless ground bar stock in the cold worked condition of each alloy. Transverse and longitudinal samples of each alloy were mounted in diallyl phthalate, ground, and polished to a final finish of 0.05μm Al_2O_3 for optical metallography. The inclusion content was evaluated on longitudinal samples according to ASTM standard "Test Methods for Determining the Inclusion Content of Steel" (E45 - 97 Method A using Plate 1-r). After examination for inclusions, the longitudinal samples were etched at 3 volts for 20 seconds in a solution of 45g KOH in 100 mL of distilled water to evaluate for free ferrite and other foreign phases. Transverse samples of alloy B were etched for grain size and grain structure determination using a solution containing 30g $FeCl_3$, 30 mL HCl, and 1.8 mL of HNO_3. Samples of alloy A and alloy C were etched in a solution of 45 % KOH solution electrolytically at 3 volts to reveal the grain structure. The values for the grain size were determined as defined by ASTM standard "Test Methods for Determining Average Grain Size" (E112 - 96) on transverse samples as defined by ASTM standards "Wrought Nitrogen Strengthened -22 Chromium-12.5 Nickel-5 Manganese-2.5 Molybdenum Stainless Steel Bar and Wire for Surgical Implants" (F1314-01) and ASTM "Wrought 18 Chromium-14 Nickel-2.5 Molybdenum Stainless Steel Bar and Wire for Surgical Implants (UNS S31673)" (F138-00).

Quantitative compositional evaluation of the major alloying elements of each material was evaluated using inductively coupled plasma emission spectrometry (ICP) with a spark attachment for analysis of solid materials (Spectro ICP with LISA[3]). Each alloy was analyzed in duplicate using calibration curves developed using standard samples. Results of analysis were compared to ASTM and/or internal melt limits as applicable to ensure each alloy met specification.

Corrosion testing was performed by dynamic cyclical anodic polarization using a Gamry[4] PC3 potentiostat. Two transverse samples with a cross section of 0.5cm² were mounted in Durofast[5] epoxy resin prior to polishing and two like samples were prepared for grinding. Grinding was performed with 600 grit silicon carbide paper and polishing was performed to a final finish with 0.05μm Al_2O_3. Polished samples were photographed at 100x magnification prior to and after anodic polarization to document surface condition. Samples were placed in a corrosion cell having a standard calomel reference electrode, two carbon counter electrodes, and Ringers solution (pH 5.5) at 37°C. The cell was purged with N_2 for the two hours prior to initiation of polarization, and N_2 was continuously bubbled through the solution for the duration of the test. During the initial purging with N_2, the rest potential was allowed to equilibrate. Anodic polarization scans were initiated 200mV below the rest potential (EOC), tested at a sweep rate of 0.6V/hr, and reversed when the potential reached 3.0 volts with respect to the reference (Eref) or when the current density reached 5mA/cm². Polarization plots of potential (E) vs. log current density (A/cm²) were recorded and Tafel extrapolations were prepared to determine for E_{corr} and I_{corr} for each test.

---

[3]SPECTRO Analytical Instruments, Fitchburg, MA, USA.
[4]Gamry Instruments, Inc., Warminster, PA, USA.
[5]Durofast/Struers, Westlake, OH, USA.

Transverse samples with a 0.5cm^2 cross section were mounted in Durofast epoxy resin prior to polishing to a final finish with 0.05µm Al$_2$O$_3$ for galvanic testing.. Micrographs were taken at 100x prior to and after testing to document the surface condition. Each alloy (A, B, and C) was coupled to each of the other two alloys to determine the galvanic potential and current. Each pair was placed in a corrosion cell containing a standard calomel electrode and Ringers solution at 37°C (pH 5.5). The cell was purged with nitrogen gas for two hours prior to initiation of the test and nitrogen gas was bubbled through the solution though out the test to minimize crevice effects. After the initial two hour purge, each pair of alloys was galvanically coupled and tested using the zero ammeter technique as outlined in the ASTM standard "Guide for Conducting and Evaluating Galvanic Corrosion Tests in Electrolytes" [G71-81 (Reapproved 98)]. The rest potentials of each individual alloy were recorded immediately prior to coupling the alloys and test initiation. Duplicate coupled scans were run for a period of 48 hours on each alloy combination. This particular time period was chosen based upon initial testing which showed no changes in potential or current after the 48 hour time period. The galvanic current and couple potential were recorded over the duration of the test in accordance with ASTM G 71.

Results

ICP compositional analysis results are provided in Table 1. All alloys were found to be within ASTM specification or Carpenter internal melt limits for major alloying elements. Metallurgical evaluation found alloy A to have a 2.0 thin globular oxide and a 0.5 thin alumina type inclusion rating. Alloy B was found to have an inclusion rating of 1.0 for thin globular oxides and a 0.5 for thin alumina. Alloy C was found to have a 2.0 thin globular oxide and a 1.0 heavy globular oxide inclusion rating. Alloy A was evaluated to have the largest ASTM grain size at 5.0, followed by alloy B at 6.0, and finally alloy C at 9.0, respectively.

Anodic polarization results are listed in Table 2, and shown in Figures 1 and 2. Alloy C had the highest rest potential of the three austenitic stainless steels, followed by alloy B, and finally alloy A. The I$_{corr}$ values for all alloys tested were similar, with alloy C having a slightly more positive value than alloys A and B. Alloys A and C recorded similar breakdown potentials, which were significantly greater than those of alloy B. Potential scans for each alloy tested revealed a slight shift between the ground and polished samples. Ground samples revealed slightly more negative rest potentials, and slightly higher current density values than the polished samples. Of the three alloys, the most pronounced shift between the ground and polished conditions was observed in alloy B. Metallographic examination of the surfaces of alloys A and C (Figures 3a and 3c) revealed significantly less evidence of pitting attack than those of alloy B (Figure 3b).

Galvanic couple results for each alloy combination of the stainless steels tested are provided in Table 3 and Figures 4 and 5. The coupling of each combination of alloys created an initial over-potential due to a net current caused by the differences in the rest potentials of the individual alloys. This change in potential and current density, for the coupled alloy combinations, stabilized over the first 24 hours of the test (Figures 4 and 5). After the first 24 hours of the tests, the coupled current densities continued to approach zero and the coupled potentials maintained a stable value. Metallographic examination of

Table 1 - Compositional Analysis of BioDur Alloys (%) (n=2)

Alloy	Fe	Cr	Ni	Mo	Mn	Si	S	P	Cu	C[1]	N[1]
Alloy A	Bal.	20.95	0.03	0.75	23.48	0.33	0.006	0.005	--	0.038	1.06
Alloy B	Bal.	17.78	14.09	2.78	1.74	0.50	0.005	0.020	0.050	0.017	0.037
Alloy C	Bal.	21.42	13.41	2.31	5.06	0.42	0.002	0.020	--	0.017	0.33

[1] Analysis performed by Carpenter Technology Corporation

Table 2 - Anodic Polarization Data vs SCE (Ringer's @ 37 °C, n=2)

Material	Condition	Open Circuit Potential (mV)	Icorr (A/cm^2)	Passivation Potential (mV @ A/cm^2)	Breakdown Potential (mV @ A/cm^2)
Alloy A	Polish to 0.05 Micron Alumina	-365.5	8.72E-08	-178@3.45E-07	1120@1.54E-04
		-366.5	5.35E-08	-133@2.73E-07	1090@1.55E-05
	Polish to 600 Grit SiC paper	-406.8	7.40E-08	-179@4.24E-07	1260@6.37E-04
		-471.1	1.40E-07	-178@1.03E-06	1200@7.32E-04
Alloy B	Polish to 0.05 Micron Alumina	-248.9	5.37E-08	-188@9.83E-08	346@7.27E-07
		-237.3	6.07E-08	-184@1.31E-07	254@5.56E-07
	Polish to 600 Grit SiC paper	-298.1	6.35E-08	-205@1.77E-07	171@7.56E-07
		-311.1	9.48E-08	-233@2.42E-07	263@7.86E-07
Alloy C	Polish to 0.05 Micron Alumina	-224.2	1.00E-07	-42@3.59E-07	1030@3.10E-06
		-220.8	7.71E-08	-5.5@4.05E-07	998@2.58E-06
	Polish to 600 Grit SiC paper	-224.0	1.24E-07	-29@4.39E-07	1070@5.96E-06
		-271.1	1.15E-07	-58@6.20E-07	1050@3.13E-05

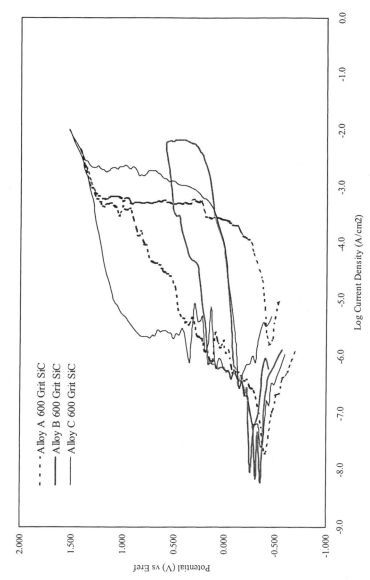

Figure 1 - *Representative anodic polarization scans of each alloy ground to a 600 grit SiC surface finish in Ringer's solution at 37 °C.*

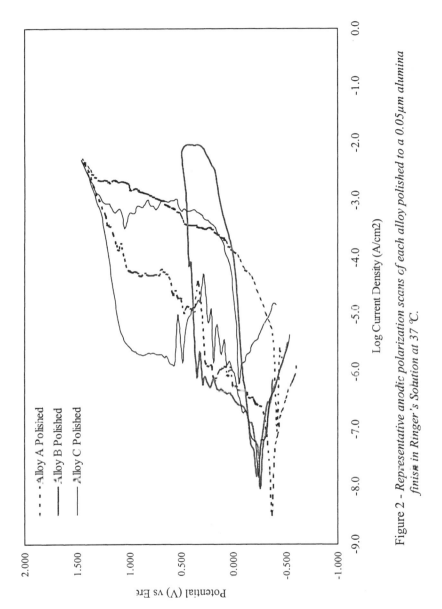

Figure 2 - *Representative anodic polarization scans of each alloy polished to a 0.05μm alumina finish in Ringer's Solution at 37 °C.*

Figure 3a - *Representative micrograph of the post-anodic polarization surface of alloy A (100X).*

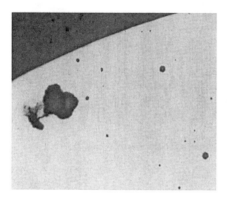

Figure 3b - *Representative micrograph of the post-anodic polarization surface of alloy B (100X).*

Figure 3c - *Representative micrograph of the post-anodic polarization surface of alloy C (100X).*

Table 3 - *Galvanic Corrosion Coupling Results (n=2)*

Coupled Alloys #1 - #2	Initial Uncoupled Potential #1 (mV)	Initial Uncoupled Potential #2 (mV)	Initial Coupled Potential (mV)	Initial Coupled Current Density (A/cm2)	Final Coupled Potential (mV)	Final Coupled Current Density (A/cm2)
A - B	-319	-382	-350	1.81E-08	-142	7.81E-10
A - B	-264	-335	-288	-2.88E-08	-215	-5.78E-10
A - C	-333	-318	-332	-1.55E-09	-210	1.66E-09
A - C	-330	-315	-302	-1.36E-09	-213	1.34E-09
B - C	-243	-383	-307	-5.32E-08	-233	-7.02E-10
B - C	-359	-338	-355	9.60E-09	-330	1.28E-09

the samples after testing revealed little, if any, evidence of pitting attack on the sample surfaces of the alloys tested.

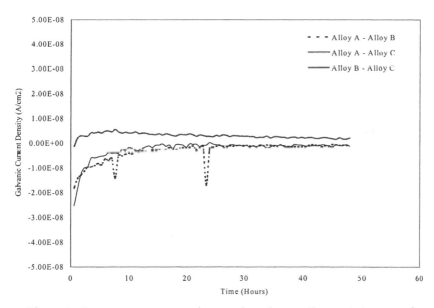

Figure 4 - *Representative scans showing the galvanically coupled current densities of the alloy combinations in Ringers solution at 37 ℃ over time.*

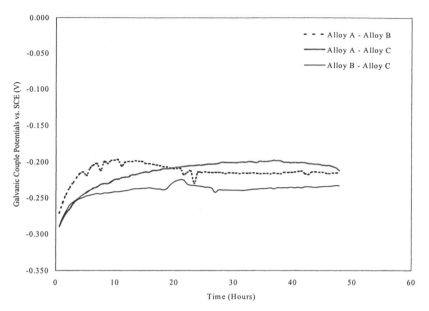

Figure 5 - *Representative scans showing the galvanically coupled potentials of the alloy combinations in Ringers solution at 37 °C over time.*

Discussion and Conclusions

The anodic polarization results of the current study are in agreement with previous investigations by other researchers documenting a substantially higher breakdown potential and a larger stable passive region in physiological solutions for 22Cr-13Ni-5Mn stainless steel (alloy C) as compared to implant quality 316L stainless steel (alloy B) [6,14]. However, these studies also reported little, if any, hysteresis between the forward and reverse potentiodynamic scans of 22Cr-13Ni-5Mn stainless steel indicating a high pitting resistance. Due to the higher scan reversal potential in the current study, which resulted in driving the potential farther into the trans-passive region, the cyclical polarization curves for alloy C exhibited a larger hysteresis. These results indicate a greater susceptibility to pitting corrosion than that noted in the above referenced study. These observations were further confirmed by post-anodic metallographic examination revealing pitting on the surfaces of alloy C (Figure 3). Nevertheless, a much heavier uniform pitting attack was shown in the post-anodic analysis of alloy B. Anodic polarization results for alloy A showed breakdown potentials and a large hysteresis similar to those for alloy C. The results shown here are in agreement with the manufacturer's material data sheets for these alloys [5,11].

It has been suggested that stainless steel to stainless steel galvanic couples are stable under static conditions [15]. The results of the zero-resistance galvanic corrosion testing between each combination of the stainless steels indicated small initial currents for galvanically coupled samples. The current diminished to a value approaching zero over the first 24-hours of testing. The galvanically coupled potentials stabilized over the first 24-hours of the couple, and maintained a near constant value for the duration of the tests. These results are in good agreement with a previous study which galvanically coupled 316L stainless steel (alloy B) to 22Cr-13Ni-5Mn stainless steel (alloy C) [14]. Under dynamic conditions leading to accelerated corrosion processes, such as fretting, electrically coupled components may experience galvanic corrosion effects [15]. In addition, studies have shown galvanic corrosion effects may be accelerated in implant situations where a small anodic area is coupled to a larger cathodic area. This effect could occur in situations such as plate and screw combinations, where the screw is anodic with respect to a much larger cathodic plate.

In conclusion, the results of the potentiodynamic portion of this study indicated that the corrosion resistance of the low-nickel alloy A is similar to alloy C, and significantly better than that of alloy B. Galvanic testing revealed little, if any, effects of coupling the individual alloy combinations. Therefore, the use of mixed combinations of these alloys appears to be adequate for many implant applications. However, the dynamic effects encountered during fretting corrosion on these alloy combinations is still a potential concern and is currently under investigation.

Acknowledgment

This research was supported by a grant from Carpenter Technology Corporation.

References

[1]   Disegi, J.A. and Eschbach, L., "Stainless Steel in Bone Surgery," *Injury*, Vol. 31, Suppl. 4, 2000, pp. D2-D6.

[2]   Zardiackas, L. D., Roach, M., Williamson, S., Bogan, J. A., "Comparison of Notch Sensitivity and Stress Corrosion Cracking of a Low-Nickel Stainless Steel to 316LS and 22Cr-13Ni-5Mn Stainless Steels," *Stainless Steels for Medical and Surgical Applications*, ASTM STP 1438, G. L. Winters and M. J. Nutt, Eds., ASTM International, West Conshohocken, PA 2003.

[3]   Xulin, S., Atsuo, I., Tetsuya, T., and Hosino, A., "Fretting Corrosion Resistance and Fretting Corrosion Product Cytocompatability of Ferritic Stainless Steel," *Journal of Biomedical Materials Research*, Vol. 34, 1997, pp. 9-14..

[4]   Gebeau, R.C. and Brown, R.S., "Tech Spotlight - Biomedical Implant Alloy," *Advanced Materials and Processes*, Vol. 159, No. 9, 2001, pp. 46-48..

[5]   Carpenter Technology Corporation Alloy Data, BioDur 108 Alloy, Carpenter Technology Corp., Reading, PA. 2000.

[6]   Shetty, R.H., Ottersberg, W.H., "Metals in Orthopedic Surgery," *Encyclopedic Handbook of Biomaterials and Bioengineering*, Vol. 1, 1995, pp. 509-540.

[7]   Ogundele, G.I., White, W.E., "Polarization Studies on Surgical-Grade Stainless Steels in Hank's Physiological Solution," *Corrosion and Degradation of Implant Materials*, ASTM STP 859, 1985, pp. 117-135.

[8]   Beddoes, J., Bucci, K., "The Influence of Surface Condition on the Localized Corrosion of 316L Stainless Steel Orthopaedic Implants," *Journal of Materials Science: Materials in Medicine*, Vol. 10, 1999, pp. 389-394.

[9]   Fraker, A.C., "Corrosion of Metallic Implants and Prosthetic Devices," *Metals Handbook*, Ninth Edition, Vol. 13, 1987, pp.1324-1335.

[10] Sedriks, J.A., "Galvanic Corrosion," *Stainless Steels*, John Wiley and Sons, 1992, pp. 344-347.

[11] Carpenter Technology Corporation Alloy Data, Carpenter 22Cr-13Ni-5Mn, Carpenter Technology Corp., Reading, PA., 1987.

[12] Baboian, R., "Electrochemical Techniques for Predicting Galvanic Corrosion," *Galvanic and Pitting Corrosion - Field and Laboratory Studies*, ASTM STP 576, 1976, pp. 5-19.

[13] Black, J., *Biological Performance of Materials: Fundamentals of Biocompatibility*, Marcel Dekker, Inc., 1992.

[14] Shetty, R.H., Jacobs, C.H., "Galvanic Corrosion Properties of 22-13-5/316L Stainless Steel Couple in Physiologic Solution," [abstract] *Transactions of the Society of Biomaterials*, Volume 10, 1987, p. 231.

[15] Jacobs, J.J., Gilbert, J.L., Urban, U.M., "Current Concepts Review: Corrosion of Metal Orthopaedic Implants," *The Journal of Bone and Joint Surgery*, Vol. 80 (2), 1998, pp. 268-282.

Tikhovski[1], Holger Brauer[1], Martina Mölders[2], Martin Wiemann[2], Dieter Bingmann[2],
 Ifons Fischer[1]

Fatigue Behavior and In-Vitro Biocompatibility of the Ni-Free Austenitic High-Nitrogen Steel X13CrMnMoN18-14-3

Reference: Tikhovski, I., Brauer, H., Mölders, M., Wiemann, M., Bingmann, D., and Fischer, A., **"Fatigue Behavior and In-Vitro Biocompatibility of the Ni-Free Austenitic High-Nitrogen Steel X13CrMnMoN18-14-3,"** *Stainless Steels for Medical and Surgical Applications, ASTM STP 1438*, G. L. Winters and M. J. Nutt, Eds., ASTM International, West Conshohocken, PA, 2003.

Abstract: Austenitic stainless steels generally have a favorable combination of strength and ductility as well as a sufficient resistance against corrosion. This and the reported biocompatibility lead to the use of 304- and later 316 L-type steels in medical applications. Especially in orthopedics these steels were applied as implants for e.g. fracture fixation as bone plates, intermedullary nails, and screws. But these steels contain a high amount of Ni, which was attributed to cause Ni-allergies for an growing amount of patients. Thus, alternatives were needed and - beside the already known CoCrMo-alloys - implants of Ti and its alloys emerged increasingly into the medical market. The aim of this paper is to introduce a new austenitic Ni-free CrMnMo-steel X13CrMnMoN18-14-3 (Material No.: 1.4452, brand name: P2000), which makes use of about 1 % N in order to gain a combination of high strength, high ductility, and a superior corrosion resistance.

In a first step the cyclic fatigue behavior in air and in Ringer solution in the solution annealed state is investigated. This is accompanied by electrochemical testing in Ringer solution as well as in-vitro cytotoxicity tests against MC3T3 cells in bovine serum.

The tests revealed that the solution annealed X13CrMnMoN18-14-3 at 5 Hz has an 50 % endurance limit of 346 MPa in air and of 302 MPa in Ringer solution, which is markedly higher compared to solution annealed CrNiMo-steels. In addition it was found that the CrMnMoN-steel shows no distinct susceptibility to stress-corrosion cracking in the entire region of finite life between stress amplitudes of 400 to 550 MPa. The pitting potential in Ringer solution was measured to be 1.1 V, which is in the range of common

[1] Dipl.-Ing. and Research Scientist, Dipl.-Ing. and Research Scientist, Prof. Dr.-Ing., respectively, Werkstofftechnik, Universitaet Essen, Universitaetsstr. 15, 45117 Essen, Germany

[2] Research Scientist, PD Dr. and Research Scientist, Prof. Dr., respectively, Institut fuer Physiologie, Universitaetsklinikum, Universitaet Essen, Hufelandstr. 152, 45122 Essen, Germany

Ni-containing high-Nitrogen steels as well as of CoCr20Mo6 alloys. No reduction of MC3T3 cell adhesion could be observed.

Thus, the Ni-free CrMnMoN-steels might be a promising alternative to the CrNiMo-steels in medical applications.

Keywords: High-Nitrogen Steel, Fatigue, Biocompatibility, Cytotoxicity

Nomenclature

$\varepsilon_{a,t}$	total strain amplitude	%
$\varepsilon_{a,pl}$	plastic strain amplitude	%
$\varepsilon_{m,pl}$	cyclic mean plastic strain%	
ΔT	temperature change	K
σ_a	stress amplitude	MPa

HNS	high Nitrogen steel X13CrMnMoN18-14-3
MTT	Methylthiazoltetrazolium
AM	Acetoxymethylester

Introduction

Austenitic stainless steels generally have a favorable combination of strength and ductility as well as a sufficient resistance against corrosion. This and the reported biocompatibility lead to the use of 304- and later 316 L-type steels in medical applications. Especially in orthopedics these steels were applied as implants for e.g. fracture fixation as bone plates, intermedullary nails, and screws. However, any implant brings about a reaction within the adjacent tissue and the surrounding media leads to a reaction of the implant surfaces [1]. Thus, these steels may corrode under combined chemical-mechanical loads and release their metal ions into the body fluid. Due to the fact, that they contain a high amount of Ni, this is attributed to cause Ni-allergies for a growing amount of patients [2-7]. Thus, alternatives were needed. One way is to increase the chemical stability of passive layers of Cr_2O_3-type on steels by adding Cr, Mo, and N [8, 9]. The other way is to choose materials which have no Ni as alloying element like most of the CoCrMo- and Ti-base alloys. The latter make use of a passive layer of TiO_2-type. This is chemically much more stable and has an excellent biocompatibility [10-12]. But, due to the fact that under fatigue and wear all these passive layers will crack there will be a release of metal ions in any case. Thus, beside the already known Ni-free CoCrMo-alloys implants of Ti and its alloys emerged increasingly into the medical market. Parallel Ni-free stainless steels have been developed, which combine a high strength and an ductility with good corrosion properties [13].

The aim of this paper is to introduce the fatigue properties of solid solution annealed austenitic high-Nitrogen Ni-free CrMnMoN-steel X13CrMnMoN18-14-3 (HNS, Material

No.: 1.4452), which makes use of about 1 % N in order to gain a combination of high strength, high ductility, and a superior corrosion resistance. In addition the results of in-vitro cytotoxicity tests are shown and discussed.

Experimental Procedures

Material

The material investigated was delivered as drawn, solution annealed and ground bars with a diameter of 30 mm. From these all specimens were cut either by sawing or by wet cutting. The range of the typical chemical compositions of the high-nitrogen steel is given in Table 1.

Table 1 - *Chemical Composition of X13CrMnMoN18-14-3*

Fe	Cr	Mn	Mo	Nb	C	N
bal.	16-20	12-16	2.5-4.2	≤0.25	≤0.15	0.75-1.0

Tensile tests at strain rates between 0.016 and 10 %/s (Figure 1) of the solution annealed state revealed no distinct strain rate sensitivity. For a strain rate of 0.1 %/s the mechanical

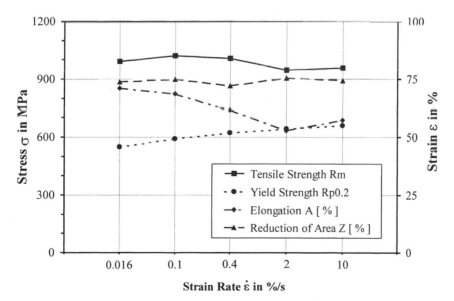

Figure 1 - *Tensile Properties of the HNS under different Strain Rates*

properties are listed in Table 2.

Table 2 - *Tensile Properties of X13CrMnMoN18-14-3*

yield strength in MPa	tensile strength in MPa	elongation to fracture in %	reduction of area in %
590	1030	70	75

Metallography and Microscopy

For the light microscopical analyses of grain size and hardness eight discs of 30 mm diameter and 5 mm thickness were cut from the bars. These specimens were ground down to 1200 mesh size SiC followed by polishing with diamond paste (ATM, Altenkirchen, Germany) down to 6 μm. The hardness testing was done according to Vickers with a load of 98.0665 N leading to HV10 hardness numbers. On every disc up to 30 measurements were taken along a line for the determination of the mean value and the standard deviation. The average hardness was measured being 259 ± 14 HV10.

After this the specimens were cleaned and further polished with diamond paste down to 1 μm. Etching was done for 120 s at 55°C in V2A etchant (100 mL distilled water, 100 mL hydrochloric acid, 10 mL nitric acid, 0,3 mL pickling inhibitor). Polishing and etching cycles were repeated three times in order to gain a preparation result which is suitable for automated image analyzing (Figure 2). From these specimens the grain size was derived according to ASTM Standard "Grain Size, Average, Using Semiautomatic and Automatic Image Analysis" (E 1382-91) using ImageC Software (Imtronic GmbH, Berlin, Germany) attached to a digital camera DIC1300 (Micromotion, Landshut, Germany), which was mounted on a light microscope METALLUX 2 (Leitz, Wetzlar, Germany). The intersections between the measuring grit and the twin boundaries were deleted manually in order to get measuring values solely from the austenite grain boundaries. This revealed an average grain size of 100 ± 13 μm. ASTM grain size ranges from 3 to 4.

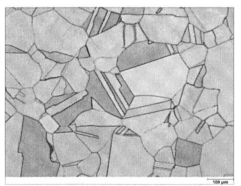

Figure 2 - *Austenite Grain Structure of the Solid Solution Annealed HNS*

For transmission electron microscopy (TEM) small discs of 3 mm diameter and

0.2 mm thickness were cut out (ATM, Altenkirchen, Germany) of the bigger specimens and ground to a thickness of 0.1 mm. Afterwards the center of these discs were thinned electrolytically (Tenupol, Struers, Willich, Germany) at 40 V and 100 mA in A8 (950 mL acetic acid, 50 mL perchloric acid) at 8 to 10°C in until a small hole was generated suitable for TEM investigations.

Corrosion

Potentiodynamic corrosion tests according to ASTM Standard "Standard Reference Test Method for making Potentiostatic Anodic Polarization Measurements" (G5-94) at 37°C in Ringer solution showed a pitting potential at 1.1 V. In order to achieve this cylindrical specimens were ground down to 6 μm diamond paste and afterwards electro polished. The Ringer solution was continuously irrigated with N so that the O_2 content was below 1 mg/L. The resting potential was measured until there was no change of the potential bigger than 1 mV over a 300 s time period. Subsequently the specimens were activated at -2 V for 60 s. Then the potentiodynamic test was started at 50 mV below the resting potential with 600 mV/h until the transpassive region was reached. Afterwards the potential was decreased with the same speed in order to measure the repassivation behavior. In comparison a standard 316L-type of steel X2CrNiMo18-15-2 (Material-No.: 1.4441) was investigated in the solid solution annealed state as well.

Cytotoxicity

In-Vitro Biocompatibility - A total of 30 discs (diameter 5.5 mm, thickness 1+/-0.3) manufactured from HNS were electro polished (Polier- und Entgratungselektrolyt, Graul, 75417 Mühlacker, Germany), cleaned in 5% HNO_3 (80°C for 2 h), defatted in acetone (3 times, 10 min each) and ethanol (70%, v/v) and finally heat sterilized at 220°C for 3 h. All further handling was under sterile conditions. Size matched discs made from copper (defatted and sterilized) were used as negative control material in some experiments. Size and shape of all metal discs allowed them to be inserted into moulds of a 96-well cell culture plate, such that the vessel wall tightly fitted the metal. This was advantageous for all cell culture testing procedures performed under conditions of direct cell-material contact.

Cell Line - The well-established osteoblast-like cell line MC3T3-E1 [14] was used throughout (passage number 5-9). Cells were maintained at 37°C in a humidified 5% CO_2 atmosphere using αMEM (ICN Biomedicals Inc., Aurora, OH, USA) supplemented with 20 % fetal calf serum, 2 mmol/L glutamine, penicillin (5,000 I.U./mL), and streptomycin (5,000 μg/mL).

Cell Morphology - Live cells were loaded with calcein AM (5 μmol/L for 1 h) (Molecular Probes Europe, Leiden, The Netherlands), washed once with Hanks balanced solution (HBS) and observed within the same solution with an upright epifluorescence microscope (Olympus Bx50Wi, Hamburg, Germany) equipped with a 20x water immersion objective [15].

MTT Assay - Confluent cultures were trypsinized according to standard methods. To establish representative growth curves, $1,5 \times 10^3$ freshly trypsinized cells were seeded into each well of a 96-well plate either in the presence or absence of the testing materials. Tests were run for 7 days. At the time points indicated, 20 μL of a Thiazolyl Blue (MTT, Sigma, Taufkirchen, Germany) stock solution (0,5 mg MTT per mL HBS) was added to 200 μL culture medium. Cells were allowed to form the reduced formazan dye for 2 h under cell culture conditions. Thereafter, wells were briefly washed with 200 μL HBS before the fluid was completely withdrawn. Dried cells were kept on the plate until formazan formed inside mitochondria was dissolved with an acid dimethyl sulfoxide containing lysis buffer [16]. A volume of 100 μL was used to measure the optical density (570/630nm) with a Dynatech MRX plate reader (Dynatech Labs., Billingshirt, UK). Background corrected OD values were converted into absolute cell numbers by means of a linear standard curve (not shown) obtained from serially diluted MC3T3-E1 cells.

Controls - For positive control we used cell culture tested polystyrene material (Falcon, Becton Dickinson Labware, Franklin Lakes, NJ, USA). For negative controls wells received 0,05% NaN_3 which induced cell death within 1 day. The latter procedure was carried out because copper discs could not be used together with the MTT reagent.

Induction of Alkaline Phosphatase (ALP) with Bone Morphogenetic Protein 2 (BMP-2) - Confluent MC3T3-E1 cells (ca. 8×10^4 cells/well) were incubated with BMP-2 (Biochrom, Berlin, Germany, 0.025-1 μg/ml) for 3 days. FCS concentration was reduced to 1% (v/v) during the incubation period, such that further cell growth and cellular protein increase was inhibited [17]. At the end of the experiments, cells were washed twice with Hanks balanced solution and cell bound ALP was determined as described [18] using 4-nitrophenyl-phosphate (Sigma, Taufkirchen, Germany) at a pH of 10.3 as a soluble chromogen for ALP. Color intensity was measured as optical density 405 nm and used as a measure for cell bound ALP. All tests were run in triplicates.

Fatigue

Round specimens (Figure 3) with cone ends were machined from the bars. The surfaces were ground by hand and afterwards electrolytically polished until the surface roughness reached values of R_a at 0.3 µm. The fatigue tests were carried out under force control with an R-Value of -1 using a MTS-BIONIX 858 (MTS Systems Corp., Minneapolis, MN, USA) at 0.5, 5, and 20 Hz under laboratory air (20°C) and Ringer solution (37°C, Figure 4). The statistical analyses of the S-N curves according to arcsin-$\sqrt{P}$ brings about a range for the average endurance limit [19].

In order to measure the stress-

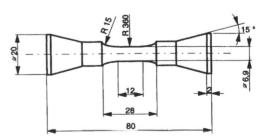

Figure 3 - *Scheme of the Specimens for Axial Fatigue Testing*

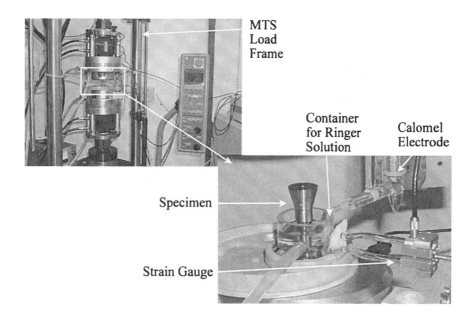

Figure 4 - *Test Set-Up for Axial Fatigue Testing in Ringers Solution*

strain curves (Figure 5) continuously at 0.5 Hz a strain gauge MTS Extensometer 10 mm (MTS Systems Corp., Minneapolis, MN, USA) with a measuring range of 2.5 % and a resolution 0.001 % was fixed to the specimens. This revealed the stress-strain hysteresis of which the total cyclic strain amplitude ($\varepsilon_{a,t}$) as well as the plastic strain amplitude ($\varepsilon_{a,pl}$) could be derived according to standard methods [20]. In addition the change of

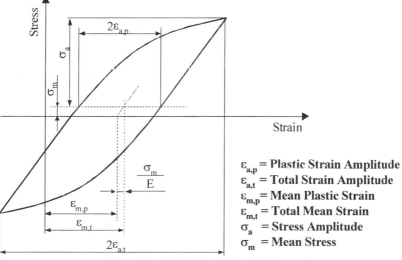

$\varepsilon_{a,p}$ = **Plastic Strain Amplitude**
$\varepsilon_{a,t}$ = **Total Strain Amplitude**
$\varepsilon_{m,p}$ = **Mean Plastic Strain**
$\varepsilon_{m,t}$ = **Total Mean Strain**
σ_a = **Stress Amplitude**
σ_m = **Mean Stress**

Figure 5 - *Cyclic Stress Strain Hysteresis*

temperature within the measuring length of the specimen was measured in air.

Results and Discussion

Corrosion

The current density potential curves of HNS and 316L are shown in Figure 6. It is obvious that the corrosion and the repassivation behavior of the HNS is distinctly better

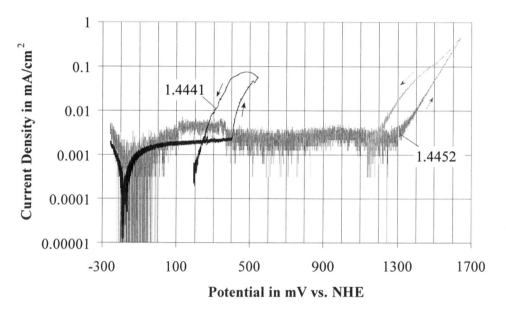

Figure 6 - *Current Density Potential Curves of HNS (1.4452) and Standard 316L-Type (1.4441)*

than that of the 316L type. This can be attributed to the higher content of Mo and N, which increases the pitting resistance equivalent [9, 21]. Thus, the pitting potential of the HNS reaches values, which are similar to that of the 0.4 % Nitrogen containing steel X5CrNiMoN22-10-3 (ISO5832-9) 1.1 [8] and slightly better than that of CoCr29Mo6 alloy at 0.8 V [22]. It should be mentioned here, that under similar conditions Ti-base materials like cp-Ti and TiAl6V4 have a pitting potential above 2 V [22].

Cytotoxicity

Epifluorescence microscopy of calcein-AM loaded MC3T3-E1 cells revealed no hints for a cytotoxic effect of HNS when cells were kept on the cleaned and electropolished material for up to 7 days. The degree of confluence, cell shape, and appearance of fine processes were all unchanged as compared to cells on positive control

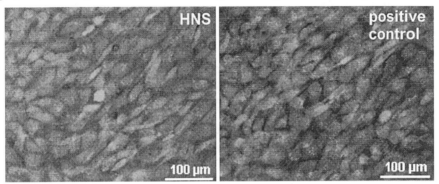

Figure 7 - *Live MC3T3-E1 Cells loaded with Calcein-AM were viewed under Water Immersion on HNS and on Cell Culture Tested Control Material. Morphological Differences are Missing. Note that some Image Distortion results e.g. from Scratches and Irregularities of the Metal Surface. The lower Contrast on HNS is due to some Light Back Scattering from the Metal Surface*

material which was the bottom of the cell culture tested plastic material (Figure 7). Comparison of growth curves (Figure 8A) also revealed no difference between cells on culture tested polystyrol material and cells on HNS. In these experiments, cells were in the phase of exponential growth as it is requested by the standard "Biologische Beurteilung von Medizinprodukten. Teil 5: Prüfungen auf in vitro Zytotoxizitaet" (DIN

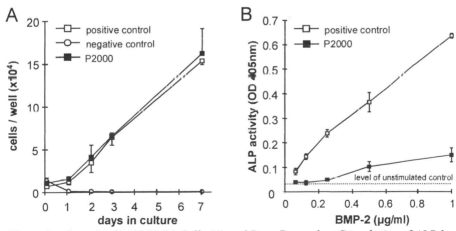

Figure 8 - *Growth of MC3T3.E1 Cells (A) and Dose Dependant Stimulation of ALP by BMP-2 (B). HNS: Cells growing directly on HNS Discs completely covering the Bottom of the Culture Vessel. Positive Control: Cells on Cell Culture Tested Polystyrol. Negative Control: Cells after Addition of 0.05% NaN₃ to the Medium.*

ISO 10993-5, 1999). Treatment with NaN₃, in contrast, led to a complete destruction of the cells within one day. Based on these in vitro results HNS should be classified as a fully biocompatible material.

Since HNS may be used as implant material in hard tissue, a typical feature of MC3T3-E1 cells, namely their inducible differentiation into osteoblasts, was included into our tests as well. We performed a stimulation with recombinant BMP-2 to induce an increase in cellular alkaline phosphatase, which is an early marker of osteoblast differentiation [18]. Also, in vivo BMP-2 stimulation is believed to be of large relevance for bone cell differentiation and clinical studies are currently under way to use this peptide for increased bone formation e.g. during fracture healing. To test whether or not the BMP-2 signaling pathway was impaired when cells were in intimate contact with HNS we applied BMP-2 to MC3T3-E1 cells adhering to a HNS surface. Figure 8B shows that cells under these conditions could be successfully stimulated with BMP-2. The efficacy of BMP-2 stimulation was, however, reduced, such that about a 5-fold higher concentrations of BMP-2 was required to yield the same amount of ALP. Besides the slope also the shape of the dose response curve was changed (Figure 8B). Further studies have to elucidate underlying mechanisms, which may encompass changes in receptor expression, BMP-2 binding to the receptor and/or subsequent intracellular signaling pathways.

Fatigue

Figure 9 shows the S-N curves at 5 Hz of the solid solution annealed HNS in ambient air and in Ringer solution. The arcsin-$\sqrt{P}$ method reveals 50% endurance limits at 346 MPa in ambient air and 302 MPa in Ringer solution.

Fatigue life and endurance limit depends strongly on the parameters under which

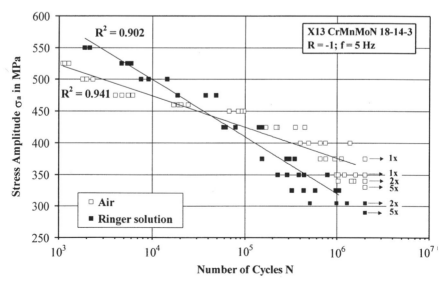

Figure 9 - *S-N curves of Solid Solution Annealed HNS in Air and in Ringers Solution*

these values were measured. Thus, any comparison between e.g. axial and rotating bending results is questionable. This is also true for tests run at different frequencies, which today might range from 0.5 Hz to 100 kHz. Another factor is the reported notch sensitivity of materials, which will have a distinct influence on the fatigue life of implants [23]. Thus, in this paper the fatigue life of the investigated HNS is compared only to literature data of other unnotched metallic implant materials. The evaluation of S-N curves is just a first step in the investigation of the fatigue behavior of any material. But due to the fact that they just represent the numbers of cycles to fracture it is important to notice that fractography as well as the metallographical analyses of the changes within the microstructure enlight the findings of mechanical testing. In order to get some information about the behavior of materials before fracture cyclic stress-strain hystereses have been measured as well as the temperature of the specimens. Both bring about information on the dissipation of energy and, therefore, on the amount of plastic deformation before crack initiation as well as in addition to the compliance of the specimen after crack initiation [24].

Fatigue in Ambient Air - Figures 10 and 11 show the plastic strain amplitude $\varepsilon_{a,pl}$ and

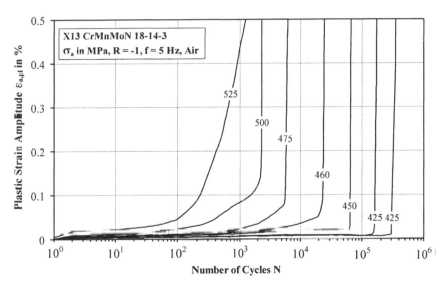

Figure 10 - *Plastic Strain Amplitude $\varepsilon_{a,pl}$ vs. Numbers of cycles N of Solid Solution Annealed HNS in Air*

the temperature change ΔT plotted vs. the numbers of cycles for constant stress amplitudes σ_a, respectively. For a high constant stress amplitude of 525 MPa obviously $\varepsilon_{a,pl}$ increases during the first two cycles and reaches a constant value for about 10 cycles. Afterwards it increases progressively until the specimen fractures. This characteristic behavior is more or less true for all $\varepsilon_{a,pl}$-N curves, even though the numbers of cycles of constant $\varepsilon_{a,pl}$ increase with decreasing σ_a. In comparing Figures 10 and 11 one can see that the temperature change, which is a measure of the dissipated plastic work, shows a similar

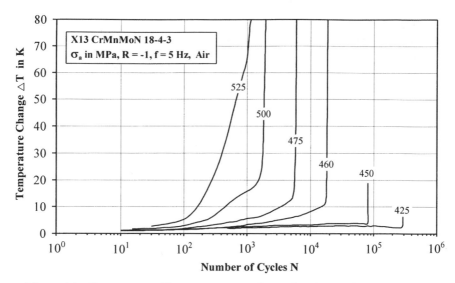

Figure 11 - *Temperature Change ΔT vs. Numbers of cycles N of Solid Solution Annealed HNS in Air*

behavior. Due to the fact that during cyclic hardening and softening before crack initiation as well as during the plastic work dissipated within the plastic zone during stable crack propagation both plots do not allow a precise definition of the crack initiation phase. In order to achieve this, the electrical resistance of the specimens should have been measured as well [25]. But nevertheless it is obvious that there is no distinct cyclic hardening. The constant values of $\varepsilon_{a,pl}$ are brought about by the compressive residual stresses, which are introduced during the compression phase of the load cycle. In Figure 12 the mean plastic strain $\varepsilon_{m,pl}$ is plotted versus the numbers of cycles N. Depending on the stress amplitudes compressive values of $\varepsilon_{m,pl}$ are introduced for σ_a values between 450 and 525 MPa, bringing about a shift in the effective strain amplitudes to smaller values. If σ_a is equal to 425 MPa or smaller no distinct plastic work is dissipated neither due to introduction of compressive residual stresses nor by tensile fraction of the load cycles. Thus, neither $\varepsilon_{a,pl}$ nor $\varepsilon_{m,pl}$ nor ΔT change distinctly during fatigue life at 5 Hz. At no stress amplitude levels any decrease of $\varepsilon_{a,pl}$ could be noticed. Thus, no cyclic strengthening of these steels could be observed.

Fatigue in Ringer Solution - During the fatigue in Ringer solution the mechanical behavior is mostly influenced after the first cracks have been initiated. Due to the action of H^+-Ions at the crack tip, the stable crack propagation is accelerated and the fatigue life as well as the endurance limit decreases. But, for the solution annealed HNS the detrimental effect of corrosion is not as pronounced as it is for a standard 316L type of steel under similar conditions [25]. For the HNS the S-N curve is very close to that in ambient air and the endurance limit is just about 8 % lower. For e.g. 316L under the same testing conditions the endurance limit in Ringer solution is lowered by 14 % [25]. The open corrosion potential, which is a measure for the ongoing corrosion processes and

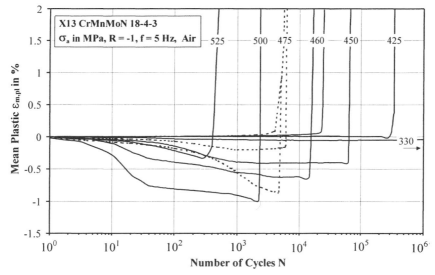

Figure 12 - *Mean Plastic Strain $\varepsilon_{m,pl}$ vs. Numbers of cycles N of Solid Solution Annealed HNS in Air*

increases markedly with existing cracks, stays at a constant value until a crack has been initiated. Now the characteristic corrosion mechanisms of HNS play a dominant role. Due to the fact that N bring about certain surface reactions [21] the concentration of H^+-ions is lowered and, therefore, the embrittlement within the plastic zone at the crack tip does not take place or at least is not as pronounced as it is for N-free steels.

Evaluation of the Fatigue Behavior - The investigation of the specimens surfaces reveals a crack initiation pattern, which is typical for austenitic steels. Small crack initiation is governed by the orientation of the sliding bends within the austenitic grains

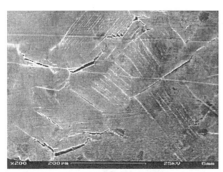

Figure 13 - *Crack Initiation on the Surfaces of Fatigue Specimens of a Solid Solution Annealed HNS tested at a Stress Amplitude of 500 MPa in Ambient Air*

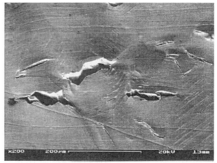

Figure 14 - *Crack Initiation on the Surfaces of Fatigue Specimens of a Solid Solution Annealed HNS tested at a Stress Amplitude of 500 MPa in Ringers Solution*

(Figure 13). It has been reported that for N-free 316L steels in Ringer solution just one crack initiates becoming the main fatigue crack of the specimens [25]. But for the HNS many cracks initiated in Ringer solution as well (Figure 14) indicating that the influence of corrosion on crack initiation and stable crack propagation is by far not as pronounced

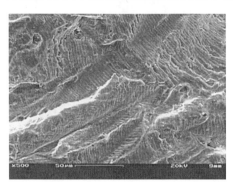

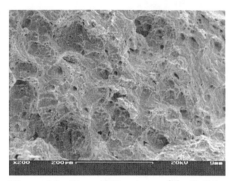

Figure 15 - *Fatigue Fracture of the Solid Solution Annealed HNS tested at a Stress Amplitude of 500 MPa in Ringer Solution*

Figure 16 - *Forced Fracture of the Solid Solutions Annealed HNS tested at a Stress Amplitude of 500 MPa in Ringer Solution*

as it is for N-free steels. In addition the fatigue (Figure 15) as well as the forced fracture (Figure 16) surface did not show any marked differences compared to those of the specimens tested in ambient air.

Even though HNS have a low stacking fault energy and tend to strain harden under static loads much more pronounced than N-free austenitic steels [13], under fatigue loads no cyclic hardening could be observed. Degallaix et al. [26] showed that cyclic softening is brought about by the reversibility of planar slip while cyclic hardening is promoted by subcell structures. Thus, depending on the predeformed state and the cyclic stress or strain amplitudes both types of cyclic behavior could be observed [13, 25]. N brings about a short range order pinning effect due to the formation of strongly bound Mo-N pairs or clusters within solid solution [27]. Thus any dislocations moving through the lattice must destroy the Mo-N bonding, which works as a very strong obstacle to dislocation motion similar to small precipitates. Now it is under discussion whether this or the low stacking fault energy has the most pronounced influence on the planarity of dislocation slip. Nevertheless it might be concluded that despite their amount of influence both mechanisms lead to the same direction. This results in the fact that cyclic hardening is just observed at high strain

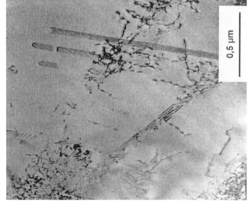

Figure 17 - *Dislocation Structure of HNS Fatigued at a Stress Amplitude of 460 MPa for 19040 Cycles in Air*

amplitudes and low N contents. At a high N-content - like it is with the investigated steel - the dislocation structure is characterized by the absence of cross slip [28]. This supports the authors' findings, which are characterized by a low density of dislocations and stacking faults as well as their planar distribution even at high stress amplitudes (Figure 17).

The endurance limits of the solution annealed HNS as well as of other metallic materials for implants is listed in Table 3. It should be noted, that the measured endurance limits strongly depend on all parameters (type of cyclic loading, frequency, grain size, etc.), which were chosen individually.

Table 3 - *Endurance Limits of Solution Annealed Metallic Materials for Implants in Physiological Media*

X13CrMnMoN 18-14-3	316L	ISO5832-9	CoCr29Mo6	cp-Ti Grade 2	TiAl6V4
302	250-320	400-420	200-280	230-280	400-450
this work	[29]	[30]	[29]	[29]	[29]

The HNS X13CrMnMoN18-14-3 shows fatigue properties in physiological media, which are in the range of other metallic materials being already applied in daily clinical practice.

Conclusion and Outlook

The austenitic high-Nitrogen steel X13CrMnMoN18-14-3 has been evaluated in the solution annealed state as to its corrosion and fatigue properties. In addition cytotoxicity was tested in-vitro. This brought about the following results:

1. The HNS investigated can be designated being biocompatible in the presence of MC3T3 bone like cells.

2. The corrosion behavior in Ringer solution is much better than 316L, slightly better than that of CoCr29Mo6, and comparable to that of N-containing ISO5832-9.

3. The fatigue properties of the HNS X13CrMnMoN18-14-3 in Ringer solution are better than that of 316L.

4. In order to understand the fatigue properties better and derive additional data rotating bending tests in Ringer solution should be carried out as well as constant strain amplitude tests. Due to the fact that many implants are not applied in the solution annealed state the investigations should be extended to different degrees of cold working.

5. Concerning the reported [9, 31] excellent tribological behavior of HNS it can be designated as a material suitable for implants. Before application further animal tests have to be carried out.

Acknowledgments The authors would like to thank VSG Energie- und Schmiedetechnik GmbH, Essen, Germany for financial sponsorship. We are in debt to Ms. B. Gleising and Dr.-Ing, S. Weiß, Werkstofftechnik, Universitaet Essen, Germany together with Prof. Dr.-Ing. W. Dudzinski, Institute of Materials Science and Applied Mechanics, TU Wroclaw, Poland for their TEM investigations. Special thanks goes to Prof. Dr. D. Nast-Kolb and Dr. G. Täger, Unfallchirurgie, Universitaetsklinik, Universitaet Essen, Germany for their important information on the future needs and constraints of implants in daily clinical practice.

References

[1] Puleo, D.A., Nanci, A.; "Understanding and Controlling the Bone-Implant Interface," *Biomaterials,* Vol. 20, 1999, p.2311-2321.

[2] Hildebrand, H.F., Hornez, J.C.; "Biological Response and Biocompatibility," in *Metals as Biomaterials*, J. A.Helsen and H. J.Breme, Eds., Wiley & Sons, Chichester, UK, 1998, p.265-290.

[3] Hildebrand, H.F., Veron, C., Martin, P.; "Ni, Cr, Co Dental Alloys and Allergic Reactions: An Overview". *Biomaterials,* Vol. 10, 1989, p. 545-548.

[4] Goh, C.L.; "Prevalence of Contact Allergy by Sex, Race and Age." *Contact Dermatitis,* Vol. 14, 1986, p. 237-240.

[5] Möller, H.; "Nickel dermatitis: Problems Solved and Unsolved." *Contact Dermatitis*, Vol. 23, 1990, p.217-220.

[6] Peltonen, L.; "Nickel Sensitivity in the General Population." *Contact Dermatitis,* Vol. 5, 1979, p.27-32.

[7] Kiec-Swierczynska, M.; "Allergy to Chromate, Cobalt and Nickel in Lodz 1977-1988." *Contact Dermatitis,* Vol. 22, 1990, p.229-231.

[8] N.N.; "REX734 High Nitrogen Austenitic Steel", Brochure, SMP Ltd., Sheffield, UK, 1999.

[9] Thomann, U.I., Uggowitzer, P.J.; "Wear-Corrosion Behaviour of Biocompatible Austentic Stainless Steels" *Wear*, Vol. 239, 2000, p.48-58.

[10] Breme, H.J., Helsen, J.A.; "Selection of Materials". in Metals as Biomaterials, J. A. Helsen and H. J.Breme, Eds., John Wiley & Sons, Chichester, UK, 1998, p.1-36.

[11] Steinemann, S.G.; "Corrosion of Titanium and Titanium Alloys for Surgical Implants" in Titanium, Science and Technology (Proc. Conf.) Lütjering, G., Zwicker, U., and Bunk, W., Eds., 5th Internation Conference in Titanium, September, 10th - 14th, 1984, Munich, Germany, Deutsche Gesellschaft für Materialkunde e.V., Hamburger Allee 26, 60486 Frankfurt, Germany, 1984, p.1373-1379.

[12] Oshida, Y., Miyazaki, S.; "Corrosion and Biocompatibility of Shape Memory Alloys." *Corrosion Engineering*, Vol. 40, 1991, p.1009-1025.

[13] Gavriljuk, V.G., Berns, H.; "High Nitrogen Steels" Springer, Berlin, Heidelberg, New York, 1999, p.135-183.

[14] Sudo, H., Kodama, H.A., Amagai, Y., Yamamoto, S., Kasai, S.; "In vitro Differentiation in a New Clonal Osteogenic Cell Line Derived from Newborn Mouse Calvaria." *Journal of Cell Biology*, Vol. 96, 1983, p.191-198.

[15] Wiemann, M., Winkler, L., Bingmann, D.; "Light Microscopic Methods to Study Cells on Non-Transparent Materials." *Materialwissenschaft und Werkstofftechnik*, Vol. 32, 2001, p.976-983.

[16] Lindl, T.;"Zell- und Gewebekultur" Spektrum Akademischer Verlag, Heidelberg, Berlin, 2000.

[17] Wiemann, M., Rumpf, H.M., Bingmann, D., Jennissen, H.;"The Binding of rhBMP-2 to the Receptors of Viable MC3T3-E1 Cells and the Question of Cooperativity." *Materialwissenschaft und Werkstofftechnik*, Vol. 32, 2001, p.931-936.

[18] Hazama, M., Aono, A., Ueno, N., Fujisawa, Y.;"Efficient Expression of a Heterodimer of Bone Morphogenetic Protein Subunits using a BaculoVirus Expression System." *Biophysical and Biochemical Research Communications*, Vol. 209, 1995, p.859-866.

[19] Dengel, D.; "Planung und Auswertung von Dauerschwingversuchen bei angestrebter statitischer Absicherung der Kennwerte." in *Verhalten von Stahl bei schwingender Beanspruchung, Kontaktstudium Werkstoffkunde Eisen und Stahl III*, Dahl, W., Ed., Verlag Stahleisen, Düsseldorf, Germany, 1978, p.23-46.

[20] Suresh, S., "Fatigue of Materials", Cambridge University Press, Cambridge, UK, 1992, p.30-96.

[21] Hänninen, H.;"Corrosion Properties of HNS." *Materials Science Forum*, Vols. 318-320, 1999, p.479-488.

[22] Williams, D.F.; "Biocompatibility of Clinical Implant Materials. Vol.I" CRC Press, Boca Raton, Florida, USA, 1981, p.26.

[23] Bensmann, G., "An Attempt to Assess Material Suitability taking the Example of Hip Endoprotheses." *Materialwissenschaft und Werkstofftechnik*, Vol. 30, H.12, 1999, p.733-745.

[24] Middeldorf, K., Harig, H.; "Thermometrische Bewertung mikrostruktureller Änderung bei zyklischer Beanspruchung von Stählen." *Zeitschrift für Metallkunde*, Bd.77, H.9, 1986, p.564-570.

[25] Göbbeler, P.;"Untersuchungen zum Ermüdungsverhalten des kaltumgeformten austenitischen Implantatwerkstoffes X2CrNiMo18-15-3 - 1.4441" Ph.D.THesis, Universitaet Essen, Germany, Werkstofftechnik, 1998, see also *Fortschritt-Berichte Verein Deutscher Ingenieure, VDI-Verlag, Düsseldorf, Germany*, Reihe 5, Nr. 513, 1998.

[26] Degallaix, S., Foct, J., Hendry, A.; "Mechanical Behavior of High-Nitrogen Steels." *Material Science and Technology*, Vol. 2, No. 9, 1986, p.946-950.

[27] Murayama, M., Hono, K., Hirukawa, H., Ohmura, T., Matsuoka, S.; "The Combined Effect of Molybdenum and Nitrogen on the Fatigued Microstructure of 316 Type Austenitic Stainless Steels." *Scripta Materialia*, Vol. 41, No. 5, 1999, p.467-473.

[28] Zlateva, G., Kemanova, T., Ilieva, M.; "Dislocation Structure of Austenitic Nitrogen Steel during High Cycle Fatigue." *Praktische Metallographie*, Vol. 34, H.10, 1997, p.508-518.

[29] Breme, H.J., Helsen, J.A.; "Selection of Materials". in *Metals as Biomaterials*, Helsen, J. A. and Breme, H. J., Eds., Wiley & Sons, Chichester, UK, 1998, p.1-71.

[30] Kramer, K.H.; "Metallische Implantatwerkstoffe - ein Überblick" *Biomaterialien*, Vol. 2, H.4, 2001, p.187-197.

[31] Buescher, R., Krause, A., Fischer, A.; "Sliding Wear Behavior of Wet-Chemically Modified High-Nitrogen Steels". in *Lubricants, Materials , and Lubrication Engineering,* Bartz, W.J., Ed., 13th International Colloquium. January 15 – 17, 2002, Stuttgart /Ostfildern, Germany Technische Akademie, Ostfildern, Germany, 2002, p.1297-1306.

Suzanne H. Parker,[1] Hsin-Yi Lin,[1] Lyle D. Zardiackas,[2] and Joel D. Bumgardner[1]

Influence of Macrophage Cells on 316L Stainless Steel Corrosion

Reference: Parker, S.H., Lin, H-.Y., Zardiackas, L.D., and Bumgardner, J.D., *"Influence of Macrophage Cells on 316L Stainless Steel Corrosion,"* Stainless Steels for Medical and Surgical Applications, ASTM STP 1438, G. L. Winters and M. J. Nutt, Eds., ASTM International, West Conshohocken, PA, 2003.

Abstract: In vitro corrosion tests have not evaluated the role of cells on the corrosion of implant quality 316L stainless steel. A new cell-culture corrosion cell was used to simulate the clinical condition of cells attached to and growing on the alloy to evaluate the effects of cells on alloy corrosion and the effect of corrosion products on cells. The corrosion potential, charge transfer, and surface composition of the alloy were measured in the presence and absence of macrophage cells (RAW 264.7) or cells stimulated to release NO over 72 hours. Whereas there was no statistical difference in the corrosion of 316L stainless steel in the presence of macrophage cells as compared to culture media alone, there was a trend for higher corrosion to occur in the presence of the cells. Corrosion was further reduced when cells were stimulated to release NO which may have oxidized the implant and contributed to an enhancement of its surface oxide. These data suggest that cells may alter alloy surface oxides and affect alloy corrosion.

Keywords: 316L stainless steel, corrosion, surface analysis, biocompatibility, cell culture, macrophages

Introduction

Implant quality 316L stainless steel (316L SS) is widely used in orthopaedic, craniofacial and cardiovascular implant devices. The alloy depends on a chromium oxide surface layer for corrosion resistance and biocompatibility. Nevertheless, when implanted, the alloy may corrode, releasing constituents of the alloy into the body. For example, Walczak et al. [1] observed significant amounts of corrosion in 9 of 11 stainless steel hip implants retrieved from patients after 9-21 years.

While most implanted 316L stainless steel devices perform well, release of elements, particularly chromium and nickel, may be of concern due to their potential for

---

[1]Graduate Student, Graduate Student, and Associate Professor, respectively, Department of Agricultural and Biological Engineering, Biomedical Engineering Program, Mississippi State University, MS State, MS, 39762.
[2]Director, Biomaterials Division, University of Mississippi Medical Center, Jackson, MS, 39216.

inducing chronic inflammatory, toxicity, hypersensitivity or other reactions over the lifetime of the implant. Vieweg et al. [2] recently reported extensive fibrosis, foreign body reactions, and chronic inflammation in 5 of 13 spinal fixator systems implanted in patients for 10 months. Evaluating the biocompatibility of materials in a rabbit brain model, Mofid et al. [3] observed the greatest inflammatory responses for 316L stainless steel wires as compared to titanium, cobalt-chromium or silicone elastomer. Savarino et al. [4] observed significant increases in serum chromium and nickel levels, and in sister chromatid exchanges, an indicator of genotoxicity, in circulating lymphocytes for patients with stainless steel fracture fixation devices as compared to patients without implants. Several studies have implicated the development of hypersensitivity reactions to nickel-containing devices, including stainless steel as a cause for device failure and loss [5-6]. In vitro cell culture studies have indicated that components of 316L stainless steel released as corrosion products, such as chromium and nickel ions or alloy particulate, are capable of activating cultured macrophage cells to release pro-inflammatory cytokines and alter the metabolism of cultured cells at sub-cytotoxic levels [7-11]. These data suggest that alloy corrosion products may stimulate macrophages and induce an inflammatory response, which may further aggravate corrosion, thereby setting up a corrosion-inflammation-corrosion-inflammation feed-back loop.

In vitro and in vivo studies have been used widely to assess the corrosion resistance of stainless steels [12-21]. In vitro corrosion tests have typically used physiological salt solutions and have shown that while stainless steels, including 316L, exhibit low corrosion rates, they are susceptible to accelerated corrosion processes such as pitting and crevice corrosion [12,13,15,18,19]. For devices like spinal fixation systems and bone plates and screws, relative motion may occur between components, mechanically removing the protective oxide film and resulting in fretting corrosion [12,17,19]. Furthermore, when proteins are present in the electrolyte or stresses applied, corrosion resistance of 316L stainless steel may be reduced and corrosion increased [13-17]. In vivo corrosion tests have shown qualitative correlations with in vitro corrosion tests [12-14], however, differences between are apparent. Brown and Simpson [12] observed more fretting corrosion in vitro with saline solutions than in vivo, which may have been due in part to differences between in vitro and in vivo loading. While Bundy et al. [13] reported that stress-corrosion cracking of 316L stainless steel was more severe in vivo than in vitro, others have disputed these findings, claiming that biological conditions are not severe enough [18]. Williams et al. [17] later reported that while proteins increased passive corrosion rates of stainless steel, they decreased in vitro fretting corrosion. Additional research by Powell [20] reported that the negative effect of Ringers solution on 316L stainless steel corrosion fatigue was neutralized when 0.25% of clottable fibrinogen was added to the solution. Hence, it has been speculated that in vitro corrosion tests with simple salt solutions may not be a true measure of in vivo corrosion, and that organics, cells, mechanical loading and bioelectric effects may play an important role [13, 21].

It is important that in vitro corrosion tests closely simulate the in vivo environment to provide accurate data on the in vivo corrosion behavior of implant alloys. To date, in vitro corrosion tests have not considered the role of cells in the corrosion behavior of biomedical alloys. Cells may affect alloy corrosion by limiting oxygen diffusion through the release of reactive metabolites, altering dissolution kinetics, and or changing the surface oxide. Increases in oxide thickness and incorporation of calcium, phosphorous, and sulfur into surface layers were reported for stainless steel devices in bony or oral soft tissues implanted in humans for up to 128 days [22]. Therefore, the aim of this study was to investigate the hypothesis that the corrosion rate of 316L stainless steel is increased when macrophage cells are attached and growing on the alloy surface. Macrophages were chosen since they are often observed adjacent to implants, have been reported to be stimulated by corrosion or degradation products in vitro, and are capable of releasing a variety of inflammatory agents including nitric oxide (NO). NO is a molecular mediator of many physiological processes, such as vasodilation, inflammation, and thrombosis, which are essential for proper wound healing and immune reactions. NO will spontaneously oxidize in the physiological environment to form nitrite. Due to its highly reactive nature, NO may also further aggravate corrosion.

Materials and Methods

316L stainless steel [ASTM Standard Specification for Wrought-18 Chromium-14 Nickel-2.5 Molybdenum Stainless Steel Sheet and Strip for Surgical Implants (F139)] plates, 4.0cm X 4.0cm X 0.2cm were prepared by wet grinding through a series of SiC papers up to 1500 grit. The plates were cleaned ultrasonically for five minutes in acetone, then rinsed with 70% ethanol, and rinsed again with distilled water. The surfaces were then passivated according to ASTM (F86) Standard Practice for Surface Preparation and Marking of Metallic Surgical Implants to simulate clinical conditions, sterilized by immersion in 70% ethanol for two hours and then air dried under a UV light in a sterile hood.

TIB-71 murine alveolar macrophages (RAW 264.7) were obtained from American Type Culture Collection, ATCC, (Manassas, VA) and cultured in a humidified 5% CO_2 atmosphere at 37C. Cells were cultured in medium specified by ATCC [Dulbecco's Modified Eagle's Medium (DMEM) supplemented with 1 mM sodium pyruvate, 4 mM L-glutamine, 1.5 g/L sodium bicarbonate, 100 units/mL penicillin, 100 µg/mL streptomycin, and 0.25 µg/mL amphotericin with a final concentration of 10% FBS], which will be referred to as complete media. For tests requiring stimulated cells (i.e., cells induced to release NO as in an inflammatory reaction), growth medium supplemented either with 50 µg/ml lipopolysaccharide (LPS: Sigma, St. Louis, MO, serotype 0127:B8) or 5 µg/mL LPS plus 0.05 µg/mL interferon-γ (IFN-γ: R&D Systems, Minneapolis, MN) was added to the cells after a 4-hour attachment period [23,24]. The combination of LPS+IFN-γ used was determined from three-day dual dose-response curves (0 LPS + 0.5 µg/ml interferon to 50 µg/ml LPS + 0 interferon) and shown in pilot studies to be necessary to induce detectable levels of NO to be produced by the cells growing on the alloy surfaces [24].

Cell-Culture Corrosion Plate

Corrosion tests were conducted in an electrochemical cell culture corrosion cell designed to simulate the in vivo condition of cells growing on implant surfaces (Figure

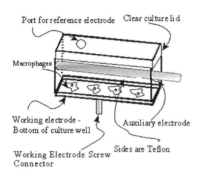

Figure 1- Schematic of electrochemical cell culture corrosion cell.

1). The bottom of the box consisted of the test alloy, the sides were composed of virgin electrical grade polytetrafluoroethylene, and the lid was plexiglass. The metal plate was held to the bottom of the box by a polytetrafluoroethylene plate screwed to the sides of the box. A stainless steel screw was inserted through the polytetrafluoroethylene bottom of the box to make an electrical contact with the stainless steel working electrode. Graphite rods (2) were inserted through ports on the side of the box and served as auxiliary electrodes. A glass bridge tube with a Vycor® tip (Princeton Applied Research, Oak Ridge, TN) was inserted through a port in the lid to hold the standard calomel reference electrode (SCE). All corrosion box components, except the bridge tube and reference electrode, were sterilized by immersion in 70% ethanol for 24 hours. The bridge tube and SCE were rinsed profusely with 70% ethanol and fresh media immediately before use. For corrosion tests, the corrosion box was placed inside a 5% CO_2, humidified cell culture incubator at 37°C, and the reference, auxiliary, and the working electrode leads were connected to the potentiometer (Princeton Applied Research, Model 6310, Oak Ridge, TN) by running the leads between the seal and glass door of the incubator. Cell density for both controls and the cell culture corrosion box was $1X10^5$ cells/cm², with a 1:1 ratio of media (mL): area (cm²).

Corrosion Experiments

A series of corrosion experiments were conducted to determine the open circuit potential (E_{corr}) and corrosion current at 0.0 mV vs. SCE over 24, 48 and 72 hour time intervals in: 1] complete media only, 2] with macrophages attached and growing on the test alloy, and 3] with macrophages stimulated with LPS or LPS+INF-γ. Using the Princeton Applied Research M352 Corrosion software (version3.04), E_{corr} was monitored for 4 hours to allow the potential of the system to stabilize, and then the corrosion rate (μA/cm²) at 0.0V vs. the SCE reference electrode was recorded for 20 hours. The test sequence was repeated at 24 hour intervals to provide E_{corr} and corrosion current data over a 72 hour period. Each test was repeated at least five times for each test electrolyte except for LPS stimulated cells, which was run only three times. The M352 software was used to calculate the charge transfers from the area under the current vs. time curves. For tests with stimulated cells, the cells were allowed to attach for 4 hours before stimulation since early tests indicated that seeding cells with LPS in the media inhibited cell attachment.

After corrosion testing, plates were cleaned and sonicated in methanol to remove cells, proteins and associated debris. Photomicrographs of freshly polished and anodized plates and plates after corrosion testing in media, and with cells were qualitatively compared to assess any surface damage due to corrosion by the cells using a JEOL JSM-35CF scanning electron microscope.

Evaluation of Macrophage Cultures

Viability/Morphology - The viability of the cells on the plate after three days of testing was qualitatively determined using a Leica laser scanning confocal microscope and the LIVE/DEAD® viability stain (Molecular Probes, Inc., Eugene, OR). Live cells fluoresced green and dead cells fluoresced red. Viability of the cells was qualitatively compared to control cells grown on glass coverslip slides in six well culture plates.

Cell morphology at the end of the three-day test period was observed via scanning electron microscope (SEM). The cells attached to the plate were rinsed twice with PBS for 10 minutes each, fixed with 2.5% glutaraldehyde in 0.1M potassium phosphate buffer (KPB) supplemented with 0.1M sucrose at pH=7.0 for 30 minutes, rinsed twice in 0.1M KPB for 30 minutes each, dehydrated through a series of alcohol washes, washed twice in hexamethyldisilazane, HMDS (Polysciences, Inc., Warrington, PA), for 10 minutes each, and then allowed to air dry in a desiccator. The cells were sputter-coated with Au/Pd for three minutes in a Polaron E5100 sputter coater and viewed from various tilt angles in the SEM operated at 15 kV beam voltage. The morphology of the cells was qualitatively compared to control cells grown on glass coverslip slides.

NO Production via Nitrite Quantitation - Stimulation of cells growing on the test alloy in the electrochemical cell culture corrosion plate was measured at 24-, 48-, and 72-hour intervals by the Griess reagent kit (Molecular Probes, Inc, Eugene, OR) using a µQuant plate reader (Biotek Instruments, Inc.,Winooski,VT). The detection limit for this test is 0.5 µM nitrite. Three 150 µl aliquots of the cell supernatant were collected from the plate on each day of the three-day tests. Each aliquot was combined with 130 µL of distilled water and 20 µL of Griess reagent in a 96-well plate. After incubating for 30 minutes at room temperature, the absorbance of each well was read at 548 nm. Absorbance values were converted to µM nitrite concentration. Cells grown in glass Petri dishes with the same growth area as the corrosion plate were used as controls.

Surface Analyses - The chemical composition of the surface oxide of the stainless steel samples in the polished and anodized condition and after corrosion testing in media, with cells and with LPS+INF-γ stimulated cells was determined via X-ray photoelectron spectroscopy, XPS. Experiments were conducted with a Physical Electronics Model 1600 surface analysis system (Eden Prairie, MN) with Mg Kα radiation (1253.6 eV) at 200 W. The analysis area was a circle approximately 800 µm in diameter. XPS spectra were referenced to the peak position of adventitious C. Survey spectra were obtained using a pass energy of 46.95 eV. High resolution spectra were acquired using a pass energy of 23.5 eV. Two spots were evaluated on each sample and two samples per test condition were evaluated.

Statistical Analyses

Factorial analysis of variance was used to determine if statistical differences existed in E_{corr} and charge transfers for the alloy in media, with cells and with stimulated cells at the 24-, 48- and 72- hour test periods. When analysis of variance tests detected differences, least significant difference (LSD) multiple comparison procedures were used to determine where statistical significances existed. Statistical analyses were conducted using Statlets v.1.1B at the 95% significance level.

Results

Corrosion Analyses

The E_{corr} values of 316L stainless steel in media, with macrophages and with stimulated macrophages over the three-day test period, are shown in Table 1. Factorial analysis of variance indicated that there were no significant interactions between the test conditions and time periods (p=0.9). Differences were detected in E_{corr} values over time (p=0.0001) but not between conditions (p=0.2) in post-hoc individual analyses. LSD comparisons indicated that for each test condition, there was a significant ennoblement of the E_{corr} potential of the alloy from the 24 hour period to the 48 hour period (p<0.05), but not from 48 to 72 hours (p>0.05).

Table 1- Ecorr potential (mV vs. SCE) of 316L stainless steel with and without macrophage cells.

Condition	24 Hr	48 Hr	72 Hr
Media	-183.7±23.3	-96.3±27.6[a]	-93.6±19.5[a]
Media + cells	-158.6±32.2	-118.0±21.5[b]	-105.9±22.6[b]
Media + cells stimulated with LPS	-161.7±17.9	-113.8±10.6[c]	-102.7±13.6[c]
Media + cells stimulated with LPS+INFγ	-174.4±27.8	-129.4±8.3[d]	-121.8±13.8[d]

Letter superscripts indicate statistically similar values within test conditions. There were no differences between test conditions.

Corrosion current versus time curves at 0.0 mV vs. SCE reference in all three test electrolytes and at each test period were very similar; initial currents rapidly decayed to very low values (Figure 2). The average calculated charge transfers at each time period in each test condition and the total cumulative charge transfers calculated are shown in Table 2. Factorial analysis of the charge transfer data indicated that there were no significant interactions between the test conditions and time (p=0.3). Analyses detected statistical differences in the charge transfers over time (p=0.0001) and between test conditions (p=0.0007). LSD comparisons indicated that for each test electrolyte condition, there was a significant decrease in the charge transfer values from the 24 hour period to the 48 hour period (p<0.05), but not from 48 to 72 hours (p>0.05). For each day, only charge transfers in media with LPS+IFN-γ stimulated cells were different from the other test conditions (p<0.05). Sum total charge transfers in the presence of cells and LPS stimulated cells were greater than with LPS+IFN-γ stimulated cells (p<0.05), but there were no differences between the media test condition and those with cells (p>0.05).

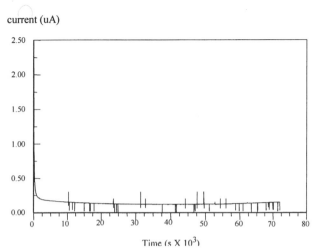

current (uA)

Time (s X 10³)

Figure 2: Current versus time for macrophage cells growin on 316L stuface on day 1. Curves were similar for days 2 and 3 and for the other test conditions.

SEM Analyses

Surfaces of polished and anodized samples exhibited only fine scratches due to the polishing procedure. After removal of non-stimulated and stimulated cells from the test plates, some protein material remained. However, no evidence of surface deterioration was observed.

Table 2- Charge Transfer (mC) for 316L stainless steel in the presence and absence of macrophage cells.

Condition	Day1	Day2	Day3	Total
Media	12.24±3.86 ⌉	3.64±1.36ᵃ ⌉	3.02±1.63ᵃ ⌉	18.91±5.92[#][^]
Media + macrophage cells	13.01±3.73 ⏐	6.41±2.45ᵇ ⏐	5.18±2.56ᵇ ⏐	24.60±7.96 [^]
Media + macrophage cells stimulated with LPS	13.69±2.68 ⌋	5.90±0.48ᶜ ⌋	5.048±0.23ᶜ ⌋	24.63±2.55 [^]
Media + macrophage cells stimulated w/ LPS+IFN-γ	5.81±0.87	3.40±1.2ᵈ	2.24±0.96ᵈ	10.73±2.12[#]

Letter superscripts indicate statistically similar values over time for an individual condition
Brackets,], indicate statistically similar values between conditions at each time period
Symbols indicate statistically similar values for total charge transferred over the three-day test period

Cell Culture Analyses

Visual observations using the confocal microscope indicated that the viability of the non-stimulated macrophage cells attached and growing on the stainless steel alloy in the corrosion plate for three days was high and indistinguishable from the viability of control cells attached and growing on glass coverslips. Nor were differences observed between the morphology of non-stimulated cells grown in the corrosion plate and on the glass coverslips seen in the SEM (Figure 3a, b). Non-stimulated cells cultured on glass slips and 316L SS plates appeared to be large and round with rough exteriors in confluent layers. However, when cells attached to 316L alloy in the corrosion plate or the glass coverslips were stimulated with LPS, the numbers and viability of the cells remaining after three days was obviously less than in the non-stimulated condition. However, the number and viability of the stimulated cells on the glass coverslip were greater than on the alloy based on visual observations. The morphology of the stimulated cells on the alloy and glass coverslips were similar to each other but different from non-stimulated cells. The stimulated cells exhibited a smooth, ball-shaped morphology with few attachments in sparsely populated patches (Figure 3c, d). When the cells were stimulated with LPS+IFN-γ, number and viability of cells appeared to be greater than with LPS alone, particularly on the 316L stainless steel surfaces, though numbers of cells still appeared to be less than nonstimulated cells. Morphology of the LPS+IFN-γ stimulate cells were similar to those of the LPS stimulated cells (Figure 3e, f).

NO Production - The results of the tests for the production of NO by the cells are shown in Table 3. Factorial analysis indicated that there were significant interactions between the condition of the cells, the growth surfaces, and the time period for the production of NO by the cells ($p=0.0001$). For glass surfaces, LPS and LPS+IFN-γ stimulated cells resulted in higher levels of NO production than the nonstimulated cells. Levels of NO production were greater on Days 2 and 3 than on Day 1 for the LPS stimulated cells on glass. For cells grown on the stainless steel surfaces, there was no difference in the levels of NO produced by nonstimulated and LPS stimulated cells, and these levels were significantly lower than for the LPS+IFN-γ stimulated cells. Only for the LPS stimulated cells were the levels of NO production different between the control glass and stainless steel surfaces.

Table 3- NO release (µM) by macrophage cells on glass and 316L stainless steel.

Condition	Surface	Day1	Day2	Day3
Macrophage cells	Glass^	0.6±0.9	0.9±0.2	0.6±1.2
	316L^	0.4±0.8	1.8±2.2	0.8±1.5
Macrophage cells stimulated w/ LPS	Glass	13.7±1.3	36.8±5.7[a]	50.9±7.6[b]
	316L^	1.5±1.4	1.4±1.4	1.4±1.3
Macrophage cells stimulated w/ LPS+IFN-γ	Glass[#]	7.0±4.4	12.8±2.7	13.6±3.2
	316L[#]	5.4±3.6	10.2±4.3	11.3±5.6

Symbols indicate similarities between conditions and letters indicate differences over time

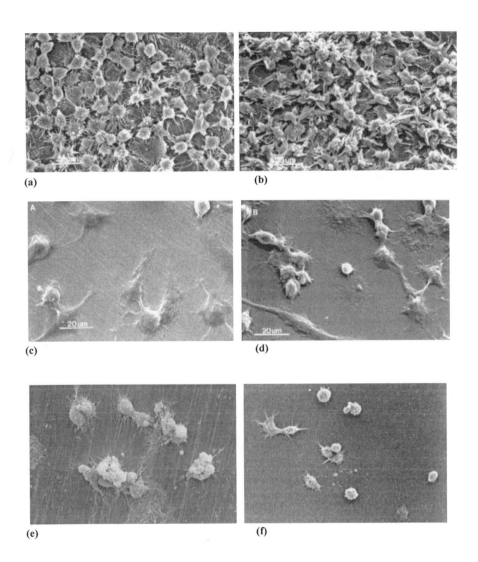

(a)

(b)

(c)

(d)

(e)

(f)

Figure 3- Photomicrographs of macrophage cells. Cells exhibit normal rough/textured morphology with many attachments on (a) 316L stainless steel and (b) glass coverslip. Cells stimulated with LPS on (c) 316L stainless steel and (d) glass or with LPS+IFN-γ on (e) 316L stainless steel and (f) glass exhibited smooth ball shaped morphology with few attachments. The number, viability, and production of NO by macrophage cells on 316L stainless steel was greater when stimulated with LPS+IFN-γ than when stimulated with LPS alone.

XPS Surface Analyses - Representative spectra of the surfaces of the stainless steel samples are shown in Figure 4. These spectra indicate that the surface of as-polished and passivated alloy was composed primarily of Cr and O, as chromium oxide/hydroxide with minor levels of Fe. After 3 days in media, sufficient protein deposition occurred to mask alloy surface elements as indicated by the large C and N peaks. After 3 days with macrophage cells or cells stimulated with LPS+IFN-γ, chromium oxide/hydroxides, as indicated by the large shoulders at 533-530 eV for O and 580-577 eV for Cr, were observed to be enhanced on the alloy's surface as well as other organic compounds. While the N detected on the surfaces was attributed primarily to proteinacious material for the cell culture media and cells, contributions to this peak from the nitric acid passivation treatments and from production of NO from the cells is possible.

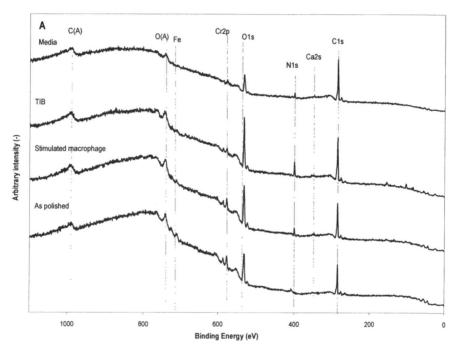

Figure 4A: XPS analyses of 316L stainless steel after three days in culture media, with TIB macrophage cells and with TIB macrophage cells stimulated with LPS+IFN-γ. As-polished and nitric acid passivated samples are also shown. Representative survey spectra [A] shows major peaks. The '(A)' designation indicates an Auger peak in the spectra.

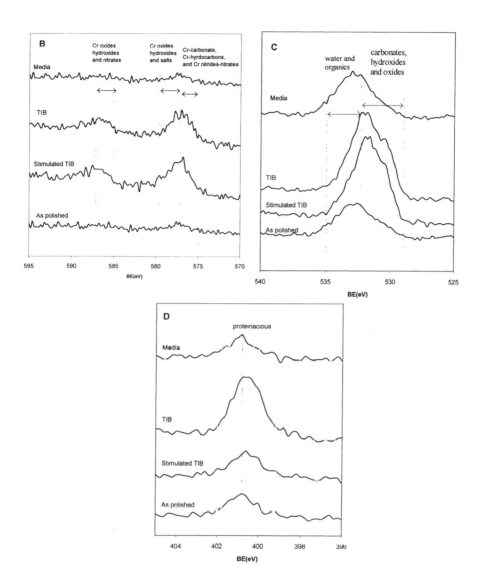

Figure 4B-C: XPS analyses of 316L stainless steel after three days in culture media, with TIB macrophage cells, and with TIB macrophage cells stimulated with LPS+IFN-γ. As-polished and nitric acid passivated samples are also shown. Representative high resolution spectra are shown for chromium [B]; oxygen [C]; and nitrogen [D].

Discussion

In this study, the E_{corr} of the alloy became more electropositive over the 3-day test period though there were no statistical differences between tests with or without cells. Similarly, corrosion rate measurements indicated that there was little difference in the amount of charge transferred when macrophage cells or LPS stimulated cells were attached and growing on the alloy's surface as compared to the media only test condition and that corrosion significantly decreased after the first 24 hours for all test conditions. These data suggest, at least initially, that when exposed to a cell culture environment, changes in the alloy's corrosion behavior are due primarily to interactions of the media with the alloy and not to the presence of cells. The ennoblement of stainless steel's E_{corr} in an aqueous environment has been attributed to the development of a chromium rich oxide layer that thickens with time [16,25]. The XPS data in this study also demonstrated the presence of a chromium rich surface oxide particularly in the presence of the cells and LPS+IFN-γ stimulated cells. Thickening and decreasing crystallinity of surface oxides and incorporation of calcium have been observed for austenitic stainless steel devices retrieved after 20-136 days, which, at least for titanium implant alloys, have been reported to reduce corrosion [14,22,26,27]. On the other hand, loss of surface oxide and significant corrosion were demonstrated for austenitic stainless steel femoral components retrieved after 9-21 years [1].

While there was a trend for increased corrosion in the presence of non-stimulated cells as compared to media only, corrosion was still low, indicating that the alloy remained in the passive state and was well tolerated by the cells. The non-stimulated cells exhibited normal morphology on the stainless steel, and were observed to have a high viability similar to controls. No evidence of surface damage or corrosion was observed. These observations agree with the clinical data indicating that 316L stainless steel devices are generally well tolerated during short-term implantation. The interpretation, though, on the long-term corrosion behavior of the alloy due to the cells is uncertain because these data were collected only from short test periods. The increase in corrosion may not be of significance within the three-day period used in these tests, but even small increases in corrosion and subsequent metal ion release may quickly become clinically relevant over the long term. Increases in Ni blood levels were reported in patients with stainless steel devices, which were associated with increased genotoxicity [4] and have been implicated in the induction of metal hypersensitivity reactions [5,6]. Small increases in the release of Ni ions from stainless steel also were observed in the presence of cultured cells as compared to media without cells [24]. Thus, the small increases in corrosion in the presence of the macrophage cells may lead to clinically relevant levels of released metal ion corrosion products. Hence, hypotheses regarding the role of cells on corrosion of 316L stainless steel still need to be investigated.

What was initially surprising was that corrosion of the alloy was not more affected when the macrophage cells were stimulated with LPS as compared to non-stimulated cells. The 50 µg/ml concentration of LPS used to stimulate the cells was determined from previous reports in the literature and dose-response curves generated in our lab with the cells in tissue culture plastic dishes [23]. This concentration gave a maximal NO production by the cells. However, it was noted that the number and viability of the macrophages on the test samples, and the levels of NO produced were greatly reduced when LPS was added to the medium to stimulate them. The reduced number of cells remaining on the alloy surface then would have limited any effect on the alloy's corrosion behavior, and thus appeared to have affected corrosion in a manner similar to non-stimulated cells. For the control LPS stimulated cells, part of the reduction in cell number and viability may be attributed to the cumulative toxic effects of NO produced and released during the three day cultures. However, the LPS stimulated cells on the alloy produced little if any NO during the tests, suggesting that NO may not account for the toxic effects. It is not clear why the stimulation of cells growing on the alloy surface lead to decreases in viability and inhibition of NO production as compared to stimulated controls. One hypothesis may be that macrophages attach to the alloy surface differently than to tissue culture plastic or glass and therefore do not receive the contact stimulus necessary for full stimulation. It has been demonstrated that there are differences in attachment of cells, e.g. osteoblasts, to different surfaces [28]. Differences in the absorption of proteins and their conformations between the metal and cell culture dish surfaces may have further affected cellular responsiveness. It has been reported that fibrinogen coated surfaces caused macrophage cells preferentially to release superoxide at the basal location of cells at the cell-material interface while albumin coated surfaces did not [29]. If the macrophage cells in this study preferentially released NO at the basal location of the cell at the cell-alloy interface, NO may have become incorporated into the alloy surface film instead of accumulating in the media. Unfortunately, due to the large amount of proteinacious material on the surface, we have not been able to determine if any of the N in the alloy surface was due to NO from the cells. Nevertheless, changes in the attachment of the cells due to the alloy surface and or absorbed proteins may have altered their responsiveness to LPS stimulation. Changes in macrophage responsiveness to antigen alone at the cell-material interface may have negative implications regarding implant associated bacterial infections.

In vivo, activated T-cells produce INF-γ to aid in macrophage activation [30]. Pruett and Higginbotham showed that a combination of LPS+IFN-γ was required to stimulate the RAW 264.7 macrophages to produce maximal amounts of NO [31]. INF-γ was not initially included in this study because cells in culture wells when stimulated with LPS alone produced NO. Titration tests in our lab determined that a combination of 5 μg/mL LPS+ 0.05μg/mL IFN-γ stimulated the cells to release detectable levels of NO without causing significant cytotoxicity [24]. When cells grown in cell culture dishes and on stainless steel samples were stimulated with LPS+IFN-γ, they produced NO in measurable quantities. The number and viability of the cells on the stainless steel samples also appeared greater than when stimulated only with LPS. The production of NO by the cells on the stainless steel though, resulted in statistically lower corrosion as compared to the non-stimulated cells and media only conditions. It is not clear as to the mechanism or how the corrosion would be reduced. It may be that NO and other reactive oxygen species produced by the cells such as H_2O_2 and O_2^- may have contributed to an enhancement of the alloy's surface oxide, as observed in the XPS analyses. This effect may be responsible for the in vivo observations that corrosion and metal ion release rates of alloys are high upon initial implantation, but then quickly subside soon after resolution of the initial inflammatory/wound healing process [32]. The reactive oxygen species released by macrophage cells close to the implant surface may facilitate the development of the implant's surface oxide and lower corrosion. The magnitude of this effect may depend in part on the type of the tissues and time in which the device is implanted. Sundgren et al. [22] noted differences in the thickness of the surface oxide of 316L stainless steel after short implantation periods in bone, bone marrow and soft tissues. For implants in bone marrow and soft tissues, oxide thickness increased 1.5 to 4 times that of the un-implanted controls and those in bone. They attributed the increase in surface oxide in the marrow and soft tissues to increased metabolic activity and inflammatory processes. These results support their hypothesis.

While this study supports the hypothesis that macrophage cells play a role in alloy corrosion, it was limited due to the short three-day test time frame. This time frame was initially chosen based on the ability to grow and maintain the cells in a monolayer under standard culture conditions. It is possible, and experiments are being planned, to increase from three days to several weeks the time frame the cells remain in culture on the test alloy samples through adjustment of culture conditions. Thus, additional data on the role of cells on the corrosion behavior of the alloy may be gained and used to further assess the long term cell-implant alloy interaction. Furthermore, it may be possible to include other factors such as mechanical loading, different surface treatments and roughness with and in addition to other cell/tissue types to more closely simulate the clinical condition. This may provide additional insights into alloy biocorrosion processes in vivo.

Conclusion

The results of this study indicated that the corrosion of 316L remained low in the presence of macrophage cells and was further reduced when cells were stimulated to release NO. NO and other reactive oxygen species can oxidize the implant and may have contributed to an enhancement of its surface oxide. These data suggest that the macrophage cells may change alloy surface oxides and affect alloy corrosion behavior. Given the trend for increased corrosion in the presence of the cells, and the potential for clinically relevant levels of metal ion corrosion products to accumulate, the investigation of hypotheses regarding the role of cells on corrosion of 316L stainless steel should continue.

Acknowledgments

Synthes (USA), Paoli, PA, for providing 316L samples. This work was supported by a grant from The Whitaker Foundation.

References

[1]   Walczak, J., Shahgaldi, F., and Heatley, F., "In Vivo Corrosion of 316L Stainless-Steel Hip Implants: Morphology and Elemental Compositions of Corrosion Products," *Biomaterials,* Vol. 19, 1998, pp. 229-237.

[2]   Vieweg, U., van Roost, D., Wolf, H.K., Schyma, C.A., and Schramm J., "Corrosion on Internal Spinal Fixator System," *Spine,* Vol. 24, 1999, pp. 946-951.

[3]   Mofid, M.M., Thompson, R.C., Pardo, C.A., Manson, P.N., and Wander-Kolk, C.A., "Biocompatibility of Fixation Materials in the Brain," *Plastic Reconstructive Surgery*, Vol. 100, 1997, pp. 14-21.

[4]   Savarino, L., Stea, S., Granchi, D., Visentin, M., Ciapetti, G., Donati, M.E., Rollo, G., Zinghi, G., Pissoferrato, A., Montanaro, L., and Toni, A., "Sister Chromatid Exchanges and Ion Release in Patients Wearing Fracture Fixation Devices," *Journal of Biomedical Materials Research*, Vol. 50, 2000, pp. 21-26.

[5]   Christiansen, K., Holmes, K., and Zilko, P.J., "Metal Sensitivity Causing Loosened Joint Prostheses," *Annals of Rheumatic Diseases*, Vol. 38, 1979, pp. 476-480.

[6]   Kerosuo, H., Kullaa, A., Kerosuo, E., Kanerva, L., and Hensten-Pettersen, A., "Nickel Allergy in Adolescents in Relation to Orthodontic Treatment and Piercing of Ears," *American Journal of Orthodontic Dentofacial Orthopaedics*, Vol. 109, 1996, pp. 148-154.

[7]   Wang, J.Y., Wicklund, B.H., Gustilo, R.B., and Tsukayama, D.T., "Titanium, Chromium and Cobalt Ions Modulate the Release of Bone-associated Cytokines by Human Monocytes/Macrophages In Vitro," *Biomaterials,* Vol. 17, 1996, pp. 2233-2240.

[8]   Haynes, D.R., Boyle, S.J., Rogers, S.D., Howie, D.W., and Vernon-Roberts, B., "Variation in Cytokines Induced by Particles from Different Prosthetic Materials," *Clinical Orthopaedics,* Vol. 352, 1998, pp. 223-230.

[9]   Charissoux, J.L., Najid, A., Moreau, J.C., Setton, D., and Rigaud, M., "Development of In Vitro Biocompatibility Assays for Surgical Materials," *Clinical Orthopaedics,* Vol. 326, 1996, pp. 259-269.

[10]   Bumgardner, J.D., Doeller, J., and Lucas, L.C., "Effects of Nickel-based Dental Casting Alloys on Fibroblast Metabolism and Ultrastructural Organization," *Journal of Biomedical Materials Research,* Vol. 29, 1995, pp. 611-617.

[11]   Schedle, A., Samorapoompichit, P., Fureder, W., Rausch-Fan, X.H., Franz, A., Sperr, W.R., Sperr, W., Slavicek, R., Simak, S., Klepetko, W., Ellinger, A., Ghannadan, M., Baghestanian, M., and Valent, P., "Metal Ion-induced Toxic Histamine Release from Human Basophils and Mast Cells," *Journal of Biomedical Materials Research*, Vol. 39, 1998, pp. 560-567.

[12]   Brown, S.A., and Simpson, J.P., "Crevice and Fretting Corrosion of Stainless Steel Plates and Screws," *Journal of Biomedical Materials Research,* Vol. 15, 1981, pp. 867-878.

[13]   Bundy, K.J., Marek, M., and Hochman, R.F., "In Vivo and In Vitro Studies of the Stress-corrosion Cracking Behavior of Surgical Implant Alloys," *Journal of Biomedical Materials Research,* Vol. 17, 1983, pp. 467-487.

[14]   Shih, C-.C., Lin, S-.J., Chung, K-.H., Chen, Y-.L., and Su, Y-.Y., "Increased Corrosion Resistance of Stent Materials by Converting Current Surface Film of Polycrystalline Oxide into Amorphous Oxide," *Journal of Biomedical Materials Research,* Vol. 52, 2000, pp. 323-332.

[15]   Milosev, I., and Strehblow, H-.H., "The Behavior of Stainless Steel in Physiological Solution Containing Complexing Agent Studied by X-ray Photoelectron Spectroscopy," *Journal of Biomedical Materials Research*, Vol. 52, 2000, pp. 404-412.

[16]   Omanovic, S., and Roscoe, S.G., "Interfacial Behavior of beta-Lactoglobulin at a Stainless Steel Surface: An Electrochemical Impedance Spectroscopy Study," *Journal of Colloidal Interface Science,* Vol. 227, 2000, pp. 452-460.

[17]   Williams, R.L., Brown, S.A., and Merritt, K., "Electrochemical Studies on the Influence of Proteins on the Corrosion of Implant Alloys," *Biomaterials,* Vol. 9, 1988, pp. 181-186.

[18]   Sheehan, J.P., Morin, C.R., and Packer, K.F., "Study of Stress Corrosion Cracking Susceptibility of Type 316L Stainless Steel In Vitro", *Corrosion and degradation of implant materials STP 859*, A.C. Fraker, and C.D. Griffin, Eds., American Society for Testing and Materials, West Conshohocken, PA, 1985, pp. 57-72.

[19]   Xulin, S., Ito, A., Tateishi, T., and Hoshino, A., "Fretting Corrosion Resistance and Fretting Corrosion Product Cytocompatibility of Ferritic Stainless Steel," *Journal of Biomedical Materials Research,* Vol. 34, 1997, pp. 9-14.

[20]   Powell, J. Effects of Fibrinogen on 316L Corrosion Fatigue, MS Thesis, Ohio State University, 1979.

[21]   Clark, G.C.F., and Williams, D.F., "The Effect of Proteins on Metallic Corrosion," *Journal of Biomedical Materials Research*, Vol. 16., 1982, pp. 125-134.

[22]   Sundgren, J.E., Bodo, P., Lundstrom, I., Berggren, A., and Hellem S., "Auger Electron Spectroscopic Studies of Stainless Steel Implants," *Journal of Biomedical Materials Research,* Vol. 19, 1985, pp. 663-71.

[23]   Shanbhag, A.S., Macaulay, W., Stefanovic-Racic, M., and Rubash, H.E., "Nitric Oxide Release by Macrophages in Response to Particulate Debris," *Journal of Biomedical Materials Research*, Vol. 41, 1998, pp. 497-503.

[24]   Parker, S.H., "Evaluation of the Effects of Murine Macrophage Cells on the Biocorrosion of Two Implant Alloys", MS Thesis, Mississippi State University, 2001.

[25]   Pan, J., Theirry, D., and Leygrak, C., "Electrochemical and XPS Studies of Titanium for Biomaterial Applications with Respect to the Effect of Hydrogen Peroxide," *Journal of Biomedical Materials Research*, Vol. 28, 1994, pp. 113-22.

[26]   Montague, A., Merritt, K., Brown, S., and Payer, J., "Effects of Ca and H_2O_2 Added to RPMI on the Fretting Corrosion of Ti6Al4V," *Journal of Biomedical Materials Research,* Vol. 32, 1996, pp. 519-526.

[27]   Hazan, R., Brener, R., and Oron, U., "Bone Growth to Metal Implants is Regulated by their Surface Chemical Properties," *Biomaterials*, Vol. 14, 1993, pp. 571-74.

[28]   Schmidt, C., Ignatius, A.A., and Claes, L.E., "Proliferation and Differentiation Parameters of Human Osteoblasts on Titanium and Steel Surfaces," *Journal of Biomedical Materials Research,* Vol. 54, 2001, pp. 209-215.

[29]   Tang, L., and Jiang, W-.W., "The Role of Adsorbed Proteins on the Persistence of Implant-associated Bacteria," *Transactions of the Annual Meeting of the Society for Biomaterials,* 2001, p. 1.

[30]   Janeway, C.A., and Travers, P., "Macrophage Activation by Armed CD4 T_H1 Cells," *Immuno-Biology: the immune system in health and disease.* Garland Publishing, New York: Garland, 1997, p. 737.

[31]   Pruett, S.B., Higgenbotham, J.N., and Lin, T.L., "Effect of Macrophage Activation on Killing of *Listeria monocytogenes.* Roles of Reactive Oxygen or Nitrogen Intermediates, Rate of Phagocytosis, and Retention of Bacteria in Endosomes," *Clinical Experimental Immunology,* Vol. 88, 1992, pp. 492-498.

[32]   Black, J., "Host response: Biological Effects of Implants," *Biological Performance of Materials – Fundamentals of Biocompatibility*, 2nd edition, Marcel Dekker, Inc., New York, 1992, pp. 125-147.

Lyle D. Zardiackas[1], Michael Roach[1], Scott Williamson[1], and Jay-Anthony Bogan[1]

Comparison of Notch Sensitivity and Stress Corrosion Cracking of a Low-Nickel Stainless Steel to 316LS and 22Cr-13Ni-5Mn Stainless Steels

---

Reference: Zardiackas, L. D., Roach, M., Williamson, S., and Bogan, J. -A., **"Comparison of Notch Sensitivity and Stress Corrosion Cracking of a Low-Nickel Stainless Steel to 316LS and 22Cr-13Ni-5Mn Stainless Steels,"** *Stainless Steels for Medical and Surgical Applications, ASTM STP 1438*, G. L. Winters and M. J. Nutt, Eds., ASTM International, West Conshohocken, PA, 2003.

Abstract: Recently, low-nickel stainless steels have been developed, in part due to concerns over patient hypersensitivity reactions. These alloys have been investigated and found to provide excellent mechanical and corrosion properties. This study compares the mechanical properties, notch sensitivity, and stress corrosion cracking (SCC) susceptibility of one such alloy, BioDur® 108, to 316LS and 22Cr-13Ni-5Mn stainless steels which have a long successful implant history. BioDur® 108 was found to have a tensile strength, yield strength, and notch tensile strength similar to 22Cr-13Ni-5Mn, and both had higher values of these properties as compared to 316LS. In addition, BioDur® 108 had the largest percentage elongation during tensile testing of the three alloys but lower reduction of area than 316LS. No evidence of SCC mechanisms was revealed in either the test results or fracture analysis on any of the materials tested. With these material properties and its very low nickel content, BioDur® 108 may be a useful alternative for certain medical implant applications.

Keywords: stainless steel, stress corrosion cracking, notch sensitivity

Introduction

High strength and good corrosion resistance have proven austenitic stainless steels to be useful for biomedical implant applications. Significant amounts of nickel are often added to these steels to stabilize the austenitic microstructure. Although less than 5% of the patient population have experienced metal sensitivity reactions due to implants, nickel does account for approximately 90% of the clinically observed sensitivity reactions of metals [1]. In part as a response to concerns over such sensitivity reactions, several low

---

[1]Professor and Coordinator of Biomaterials and Professor of Orthopaedic Surgery, materials engineer, senior materials engineer and senior materials engineer, respectively, University of Mississippi Medical Center, School of Dentistry/Biomaterials, 2500 North State Street, Jackson, MS, 39216-4505.

nickel stainless steels have been developed. One such alloy, BioDur® 108 from Carpenter Specialty Alloys, contains very low nickel (<0.05%) and uses a high nitrogen content (>0.90%) to stabilize its austenitic microstructure. This high nitrogen content has also been shown to strengthen the alloy as well as contribute to its corrosion resistance [2 -4].

Most studies that have documented susceptibility of austenitic stainless steels to stress corrosion cracking (SCC) have been performed in high-chloride content, caustic, or acid environments and/or at elevated temperatures. However, some studies have hypothesized chloride SCC to be at least a partial failure mechanism in stainless steel medical devices in vivo [5-7]. These hypotheses have led to a great deal of controversy among researchers over the potential of SCC to occur at the chloride concentrations, temperatures, and pH of physiological solutions. Several investigators [5,8] have noted that minimum temperatures ranging from 60°C to 80°C are needed in chloride solutions to induce SCC susceptibility of austenitic stainless steels, while others [9] have shown that a critical acidity and chloride ion combination may induce SCC even at ambient temperatures. Bundy et al. [8] also hypothesized that SCC may occur at lower temperatures when 300 series austenitic stainless steels are stressed beyond their yield point, which can happen in certain biomedical applications such as over-torqued bone screws. Sheehan et al. [10] reported no effects on the strength and ductility of smooth tensile samples subjected to slow strain rate SCC and no signs of SCC mechanisms on the fractured surfaces of 316L in Ringer's solution at 37°C in vitro. Bundy and other researchers [8,11] have hypothesized that due to possible bioelectric and biochemical effects, the human body may be more conducive to stress corrosion cracking than a simple chloride environment at 37°C. From their observations, they suggest the possibility for SCC of 316L in physiological solutions under certain extreme conditions. It has been shown by Sedriks [12] that low nickel containing stainless steels may be beneficial in resisting chloride SCC, but he also cautions that SCC susceptibility is dependent on compositional, structural, and environmental factors that should not be overlooked.

The purpose of the current study was to characterize the notch sensitivity and SCC susceptibility of BioDur® 108 (alloy A), as compared to 316LS (alloy B) and 22Cr-13 Ni-5Mn (alloy C), which have a long and successful history as implant materials.

Materials and Methods

Samples of each alloy (A, B, C) were prepared from single lots of centerless ground 8 mm round bar stock supplied by Carpenter Specialty Alloys. Quantitative compositional analyses was performed on a SPECTRO[1] inductively coupled plasma spectrometer (ICP) with LISA spark attachment to confirm that the alloys met ASTM or Carpenter internal melt limits for major elements. Compositional values, as well as, metallurgy and hardness results have been reported elsewhere for these alloys [13,14].

Mechanical testing was performed using an MTS[2] servo hydraulic test system. Five smooth and five notched tensile samples of each alloy were machined by Low Stress

---

[1]SPECTRO Analytical Instruments, Fitchburg, MA, USA
[2]MTS, Eden Prairie, MN, USA

Grind[3] (LSG) to a maximum surface roughness of 16 micro-inches (Ra=16) in the gauge. Smooth samples were prepared with a 36 mm gauge length and a 6 mm gauge diameter as shown in Figure 1a. Testing was performed at a 0.3 mm/min stroke rate to yield, and a 3.0 mm/min stoke rate from yield to failure and strain was measured using an extensometer with a 25 mm gauge length. The ultimate tensile strength (UTS), 0.2% yield strength (YS), elastic modulus (MOD), percentage elongation (%El.) to fracture, and reduction of area (%ROA) were calculated. Notched tensile samples were prepared with a K_t factor of 3.2 and a notch diameter of 6 mm as shown in Figure 1b. For many years, the ratio of the notch tensile strength to the smooth tensile strength was considered the most valid method for evaluating the sensitivity to a notch and the toughness of a material. As specified in the ASTM "Standard Test Method for Sharp-Notch Tension Testing with Cylindrical Specimens" (E602-91 [Reapproved 1997]), it is widely recognized that since the onset of plastic deformation occurs at the yield strength, the ratio of the notch tensile strength to the 0.2% yield strength may be a more useful predictor of toughness. Notch tensile testing was performed according to ASTM E602 such that the load rate did not exceed the limit of 690 MPa/min. The notch tensile strength (NTS), the ratio of NTS to UTS, and the ratio of NTS to 0.2%YS were determined. Scanning electron microscopy (SEM) was used to characterize the fractured surfaces.

There are two generally accepted methodologies that may be employed when evaluating SCC [15, 16]. The first method uses a constant strain rate. In order to perform this test accurately, a strain gauge must be attached to the sample and remain in solution for the duration of the test. This method presents a number of potentially significant problems, including retention of the gauge on the sample, corrosion of the gauge, and galvanic coupling of the gauge and the sample. The second method uses a constant extension rate as described in the ASTM "Standard Practice for Slow Strain Rate Testing to Evaluate the Susceptibility of Metallic Materials to Environmentally Assisted Cracking" (G129-00). In this method, only the sample and fixtures are in the corrosive environment. By making the fixtures out of the same material as the samples, the potential galvanic coupling effect can be eliminated. While the strain rate is not constant with this method, if it is sufficiently slow, the small change in strain rate over the test duration will not adversely affect the results. Due to the potential problems involved with the strain gauge, testing was performed by the slow extension rate method as outlined in ASTM G129. In order to use this method, a sufficiently slow or critical stain rate must be determined. Previous research in our laboratories and several investigations by other researchers as cited in the Metals Handbook [17] have determined that the appropriate strain rate for austenitic stainless steels is in the range of 10^{-5} to 10^{-6} sec^{-1}.

Smooth and notched SCC samples (K_t=3.2, Ra=16 μin) of each alloy were machined by LSG. Smooth SCC samples were machined to a gauge length of 10 mm and a gauge diameter of 4 mm as shown in Figure 2a, and notched samples were machined with a 1 mm notch width and a 4 mm notch diameter as shown in Figure 2b. The mechanical testing setup for SCC testing is shown in Figure 3. Triplicate smooth and notched SCC

---

[3]Low Stress Grind, Cincinnati, OH, USA

were tested in distilled/de-ionized water (DI) and Ringer's solution at 37°C using an MTS servo hydraulic test system. The samples in this study were tested at a constant stroke rate of 10^{-5} mm/sec, to obtain the suggested initial strain rate of samples 10^{-6} mm/mm/sec. In addition, one sample of each alloy in each solution was tested at strain rates of 10^{-5} sec^{-1} and 10^{-7}sec^{-1} to validate the critical strain rate of 10^{-6} mm/mm/sec. Critical dimensions of samples were measured prior to and after testing to an accuracy of 10^{-3} mm to calculate the %El. and %ROA. The percent elongation ratio (PER) and the reduction of area ratio (ROAR) were calculated by dividing the mean values in Ringer's solution by the mean values in distilled water. SEM was used to examine the fractured surfaces.

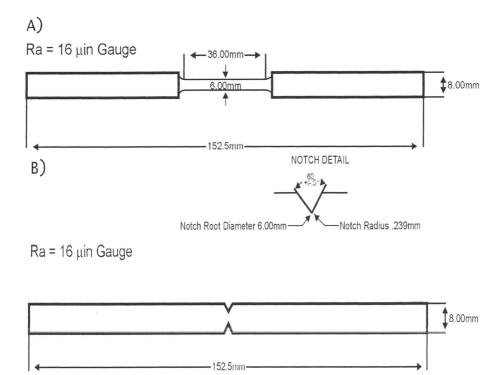

Figure 1 - *A) Sample drawing for smooth tensile samples, B) Sample drawing for notch tensile samples.*

Results

Tensile testing results for smooth and notched samples are summarized in Table 1. Alloys A and C were found to have similar ultimate tensile strengths and yield strengths, which were greater than those for alloy B. Alloy B had the greatest reduction of area, followed by alloy A, and then alloy C. Alloy A was found to have the largest percentage

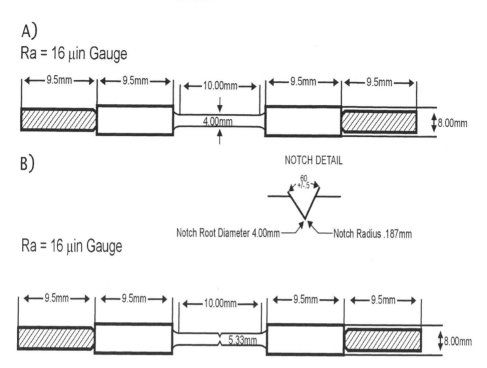

Figure 2 - *A) Sample drawing for smooth SCC samples, B) Sample drawing for notch SCC Samples.*

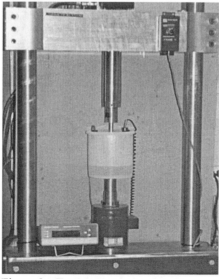

Figure 3 - *Testing apparatus for stress corrosion cracking.*

of elongation, followed by alloy B, and then alloy C. Figure 4 shows areas of the gauge length of representative samples of each alloy after tensile testing. The effect of cold-working on the surface during the tensile test is clearly observable. The smooth tensile samples for all three alloys demonstrated typical ductile cup and cone fractures (Figure 5a). Examination at higher magnifications showed a dimpled morphology normally seen in ductile metals (Figure 5b).

Table 1 - *Smooth and Notch Mechanical Testing Results (n=5)*

Alloy	Alloy A	Alloy B	Alloy C
Elastic Modulus (GPa)	188±3	167±5	186±2
UTS[1] (MPa)	1344±7	1014±0	1351±13
0.2% YS[2](MPa)	1179±21	793±7	1082±13
% ROA[3]	68±0	71±0	60±1
% Elongation	35±1	25±1	19±1
NTS[4] (MPa) (K_t = 3.2)	2255±41	1455±7	2206±41
NTS/ 0.2% YS Ratio	1.91	1.83	2.04
NTS/UTS Ratio	1.68	1.43	1.63

[1]UTS – ultimate tensile strength   [3]ROA – reduction of area
[2]YS = 0.2% yield strength   [4]NTS = notch tensile strength

Testing on notched samples revealed alloys A and C to have similar notch tensile strengths, which were greater than the values for alloy B. Both the NTS/UTS and NTS/YS ratios for all three alloys were significantly greater than 1.00, indicating that none of the materials tested were notch sensitive. SEM fracture analysis of notch tensile samples of alloys B and C showed ductile cup and cone fracture with a dimpled morphology at higher magnification (Figure 6a). The notched tensile fracture surfaces on these two alloys were very similar to that of the smooth tensile fractures. On alloy A, however, the notch tensile fracture revealed a complex morphology with areas of ductile overload dimples due to microvoid coalescence and other areas with faceted appearance of brittle cleavage as shown in Figure 6b (500X). It should be noted, however, that even with what appears to be a partial brittle cleavage fracture mechanism, alloy A had the highest notched tensile strength, percentage elongation, and NTS/UTS ratio.

Materials are considered to be susceptible to SCC if the percentage of elongation and reduction of area in an aggressive corrosion medium are significantly inferior to those properties in a non-aggressive solution. An elongation percentage ratio (PER) or reduction of area ratio (ROAR) below 0.90 is deemed indicative that SCC

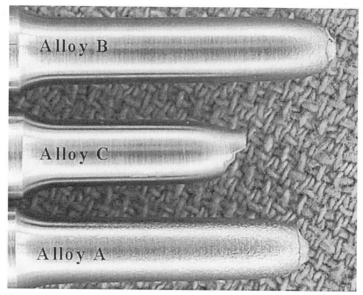

Figure 4 - *Representative samples of each alloy revealing the effect of cold-working on the surface during smooth tensile testing. Note the high level of deformation on the surface of alloy A.*

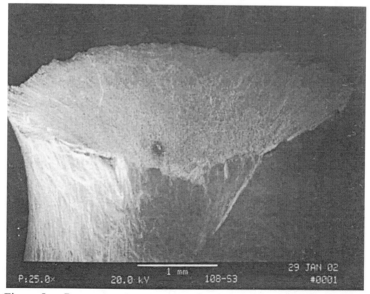

Figure 5a - *Representative scanning electron micrograph showing cup and cone fracture of alloy A.*

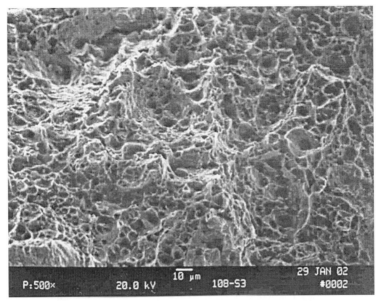

Figure 5b - *Representative scanning electron micrograph showing ductile dimples on the fracture surface of smooth tensile samples of alloy A.*

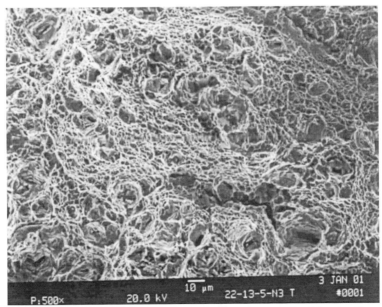

Figure 6a - *Representative scanning electron micrograph of the ductile dimpled fracture mechanism on the notched tensile samples of alloy C.*

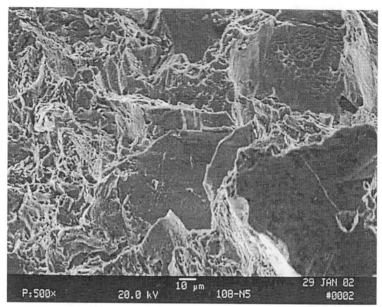

Figure 6b - *Representative scanning electron micrograph showing mixed mode fracture mechanism on the notched tensile samples of alloy A.*

mechanism may be taking place. Smooth and notched SCC results are provided in Tables 2 and 3, respectively. Percentage elongation and reduction of area values on the smooth and notched samples for all of the alloys tested revealed only minor if any differences in these values for each alloy between the aggressive Ringer's solution and non-aggressive distilled/de-ionized (DI) water. The closer the PER and ROAR values are to 1.00, the less susceptible the material is to SCC in the particular corrosive media in which testing has been performed. Because all of the PER and ROAR ratios approach 1.00, SCC of each alloy appears negligible. It is generally considered that values of PER and ROAR above .90 constitute no SCC effects.

SEM analysis on the smooth SCC samples revealed ductile cup and cone fractures with dimples evident at higher magnifications. These fracture surfaces had an essentially identical morphology to that seen on the samples tested at higher strain rates in ambient temperature air (Figures 5a and 5b). In addition, no differences in fracture morphology were seen on the smooth fracture surfaces for SCC samples pulled at the slower and faster strain rates in both solutions.

The appearance of the fracture surfaces on notched SCC samples of alloy B and alloy C were essentially identical to those of the smooth samples indicating no visual signs of SCC (Figure 7a). On notched SCC samples of alloy A, SEM analysis (Figure 7b) revealed a similar morphology to that seen for notched tensile samples tested at a higher strain rate in air (Figure 6b). These results, which once again show no detectible differences in the fracture surface morphology regardless of testing media, indicate that SCC mechanisms are not occurring regardless of the testing solution or strain rate.

Table 2 - *SCC Results of Smooth Samples (n=3)*

Alloy	Solution	% ROA[1]	% Elongation	PER[2]	ROAR[3]
Alloy A	DI[4]	56.8±2.2	26.3±0.4	1.01	1.02
	Ringer's	58.0±1.1	26.5±0.5		
Alloy B	DI[4]	71.5±1.7	18.5±0.6	1.00	1.00
	Ringer's	71.3±1.4	18.5±0.2		
Alloy C	DI[4]	55.8±0.8	14.0±0.2	0.97	1.00
	Ringer's	55.9±1.8	13.6±0.5		

[1]ROA = reduction of area   [3]ROAR = reduction of area ratio
[2]PER = percentage elongation ratio   [4]DI = distilled/de-ionized water

Table 3 - *SCC Results of Notched Samples (n=3)*

Alloy	Solution	% ROA[1]	% Notch Elongation	PER[2]	ROAR[3]
Alloy A	DI[4]	16.2±1.5	43.9±5.5	0.92	0.95
	Ringer's	15.4±1.7	40.3±1.9		
Alloy B	DI[4]	34.6±1.3	68.8±2.1	0.95	1.03
	Ringer's	35.6±0.2	65.7±9.2		
Alloy C	DI[4]	13.1±0.0	26.1±1.8	0.94	0.98
	Ringer's	12.8±0.3	24.5±0.9		

[1]ROA = reduction of area   [3]ROAR = reduction of area ratio
[2]PER = percentage elongation ratio   [4]DI = distilled/de-ionized water

Discussion and Conclusions

Two commonly accepted measures for ductility in a material are elongation and reduction of area. Normally these variables are proportional, and thus a material with more elongation will also have a greater reduction of area. In the present study, mechanical test results to determine notch sensitivity as well as SCC indicated alloy B and alloy C followed these general principles. Alloy A, which is the low Ni stainless steel, was found to have a substantially higher (~30%) percent elongation and yet 3-20% less reduction of area in the smooth tensile and SCC samples than alloy B. This large percent elongation with a somewhat lower reduction of area is believed to be a function

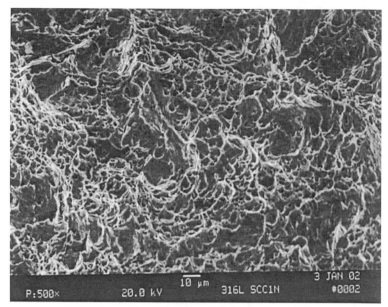

Figure 7a - *Representative scanning electron micrograph showing the ductile fracture mechanism on the notched stress corrosion cracking samples of alloy B.*

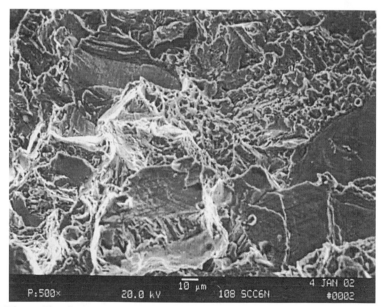

Figure 7b - *Representative scanning electron micrograph revealing mixed mode fracture mechanism on the notched stress corrosion cracking samples of alloy A.*

of the higher degree of work hardening experienced by alloy A as compared to the other two alloys. This observation is evidenced by the appearance of the surfaces of the samples as seen in Figure 4. These observations may have a direct effect on processing parameters during the fabrication of devices.

The SCC results obtained for alloy B agreed with the previous studies of Sheehan et al. [10] and Jones et al. [18], as the material exhibited typical ductile cup and cone fractures by microvoid coalescence with no evidence of stress corrosion cracking mechanisms on samples tested in physiological saline solutions. Alloy C revealed similar fractures to those of alloy B, but this alloy showed significantly higher smooth and notched tensile strengths, while testing resulted in lower percent elongation and reduction of area values. These are the results expected based upon data reported by others [19-21]. It is interesting to note that alloy A had the highest elongation percentages on the smooth tensile samples of the alloys tested, showed no signs of notch sensitivity by the NTS/UTS and NTS/YS ratios, and yet SEM fracture analysis revealed a mixed fracture mode. Areas of smooth terraces indicative of brittle cleavage intermingled with areas of dimpling were noted. This fracture mechanism is similar to some forms of SCC for other types of alloys described by others [12,22].   However, the percentage elongation and reduction of area ratios between the more corrosively aggressive Ringer's solution and distilled/de-ionized water were well above 0.90. In addition, the same complex fracture morphologies, including ductile overload and brittle cleavage, were observed on the notched samples of alloy A regardless of testing environments including air, distilled/de-ionized water, and Ringer's solution. This combined evidence indicates that SCC mechanisms are not taking place in this alloy or alloys B and C.

Results do indicate that the mixed fracture modes experienced by alloy A may be occurring as a function of localized grain orientation, and/or greater work hardening in specifically oriented grains as related to the direction of applied stress. Alloy A has a very high work hardening rate which is reportedly due to its high nitrogen content [2-4]. This mixed mechanism of fracture on the notched samples of alloy A may be a function this high work hardening rate. If localized areas of high tensile residual stress are created at the root of the notch or crack tip during testing, areas that may become highly work hardened can fracture by a brittle cleavage mechanism due to the presence of a tri-axial state of stress. Once this localized brittle fracture has occurred, these internal residual stresses are relieved. The total stress is the sum of the applied stress and these internal residual stresses. Because the residual component of the total stress is now relieved, the areas surrounding these brittle cleavage terraces are subjected to only the applied stress. Ductile fracture may then occur. On the smooth samples, the applied stress is spread over the entire gauge section and thus not concentrated at the notch. With this larger area of stress distribution, these local areas do not become as highly cold worked and thus the entire sample experiences ductile failure.

Overall, the mechanical properties for alloy A were similar to those of alloy C and superior to alloy B. Based upon these results, and with the low-nickel content of alloy A, this alloy appears to be a possible alternative for biomedical implant applications.

Acknowledgment

This research was supported by a grant from Carpenter Technology Corporation.

References

[1]   Hierholzer, S. and Hierholzer, G., *Internal Fixation and Metal Allergie*, Thieme Medical Publishers, 1992.
[2]   Disegi, J. A. and Eschbach, L., "Stainless Steel in Bone Surgery," *Injury*, Vol. 31, Suppl. 4, 2000, pp. D2-D6.
[3]   Gebeau, R C. and Brown, R.S., "Tech Spotlight - Biomedical Implant Alloy," *Advanced Materials and Processes*, Vol. 159, No. 9, 2001, pp. 46-48.
[4]   Carpenter Technology Corporation Alloy Data, BioDur® 108 Alloy, Carpenter Technology Corp., Reading, PA, 2000.
[5]   Bombara, G. and Cavallini, M., "Stress Corrosion Cracking of Bone Implants," *Corrosion Science*, Vol. 17, 1977, pp. 77-85.
[6]   White, W.E. Postlethwaite, J., May, I.L., "On the fracture of Orthopaedic Implants," *Microstructural Science*, Vol. 4, 1976, pp. 145-158.
[7]   Gray, R.J., "Metallographic Examinations of Retrieved Intramedullary Bone Pins and Bone Screws from the Human Body," *Journal of Biomedical Materials Research Symposium*, No. 5, 1974, pp. 27-38.
[8]   Bundy, K.J., Marek M., and Hochman R.F., "In vivo and in vitro studies of the stress-corrosion cracking behavior of surgical implant alloys," *Journal of Biomedical Materials Research*, Vol. 17, 1983, pp. 467-487.
[9]   Harston, J. D. and Scully, J. C., "Stress Corrosion of Type 304 Steel in H_2SO_4/NaCl Environments at Room Temperature," *Corrosion*, Vol. 25, No. 12, 1969, pp. 496-501.
[10] Sheenan, J.P., Morin C.R., and Packer K.F., "Study of Stress Corrosion Cracking Susceptibility of Type 316L Stainless Steel in Vitro," *Corrosion and Degradation of Implant Materials, ASTM STP 859*, 1985, pp 57-72.
[11] Bundy, K. J. and Desai, V.H. , "Studies of Stress-Corrosion Cracking Behaviour of Surgical Implant Materials Using a Fracture Mechanics Approach," *Corrosion and Degradation of Implant Materials, ASTM STP 859*, 1985, pp 73-90.
[12] Sedriks, J. A., "Stress Corrosion Cracking," *Corrosion of Stainless Steels*, John Wiley and Sons, 1992, pp. 267-325.
[13] Roach, M.D. et al., "Physical, Metallurgical, and Mechanical Comparison of a Low-Nickel Stainless Steel," *Proceedings of the 27th Annual Meeting of the Society of Biomaterials*, 2001 p. 343.
[14] Zardiackas, L.D. et al., "Comparison of Anodic Polarization, Galvanic Corrosion, and Fretting Corrosion of a Low-Nickel Stainless Steel to 316L and 22Cr-13Ni-5Mn," *ASTM F4 Symposium on Stainless Steels for Medical and Surgical Applications*, In Review 2002.
[15] Parkins, R.N., "Stress Corrosion Cracking - The Slow Strain Rate Technique," *ASTM STP 665*, 1979, pp. 5- .
[16] Lisagor, W.B., "Environmental Cracking - Stress Corrosion," *Corrosion Tests and Standards*, 1995, pp. 240-252.
[17] Sprowls, D.O., "Evaluation of Stress-Corrosion Cracking," *Metals Handbook*, Ninth Edition, 1987, Vol. 13, pp. 245-282.
[18] Jones R.L., Wing, S.S., and Syrett, B.C., "Stress Corrosion Cracking and Corrosion Fatigue of some Surgical Implant Materials in a Physiological Saline Environment," *Corrosion*, Vol. 34, No. 7, 1978, pp. 226-236.

[19] Black, J. *, Biological Performance of Materials: Fundamentals of Biocompatibility,* Marcel Dekker, Inc., 1992.

[20] Carpenter Technology Corporation Alloy Data, Carpenter 22Cr-13Ni-5Mn, Carpenter Technology Corp., Reading, PA, 1987.

[21] Carpenter Technology Corporation Alloy Data, Carpenter Stainless Type 316L, Carpenter Technology Corp., Reading, PA, 1986.

[22] Kerlins, V. and Phillips, A, "Fractography: Modes of Fracture" *ASM Handbook*, Vol. 12, 1999, pp.12-71.

Ruth F. V. Villamil,[1] Arnaldo H. P. de Andrade,[2] Celso A. Barbosa,[3] Alexandre Sokolowski,[3] and Silvia M L. Agostinho[4]

Comparative Electrochemical Studies of F 1586-95 and F 138-92 Stainless Steels in Sodium Chloride, pH = 4.0 Medium

Reference: Villamil, R. F. V., de Andrade, A. H. P., Barbosa, C. A., Sokolowski, A., and Agostinho, S. M. L., "**Comparative Electrochemical Studies of F 1586-95 and F 138-92 Stainless Steels in Sodium Chloride, pH = 4.0 Medium**," *Stainless Steels for Medical and Surgical Applications, ASTM STP 1438*, G. L. Winters and M. J. Nutt, Eds., ASTM International, West Conshohocken, PA, 2003.

Abstract: In this work, ASTM F 1586-95 stainless steel used for surgical implants is studied in 0.9 % NaCl aqueous solution, pH = 4.0 at 40 °C, using potentiodynamic polarization curves and optical surface analysis techniques and its performance is compared to F 138 stainless steel. F 1586-95 remains passivated until transpassivation potential above, which shows only generalized corrosion. F 138-92 presents breakdown potentials of 370 mV / SCE, with the presence of pitting corrosion. The presence of 0.40 % Nb in F 1586-95 promotes passivation currents one order of magnitude higher than that observed for F 1586-95 containing 0.28 % Nb.

Keywords: breakdown potentials, austenitic stainless steel, ASTM F 1586-95, ASTM F 138-92, orthopedic implants.

Stainless steels are extensively used in orthopedic implants [1-10]. These alloys are less expensive than cobalt and titanium alloys [1-6]. Pitting corrosion of these ferrous materials in chloride media has been one of the main reasons for the development of new stainless steel compositions for implant applications [11-23]. The nucleation and growth of pitting corrosion are related to the characteristics of oxide film formed on the metallic surface [2-5]. Two types of stainless steels have been used in surgical implants in Brazil: ASTM F 138 since 1982 and ASTM F 1586-95, more recently.

---

[1] Postdoctoral Student, Instituto de Química, Universidade de São Paulo, Av. Prof. Lineu Prestes 748. 05508-900, São Paulo, SP, Brazil.

[2] Research Scientist, Instituto de Pesquisas Energéticas e Nucleares (IPEN) Trav. R 400 - Cidade Universitária, S.P - Brazil.

[3] Manager and Research Engineer, respectively, Villares Metals S. A., Av. Alfredo Dumont Villares, 155. 13177-900, Sumaré, SP, Brazil.

[4] Professor, Instituto de Química, Universidade de São Paulo, Av. Prof. Lineu Prestes, 748. 05508-900, São Paulo, SP, Brazil.

This last stainless steel presents about 0.5 weight percent of niobium in order to reduce the chromium precipitation as chromium carbide, and also higher chromium, molybdenum and nitrogen contents to promote a higher PRE number (Pitting Resistance Equivalent). This composition also improves the mechanical properties in such material.

The purpose of the present paper is to characterize the pitting corrosion resistance of ASTM F 1586-95 samples in dearated 0.9 % NaCl aqueous solution, pH = 4.0 at 40 °C, with two different niobium contents: 0.28 % (ISO A) and 0.40 % (ISO B). The results are compared to those observed in the steel ASTM F 138-92 (F 138).

A pH = 4.0 of this solution was chosen for two reasons: its more aggressive character and establish a better comparison than the normal pH = 7.0, which is observed in human body fluids. This pH value can be attained when an inflammation process is observed [8, 22].

Experimental Procedure

The chemical compositions of the stainless steel samples studied as well as the PRE number of each alloy (Pitting Resistance Equivalent) are presented in (Table 1). One can note the higher PRE number of the steel ASTM F 1586-95. The F 1586-95 was produced with the niobium content in the lower range of the ASTM specification in order to have the minimum amount of niobium carbonitrides particles. The F 138-92 was produced using an industrial 3.5 t vacuum induction furnace plus ESR refining. The F 1586-95 material was produced starting from a 50 kg ingot in a vacuum induction furnace of the Villares R&D Center. All the ingots were homogenized at high temperatures and rolled to 30 mm diameter bars. The bars were solution annealed at 1050 °C for one hour followed by water cooling.

The stainless steel disk working electrodes were taken out from the core regions of the bars and had an area of 0.363 cm^2. A cylindrical polytetrafluoroethylene (PTFE) sleeve was fitted on the steel disk. A concentric brass rod was coupled to the steel + PTFE. The disks surfaces were grounded and polished through no 320, 400 and 600 mesh wet silicon carbide sandpaper, rinsed with distilled water and ethanol and air dried. The metallographic samples were polished through 1 μm diamond paste, rinsed with water and ethanol and air dried. A platinum foil with a large area was used as counter electrode and the saturated calomel electrode was the reference electrode.

The electrolytic cell was a boronsilicate glass with 150 mL capacity. The cell top had three entries to pass the three electrodes. The experiments were conducted at 40 °C.

Analytical grade sodium chloride and twice-distilled water were used to prepare the solutions. The electrolyte was a 0.9 % NaCl aqueous solution, pH = 4.0 adding HCl.

The solutions were dearated with previously purified N$_2$ for 1 hour. The electrodes were immersed in the solution and after 45 minutes at open circuit potential an anodic galvanostatic polarization was applied for 3 minutes at 100 mA cm^{-2} before the electrochemical measurements. Anodic polarization curves were obtained using 0.17 mVs^{-1} scan rate. A computer controlled EG&G PAR 273A potentiostat/galvanostat was used in the electrochemical measurements. This procedure is according to ASTM G5 standard.

Optical microscopy of the surfaces were conduced for the materials after polishment and anodic polarization curves. The anodic potentiodynamic polarization was followed by 15 min etching at a value 50 mV higher than the potential

Table 1. Chemical Composition of the Studied Materials and the Composition Specification According ASTM Standards, (wt %).

Sample	ASTM (UNS Designation)	ISO Designation	C	Mn	P	S	Si	Cr	Ni	Mo	N	Nb	PRE
F 138-92	F 138 - 92 Grade 2 (S 31673)	5832 - 1[A]	0.012	1.94	0.023	0.002	0.26	17.60	14.20	2.08	0.021	---	24.5[B]
Steel A	F 1586 - 95 (S 31675)	5832 - 9	0.015	4.09	0.014	0.005	0.33	20.70	9.94	2.50	0.320	0.28	29.0[C]
Steel B	F 1586 - 95 (S 31675)	5832 - 9	0.013	3.77	0.015	0.005	0.32	20.30	9.91	2.49	0.320	0.40	29.0[D]
---	F 138 - 92[E] Grade 2 (S 31673)	5832 - 1[A]	0.030 max.	2.00 max.	0.025 max.	0.010 max.	0.75 max.	17.00 19.00	13.00 15.50	2.00 3.00	0.10 max.	---	---
---	F 1586 - 95[F] (S 31675)	5832 - 9	0.08 max.	2.00 4.25	0.025 max.	0.010 max.	0.75 max.	19.50 22.00	9.00 11.00	2.00 3.00	0.25 0.50	0.25 0.80	---

[A] In ISO 5832 - 1 (1987) standard, molybdenum content is 2.25 to 3.50 %.
[B] PRE = % Cr + 3.3 % Mo.
[C,D] PRE = % Cr + 3.3 % Mo + 16 % N.
[E] Maximum, unless range or minimum is indicated. Copper content is 0.50 % max.
[F] Maximum, unless range or minimum is indicated. Copper content is 0.25 % max.

corresponding to breakdown potential (E_b), for F138-92 and to transpassivation potential (1100 mV) for ASTM F 1586-95.

The scanning electron microscopy (SEM) of the samples performed after 15 minutes attack at 50 mV above the potential corresponding to the current increase and in different surface regions were analyzed using energy dispersive spectroscopy (EDS)

Results and Discussion

The anodic polarization curves are shown in (Figure 1). All the materials are naturally passivated in the aqueous solution studied but there is a significant difference in the potential values corresponding to the current increase. F 138-92 presents breakdown potential (E_b) meanwhile for Steel A and Steel B the current increases only at the transpassivation potential values. The potential value (E_i) of current increase (breakdown potential (E_b) for F 138-92) and passivation current density values are presented in (Table 2).

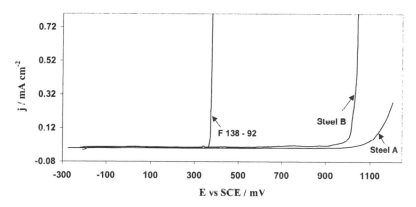

Figure 1. *Potentiodynamic polarization curves of stainless steels studied in 0.9 % NaCl, pH = 4.0 medium at 40 °C, using 0.17 mV s^{-1} scan rate.*

The Steel A shows lower passivation current values than F 138-92 and steel B. The results reveal that Steel A (with 0.28 % niobium) is the best alloy. It can be seen that Steel A and Steel B present a 600 mV potential range above F138-92 E_b, where they are passivated.

Table 2. *Potential values of current increase (E_i) and passivation current densities (j_{pass}) values for the three steels studied in 0.9 % NaCl aqueous solution, pH = 4.0 at 40 ° C.*

Stainless steel Samples	E_i vs. ECS / mV	J_{pass} / μA cm^{-2} (100mV)
F 138-92	370 ± 4 (6)	8.26 ± 4 (9)
Steel A	1150 ± 12 (7)	0.82 ± 1.3 (7)
Steel B	1050 ± 32 (7)	6.61 ± 1.8 (5)

The numbers in brackets denote the number of samples tested.

Optical microscopy of the samples polished through 1 μm diamond showed the presence of globular oxide inclusions for all materials studied, according to (Figure 2). The oxide inclusion rating was at the upper acceptable limit according ASTM F 138-92 and F 1586-92

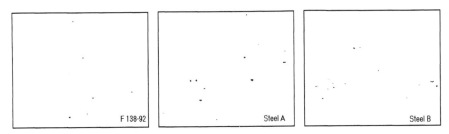

Figure 2 (a) to (c). *Optical microscopy of stainless steels samples polished through 1 μm diamond paste. Inclusion rating according to ASTM E45, method A, plate I-r. Magnification: 100 X.*

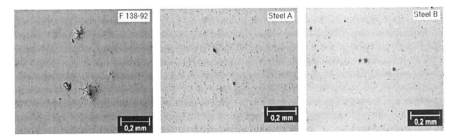

Figure 3 (a) to (c). *Optical microscopy of stainless steels samples after 15 min etching at 50 mV higher than the potential corresponding to the current increase (Eᵢ).*

The optical microscopy of the surfaces of the three steel after etching at 50 mV higher than the potential corresponding to the current increase (E_i) are shown in (Figure 3). F 138-92 presents a significative localized corrosion while Steel A and Steel B show surfaces similar to those observed when they are only polished, showing only the non metallic inclusions. In order to show the absence of localized corrosion in steel A and steel B different surface regions were analyzed using energy dispersive spectroscopy (EDS).

The scanning electron microscopy (SEM) of the samples performed after 15 minutes attack at 50 mV above the potential corresponding to the current increase are presented in (Figure 4). The delimited areas for EDS analysis and the results are shown in (Table 3). The presence of localized corrosion for F138-92 SS is confirmed from (Figure 4). The presence of more silicium in region II can be attributed to silicate microinclusions show in (Table 3). These results suggest that the pitting corrosion can begin around these inclusions, while the region I presents a composition similar to the bulk.

It can be seen for steel A and steel B that regions I and II present nearly the same chemical composition when compared to the alloy chemical composition, except in region II in relation to niobium content. These results suggest that the attach at potentials higher than the transpassivation potential is generalized. The higher niobium content can be attributed to niobium carbonitride particles present in region II.

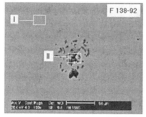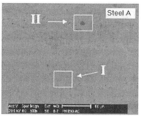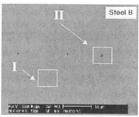

Figure 4. *Scanning electron microscopy-SEM of stainless steel samples performed after attack 15 minutes at 50 mV above the potential corresponding to the current increase.*

Table 3. *Different surface regions analyzed using energy dispersive spectroscopy (EDS).*

ASTM F 138-92	Mn	Cr	Ni	Mo	Si
F 138-92 (bulk)	1,94	16.60	14,20	2,08	0.26
Region I	1.7	17,3	10.64	2,55	0.65
Region II	2.05	16.29	12.09	2,02	10.72

ASTM F 1586-95	Mn	Cr	Ni	Mo	Nb
Steel A (bulk)	4.09	20.70	9.94	2.50	0.28
Region I	4.14	20.22	9.24	2.31	0.45
Region II	3.95	20.14	9.14	2.31	3.4

ASTM F 1586-95	Mn	Cr	Ni	Mo	Nb
Steel B (bulk)	3.77	20.30	9.91	2.49	0.40
Region I	4.39	20.7	10.04	2.56	0.42
Region II	4.75	20.35	10.1	2.59	0.7

Conclusions

Based on the tests conducted on the three Steels, the following conclusions are pertinent:

- ASTM F 138-92 and F 1586-95 stainless steel show different electrochemical behavior in 0.9% NaCl aqueous solution, pH = 4.0 at 40°C. F 138-92 presents breakdown potential at 370 mV/SCE and pitting corrosion while F 1586-95 is passivated until the transpassivation potential.

- F 1586-95 shows only generalized corrosion at 50 mV above the transpassivation potential.
- The Steel A sample, with lower niobium content (0.28 %) presents a better performance in this solution when compared to Steel B sample, containing 0.40 % niobium.

Acknowledgments

The authors acknowledge support from the Fundação de Amparo à Pesquisa do Estado de São Paulo (FAPESP) for supporting part of this work. R.F.V. Villamil also thanks FAPESP for the grant of a postdoctoral fellowship.

References

[1] Fonseca, C. Barbosa, M.A., "Corrosion behaviour of titanium in biofluids containin H_2O_2 studied by electrochemical impedance spectroscopy", *Corrosion Science*, Vol. 43, 2001, p. 547.

[2] Gonzáles, J. E. G., Mirza-Rosca, J. C., "Study of The Corrosion Behavior of Titanium and some of its Alloys for Biomedical and Dental Implant Applications", *Journal Electroanalytical Chemestry*, Vol. 471, 1999, pp.109-115.

[3] Yu, S. Y., Scully, J. R., "Corrosion and Passivity of Ti-13% Nb-13% Zr in Comparison to Other Biomedical Implant Alloys", *Corrosion*, Vol. 53, No. 12, 1997, pp. 965-976.

[4] Lausmaa J., "Surface spectroscopic characterization of titanium implant materials. *Journal of electron spectroscopy and related phenomena*", Vol. 81, 1996, p. 343.

[5] Pankuch, M., Bell, R., Melendrest, C. A., "Composition and structure of the anodic films on titanium in aqueous solutions", *Electrochemical Acta*, Vol. 38, No.18, 1993, pp. 2777-2779.

[6] Tomashov, N.D., Chernova, G. P., Ruscol, Yu.S., Ayuyan, "The passivation of alloys on titanium bases", Electrochimica Acta, Vol. 19, 1974, pp. 159-172.

[7] Lei M.K., Zhu X.M., "In vitro corrosion resistance of plasma source ion nitrided austenitic stainless steels", *Biomaterials*, Vol. 22, 2001, p. 641.

[8] Mears, D.C., "Metals in medicine and surgery", *Review 218, International Metals Reviews*, 1977, pp. 119-155.

[9] Fraker, A.C., Ruff, A.W., "Metallic surgical implants: state of art", *Journal of Metals*, 1977, pp. 22-28.

[10] Gotman I., "Characteristics of Metals Used in Implants", *Journal of Endourology*, Vol. 11, No. 6, 1997, Pp. 383-389.

[11] Walczak J. Shahgaldi F. Heatley F., "In vivo corrosion of 316 L stainless-steel hip implants: morphology and elemental compositions of corrosion products", *Biomaterials*, Vol.19, No. 1-3, 1998, pp. 229-237.

[12] Taira M, Lautenschlager EP, "In vitro Corrosion Fatigue of 316 L Cold-Worked Stainless-Steel", *Journal of Biomedical Materials Research*, Vol. 26, No. 9, 1992, pp. 1131-1139.

[13] Sobral A.V.C., Ristow Jr. W., Azambuja D.S., Costa I., Franco C.V., "Potentiodynamic test and electrochemical impedance spectroscopy of injection model 316 L steel in NaCl solution", *Corrosion Science*, Vol. 43, 2001, p. 1019.

[14] Cakir A., Tuncell S., Aydin A., "AE response of 316 L SS during SSR test under potentiostatic control", *Corrosion Science*, Vol. 41, 1999, p. 1175.

[15] Guemmaz M., Mosser A., Grob J-J, Stuck R., "Sub-surface modifications induced by nitrogen ion implantation in stainless steel (SS 316 L). Correlation between microstructure and nanoindentation results", *Surface and Coating Technology*, Vol. 100, 1998, p. 353.

[16] Rogero S.O., Higa O.Z., Saiki M., Correa O.V. and Costa I., "Cytotoxicity due to corrosion of ear piercing studs", *Toxicology in vitro*, Vol. 14, 2000, p. 497.

[17] Reclaru L., Lerrf R., Eschler P.-Y., Meyer J.-M., "Corrosion behavior of a welded stainless-steel orthopedic implant", *Biomaterials*, Vol. 22, 2001, pp. 269.

[18] Basridas J. M., Polo J. L., Torres C. L., Cano E., "A study on the stability of AISI   316 L stainless steel pitting corrosion through its transfer function", *Corrosion   Science*, Vol. 43, 2001, p. 269.

[19] Laycock N.J., Newman R.C., "Temperature dependence of pitting potentials for austenitic stainless steels above their critical pitting temperature", *Corrosion Science*, Vol. 40, No. 6, 1998, p. 887.

[20] Carranza R.M., Alvarez M.G., "The effect of temperature on the passive film properties and pitting behaviour of a Fe Cr Ni alloy", *Corrosion Science*, Vol. 38, No. 6, 1996, p. 909.

[21] Disegi J.A., Eschbach L., "Stainless steel in bone surgery", *International Journal of the Care of the Injured*, Vol. 31, 2000, S-D2-6.

[22] Raimondi M.T., Pietrabissa R., "Modelling evaluation of the testing condition influence on the maximum stress induced in a hip prosthesis during ISO 7006 fatigue testing", *Medical Engineering & Physics*, Vol. 21, 1999, p.353.

[23] Paszenda Z., Marciniak J., "The influence of base structure and carbon coating on the corrosion resistance of Co-Cr-Mo alloy", *Journal of Materials Processing Technology*, Vol. 78, 1998, p. 143.

Bernard S. Covino, Jr,[1] Charles H. Craig,[2] Stephen D. Cramer,[3] Sophie J. Bullard,[1] Margaret Ziomek-Moroz,[1] Paul D. Jablonski,[4] Paul C. Turner,[4] Herbert R. Radisch, Jr.,[2] Nev A. Gokcen,[5] Clifford M. Friend,[6] and Michael R. Edwards[6]

Corrosion Behavior of Platinum-Enhanced Radiopaque Stainless Steel (PERSS®) for Dilation-Balloon Expandable Coronary Stents

Reference: Covino, B. S., Jr., Craig, C. H., Cramer, S. D., Bullard, S. J., Ziomek-Moroz, M., Jablonski, P. D., Turner, P. C., Radisch, H. R., Jr., Gokcen, N. A., Friend, C. M., and Edwards, M. R., "**Corrosion Behavior of Platinum-Enhanced Radiopaque Stainless Steel (PERSS®) for Dilation-Balloon Expandable Coronary Stents,**" *Stainless Steels for Medical and Surgical Applications, ASTM STP 1438*, G. L. Winters and M. J. Nutt, Eds., ASTM International, West Conshohocken, PA, 2003

Abstract

Dilation-balloon expandable coronary stents are made of implant grade stainless steels, UNS S31673, e.g., BioDur® 316LS. Boston Scientific / Interventional Technologies (BS/IVT) determined that addition of platinum to UNS S31673 could produce a stainless steel with enhanced radiopacity, which made such stents more visible radiographically. A goal of the program was to ensure the platinum additions would not adversely affect the corrosion resistance of the resulting 5-6 wt % PERSS® alloys. Corrosion resistance of PERSS and BioDur 316LS was determined using electrochemical tests for general, pitting, crevice and intergranular corrosion. Experimental methods included A262E, F746, F2129, and potentiodynamic polarization. The ~ 6 wt % PERSS alloy (IVT 78) had a resistance to pitting, crevice and intergranular corrosion similar to base materials. IVT 78 was a single-phase austenitic PERSS alloy with no evidence of inclusions or precipitates; it was more resistant to pitting corrosion than the ~ 5 wt % PERSS alloys. PERSS performance was not a function of oxygen content in the range 0.01 to 0.03 wt %.

[1] Research Chemist, Materials Conservation Division, Albany Research Center, U.S. Department of Energy, 1450 Queen Ave., SW, Albany, OR 97321.

[2] Principal Engineer and Vice President for Research & Development, respectively, Boston Scientific Corporation/Interventional Technologies, 3574 Ruffin Rd, San Diego, CA 92123.

[3] Chemical Engineer, Materials Conservation Division, Albany Research Center, U.S. Department of Energy, 1450 Queen Avenue, SW, Albany, OR 97321.

[4] Metallurgist and Division Chief, respectively, Thermal Treatment Technology Division, Albany Research Center, U.S. Department of Energy, 1450 Queen Avenue, SW, Albany, OR 97321.

[5] Consultant, Thermodynamics and Inorganic Materials, Palos Verdes Estates, CA 90274.

[6] Professor and Head, and Senior Lecturer, respectively, Department of Materials and Medical Sciences, Cranfield Postgraduate Medical School, Shrivenham, Swindon SN6 8LA, UK.

Ke   ary stents, corrosion, stainless steel, platinum, alloy, Ringers solution,
p·   breakdown potential, radiopacity, x-rays

Introduc.

Stainless steels have long been used to fabricate medical devices for the human body. These devices include artificial joints and, especially during the past decade, vascular stents. It is estimated that nearly a million patients worldwide undergo interventional procedures each year with 50 % of these patients receiving coronary vascular stents [1]. The commercial, implant grade alloy BioDur® 316LS[1] (UNS S31673) has been used to fabricate such stents. The stents are inserted into diseased arteries and are designed to have adequate mechanical and corrosion properties in blood plasma environments.

Stainless steel stents as used today can often be almost radiolucent to x-rays [2] when placed in the human body. This in turn makes it difficult to locate their position with the required precision. Gold, platinum, or tantalum marker bands are sometimes affixed to catheters or coatings applied to stents to increase radiopacity for precise location of stents [2]. A new method is described in this volume for increasing stent radiopacity by modifying the composition of the stainless steel alloy used in fabricating coronary stents. This method consists of alloying precious metals, such as platinum, with a stainless steel. Such platinum additions enhance the radiopacity of stainless steel, leading to a new class of radiopaque stainless steels, PERSS®[2], for applications within the human body [3-4]. However, it must be shown that such alloying can be accomplished without significant reduction in the mechanical properties or corrosion resistance of the deployed stent.

Several studies have been conducted on the effect of precious metal additions on the corrosion performance of stainless steels. A summary of the research conducted between 1949 and 1980 is found in the reviews of McGill [5-6]. These papers report on the effects of palladium, ruthenium, iridium, osmium, and platinum additions on the corrosion resistance of stainless steels. Test environments ranged from oxidizing to reducing solutions and included solutions that cause either pitting or stress corrosion cracking. A summary of the reviews suggests: (1) a critical noble metal concentration must be reached for passivity of the steel; (2) noble metal modified steels corrode rapidly before becoming passive; and (3) the improvement in corrosion resistance with noble metal additions is less for the higher alloyed steels that contain, for example, molybdenum. There is also some evidence that noble metal modified steels are more susceptible to stress corrosion cracking. Unfortunately the results presented by McGill [5-6] are for solutions more typical of the chemical process industry than of the human body. To assess the corrosion resistance of alloys considered as biomaterials, it is necessary to work in an environment comparable to that encountered in the body. *In vitro* corrosion experiments do not normally use whole blood or blood plasma, but rather a synthetic environment that simulates the properties of blood. Corrosion studies have been conducted in a variety of simulated blood environments. Synthetic body fluid

---

[1] Registered trademark, Carpenter Technology Corporation, P.O. Box 14662, Reading PA 19612-4662.
[2] Registered trademark, Boston Scientific Corporation/Scimed Life Systems, Maple Grove, MN 55311.

(SBF) is one such solution [7]. It is compared to the composition of a synthetic blood plasma [8] in Table 1.

Table 1 – *Comparison of synthetic body fluid and blood plasma solutions*

Solution ions	Composition, mM	
	SBF [7]	Plasma [8]
Na^+	142	142
Cl^-	194	148
K^+	5.0	5.0
Mg^{2+}	1.5	1.5
Ca^{2+}	2.5	2.5
HCO_3^-	4.2	4.2
HPO_4^{2-}	1.0	1.0
SO_4^{2-}	NA	0.5

NA = Not applicable

Another environment is a synthetic blood plasma that is in conformity with the recommendations of Association Française de Normalisation (AFNOR)[9], but no details are given. ASTM Test Method for Conducting Cyclic Potentiodynamic Polarization Measurements to Determine the Corrosion Susceptibility of Small Implant Devices (F2129) offers three solutions for testing implant devices such as stents – Tyrodes, Ringers, and Hanks; the compositions of these solutions are given in Table 2.

Table 2 – *Simulated physiological solutions suggested in ASTM F2129*

Compound	Tyrodes	Ringers	Hanks
	Concentration, g/L		
NaCl	8.0	9.0	8.0
$CaCl_2$	0.20	0.24	0.14
KCl	0.2	0.42	0.4
$MgCl_2 \cdot 6H_2O$	0.10	NA	0.10
$MgSO_4 \cdot 7H_2O$	NA	NA	0.06
$NaHCO_3$	1.00	0.20	0.35
$Na_2H_2PO_4$	0.05	NA	0.10
$Na_2HPO_4 \cdot 2H_2O$	NA	NA	0.06
Glucose	1.00	NA	1.00
Solution pH	7.4	7.4	7.4

NA = Not applicable

Leclerc reviewed both *in vivo* and *in vitro* research on surgical implant materials, including UNS S31603 (AISI 316L), conducted between 1966 and 1985 [10]. The research included measurements of corrosion potential and corrosion rate under pitting, stress corrosion cracking, corrosion fatigue, fretting and crevice corrosion, galvanic corrosion, and sensitization conditions. He concluded that the basic surgical implant materials, when in their correct metallurgical condition, have adequate strength and corrosion resistance for most orthopedic applications

The primary purpose of the research reported here is to determine the effects of platinum additions on the corrosion resistance of UNS S31673-based PERSS alloys in deaerated Ringers solution representative of blood or blood plasma. A secondary purpose is to determine the effect of dissolved oxygen, introduced into alloys in the melting process, on the corrosion resistance of the UNS S31673-based PERSS alloys.

Experimental Methods

Alloy Fabrication

The materials used in this study were BioDur 316LS, the base material used to make these PERSS alloys, and PERSS alloys made by the addition of 5 to 6 wt % platinum to the base material. The ~ 6 wt % PERSS alloy (IVT 78) has more optimized processing parameters and more closely resembles a commercial product. The ~ 5 wt % alloys (IVT 30-series and 50 series), made earlier, are exploratory alloys; their processing parameters were somewhat less refined than either the BioDur 316LS or IVT 78. Corrective additions of Cr and Mo were made to all PERSS alloys to account for dilution resulting from the addition of platinum [3]. The corrections were made so the pitting resistance equivalent (PRE) of the PERSS alloys was equal to a PRE of 26 or greater; this was done by computing the corrections using the equation $PRE = [Cr] + 3.3 * [Mo]$, where the chromium [Cr] and molybdenum [Mo] concentrations of the alloy are given in weight %.

Alloys IVT 37, 38, 50 and 78 were consolidated by vacuum induction melting BioDur 316LS base with either a 5 wt% Pt addition (IVT 37, 38 and 50) or 6 wt % Pt addition (IVT 78) and enough additional Cr and Mo to return the overall composition to a PRE > 26. IVT 50 and 78 were remelted in a vacuum arc furnace to further refine the structure and provide sound material for further processing. Both IVT 54 and 56 were derived from IVT 50; they were produced to yield alloys of different oxygen content. IVT 54 and IVT 56 were vacuum induction melted under a partial pressure of argon, but they were not subsequently vacuum arc remelted. IVT 54 consisted of 1 kg of IVT 50 inductively melted in a new alumina (Al_2O_3) crucible and poured into a new conical mold. IVT 56 consisted of 1 kg IVT 50 plus 250 ppm aluminum (Al) plus 750 ppm calcium oxide (CaO) inductively melted in the same crucible as IVT 54 and poured into a conical mold.

Alloy Description and Analysis

The results of wet chemistry and inductively-coupled plasma atomic absorption spectroscopy (ICP AA) chemical analyses of the base material and the PERSS alloys are listed in Table 3. IVT 50-series alloys had higher oxygen contents than the base material. Cr, Ni, and Mo contents of the PERSS alloys were similar to those of the base material. All of the alloys (Table 4) were tested in their annealed condition. The base material and IVT 78 had similar hardness values. The IVT 78 grain size was refined by cold rolling, as compared to the grain size of the base material, which was obtained in bar form. Both alloys were single-phase austenitic alloys with no evidence of inclusions or precipitates.

Table 3 – *Chemical Analysis of alloys, wt %*

Element	BioDur[1] 316LS Heat 1	BioDur[1] 316LS Heat 2	IVT 78	IVT 50	IVT 54	IVT 56	IVT 37	IVT 38
Carbon	0.018	0.018	0.015	NA	NA	NA	NA	0.027
Silicon	0.45	0.38	0.41	0.45	0.45	0.45	0.48	0.47
Manganese	1.80	1.78	1.18	1.54	1.54	1.54	1.71	0.96
Sulfur	0.001	0.001	NA	NA	NA	NA	NA	0.0025
Phosphorus	0.015	0.017	NA	NA	NA	NA	NA	NA
Chromium	17.6	17.4	18.2	18. 7	18. 7	18. 7	17.5	17.5
Nickel	14.8	14.7	13.4	13.3	13.3	13.3	13.6	14.2
Molybdenum	2.81	2.79	2.90	2.94	2.94	2.94	2.87	2.89
Copper	0.09	0.11	0.10	0.10	0.10	0.10	0.08	0.07
Cobalt	0.07	0.05	>0.01	NA	NA	NA	NA	NA
Aluminum	0.009	0.006	>0.01	0.005	0.005	0.013	0.006	0.009
Nitrogen	0.025	0.029	NA	NA	NA	NA	NA	0.056
Titanium	0.002	<0.002	0.007	NA	NA	NA	NA	NA
Niobium	0.013	0.020	0.022	0.014	0.014	0.014	0.014	0.015
Vanadium	0.07	0.06	0.06	0.03	0.03	0.03	0.07	0.06
Platinum	0.00	0.00	6.01	5.32	5.32	5.32	4.95	4.78
Oxygen	0.0069	NA	NA	0.0205	0.0305	0.0100	NA	0.0400

[1] UNS S31673.   NA = not available.

Table 4 - *Alloy hardness and grain size*

Material	Hardness VHN (1 kg load)	ASTM grain size number
BioDur 316LS, Heat 2, annealed and electropolished	155	6.5
IVT 78, vacuum annealed and electropolished	161	10.0

Corrosion Tests

The primary test method used for evaluating corrosion susceptibility was F2129; it was used to measure pitting corrosion resistance in nitrogen deaerated Ringers solution of the alloys in Table 3, with the exception of IVT 30-series alloys. For comparison with the results from F2129 tests, potentiodynamic polarization measurements were made on selected alloys. Additional measurements were made on BioDur 316LS, Heat 1, and on IVT 37 and IVT 38, using Practice E of ASTM Practices for Detecting Susceptibility to Intergranular Attack in Austenitic Stainless Steels (A262), and ASTM Test Method for Pitting or Crevice Corrosion of Metallic Surgical Implant Materials (F746).

F2129 - This test method is for assessing corrosion susceptibility of specified metallic medical devices or components using cyclic forward and reverse potentiodynamic polarization. Examples of specified devices include coronary stents. The test method is intended to evaluate the medical device in its final form and finish, i.e., as it would be implanted. While it was not the aim of the present research to evaluate finished devices, the test method provided a valuable basis for assessing pitting corrosion resistance of PERSS alloys and comparing it to that of their base material. Most of the alloys were surface ground to a 120-grit aluminum oxide finish prior to testing. The BioDur 316LS, Heat 2, and IVT 78 alloys were prepared for testing in a manner closely approximating that used for coronary stents, i.e., polished to a 1 µm finish and then electropolished. All testing was in Ringers solution (Table 2), because this solution most closely simulates the composition of blood plasma. Samples were immersed in Ringers solution at 37 C after deaerating with high purity nitrogen. All potential measurements were made with respect to the saturated calomel electrode (SCE). The open circuit corrosion potential (E_{corr}) was measured for one hour. After one hour, the cyclic potentiodynamic scan was started in the positive (noble) direction at 10 mV/min, beginning at a potential 100 mV negative to the last measured E_{corr} value. The potential scan was reversed when current density reached a value approximately two decades greater than current density at the breakdown potential (E_b), sometimes called the pit nucleation potential, E_{np} [11]. The scan was halted when the potential reached 100 mV negative of the E_{corr} or when current density dropped below the passive current density and a protection potential (E_{prot}) was observed.

All tests were conducted in a flat cell modified to simulate the standard Avesta cell [12]. High purity water flowed through a fiber washer at 0.6 ml/min to maintain crevice-free conditions at the test sample surface. Figure 1 shows the experimental apparatus,

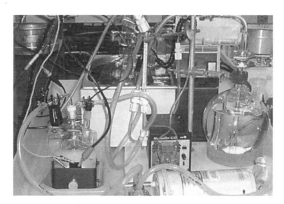

Figure 1 - *F2129 and potentiodynamic polarization experimental equipment showing the modified flat cell with an Avesta head, solution reservoir, water reservoir, and pumps*

including the flat cell fitted with an Avesta head, the solution reservoir, and the high purity water reservoir. Two or more tests were performed on each alloy.

Potentiodynamic polarization measurements were made on the two electropolished alloys, BioDur 316LS, Heat 2, and IVT 78, to show the full polarization curve, including both anodic and cathodic branches. All procedures were the same as in F2129 except that the cyclic scan was started in the positive (noble) direction at 10 mV/min, beginning at a potential of –300 mV vs SCE. The scan was reversed when current density reached a value approximately two decades greater than the current density at the breakdown potential (E_b). The scan was halted at the potential where the current density dropped below the passive current density, i.e., the protection potential (E_{prot}).

A262E – This practice is a requirement of ASTM Specification for Wrought 18 Chromium-14 Nickel-2.5 Molybdenum Stainless Steel Bar and Wire for Surgical Implants (F138) and ASTM Specification for Wrought 18 Chromium-14 Nickel-2.5 Molybdenum Stainless Steel Sheet and Strip for Surgical Implants (F139). It is intended to determine susceptibility of austenitic stainless steels to intergranular corrosion attack associated with precipitation of chromium-rich carbides.

Duplicate samples of BioDur 316LS, Heat 1, and IVT 37 and IVT 38 were tested in annealed and sensitized heat-treat conditions. The sensitized samples were heat-treated at 675 C for one hour and air cooled. All samples were ground to a 120-grit finish. They were then embedded in copper granules and exposed for 24 hours to a boiling solution of 100g/L hydrated copper sulfate ($CuSO_4 \cdot H_2O$) and 100 mL/L of concentrated sulfuric acid (H_2SO_4), Figure 2. After exposure, the samples were bent through a 180 arc over a mandrel with a diameter equal to the thickness of the samples. The bent samples were examined at 20X magnification for cracks indicative of a sensitized material.

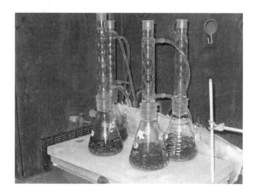

Figure 2 - *Apparatus for conducting ASTM A262, practice E*

F746 – This procedure is not a requirement of F138 and F139 for UNS S31673 alloys. It is designed solely for determining comparative laboratory indices of performance. The results are used for ranking alloys in order of increasing resistance to pitting and crevice corrosion under the specific conditions of the test method. The method is intentionally designed to produce conditions sufficiently severe to cause breakdown of UNS S31603, an alloy similar to UNS S31673 and also considered acceptable for surgical implant use.

Alloys that suffer pitting and crevice corrosion during the more severe portion of the test do not necessarily suffer localized corrosion when placed in the human body as implants.

Three samples each of BioDur 316LS, Heat 1, and IVT 38 were evaluated in the annealed condition. The surface of each cylindrical sample was first ground to a 600-grit finish. Samples were fitted with an inert tapered collar and immersed in a saline solution (consisting of 9 g/L sodium chloride (NaCl) in distilled water) at 37°C. E_{corr} was established after immersion for one hour. Localized corrosion was then stimulated by potentiostatically polarizing the sample to a potential of +800 mV vs SCE. Localized corrosion was marked by a large and generally increasing anodic current. The potential was then decreased rapidly to the original E_{corr}. If the alloy was susceptible to localized corrosion, the current remained at a relatively high value and fluctuated with time. If the pits or crevices repassivated and localized attack was halted, the current dropped to a value typical of a passive surface and continued to decrease. If the sample repassivated, it was repolarized to +800 mV vs SCE and the potential decreased to a value more noble (more positive) than E_{corr} and the current response observed. This was repeated stepwise until a potential was reached where the sample did not repassivate. The critical potential for localized attack is the most noble potential at which localized corrosion repassivated, i.e., similar to E_{prot}.

Results

F2129

IVT 78 PERSS alloy – Results of the F2129 test on the Biodur 316LS, Heat 2, and the PERSS alloy IVT 78 alloy are shown in Figure 3 and summarized in Table 5. Parameters measured in the ASTM F2129 tests were E_{corr}, E_b, E_{prot} and I_{corr}; derived values included $(E_b - E_{corr})$ and $(E_b - E_{prot})$. The heavy curves in Figure 3 are for Biodur 316LS, Heat 2. They bracket the results for IVT 78. Both the base material and IVT 78 were passive until E_b was achieved. Measured E_b values for IVT 78 were grouped between those measured for Biodur 316LS, Heat 2, Figure 3 and Table 5. No E_{prot} was measured for Biodur 316LS, Heat 2, or IVT 78 because the ASTM F2129 test did not allow potentials more negative than –100 mV below the last measured E_{corr} to be included in the scans.

Full potentiodynamic polarization curves, including both the anodic and cathodic branches, are shown in Figure 4 for Biodur 316LS, Heat 2, and IVT 78. They are typical for stainless steel-based alloys in contact with chloride solutions at moderate pH values [13] as opposed to the curves generated by ASTM F2129, Figure 3. The curves in Figure 4 show extended regions of passivity, a breakdown of the passive film due to the initiation and growth of pits, and a well-developed hysteresis loop. The presence of the hysteresis loop is an indication that the alloys are susceptible to localized corrosion. These results are summarized in Table 5. The polarization curves include both E_{corr} and E_{prot}. They show the curves for Biodur 316LS, Heat 2, and IVT 78 were similar except for the values of E_{corr}. E_{corr} for IVT 78 was higher than that for Biodur 316LS, Heat 2. Both Biodur 316LS, Heat 2, and IVT 78 were passive at potentials up to E_b. The E_b

values for the two alloys were almost the same and E_{prot} values for the two alloys were similar. However, IVT 78 repassivated at potentials below (cathodic to) E_{corr} while Biodur 316LS, Heat 2, repassivated at potentials above (anodic to) E_{corr}. Corrosion currents for the Biodur 316LS, Heat 2, and IVT 78 were low and similar.

Photomicrographs are shown in Figure 5 of the BioDur 316LS, Heat 2, and IVT 78 surfaces following the ASTM F2129 test and potentiodynamic polarization scans (the staining is not significant). In each case pitting occurred at only one or two locations on the 1 cm^2 exposed surface. There was no other population of pits distributed over the surface and there was no evidence of crevice corrosion. Results were the same for both BioDur 316LS, Heat 2, and IVT 78.

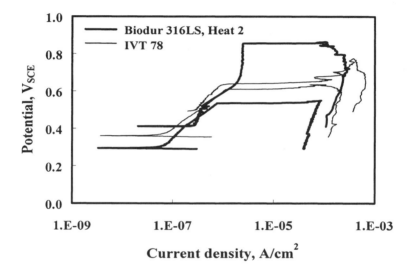

Figure 3 - *F2129 results for Biodur 316LS, Heat 2, and IVT*

IVT 50-series PERSS alloys – Figure 6 shows cyclic potentiodynamic polarization curves for BioDur 316LS, Heat 1, and IVT 56 in de-aerated Ringers solution. The curve for IVT 56 shown in Figure 6 is qualitatively similar to that for each of the IVT 50-series alloys. Pits were observed on the exposed surface of the IVT 50 series alloys, but there was no indication of crevice corrosion in the area where the sample was sealed to the test cell. Both BioDur 316LS, Heat 1, and the IVT 50-series alloys exhibited breakdown potentials more noble than their corrosion potentials. E_b for BioDur 316LS, Heat 1, was more noble than that for the IVT 50-series alloys, indicating a greater resistance to pitting corrosion for BioDur 316LS than the IVT 50-series alloys.

Table 5 – *Results of the ASTM F2129 Test*

Sample and finish	O wt %	E_{corr} V vs SCE	E_b V vs SCE	E_{prot} V vs SCE	I_{corr} µA/cm²	E_b-E_{corr} V	E_b-E_{prot} V
BioDur 316LS, Heat 1, 120-grit finish	0.007	0.150	0.742	0.154	NA	0.592	0.588
BioDur 316LS, Heat 2, electropolished	NA	0.008 [1]	0.860 [1]	0.128 [1]	0.011 [1]	0.852 [1]	0.732 [1]
			0.856				
			0.535				
IVT 78, electropolished	NA	0.217 [1]	0.939 [1]	0.021 [1]	0.042 [1]	0.722 [1]	0.918 [1]
			0.636				
			0.608				
IVT 56, 120-grit finish	0.0100	-0.098	0.340	0.103	0.378	0.438	0.237
		-0.079	0.319	0.100	0.138	0.398	0.219
IVT 50, 120-grit finish	0.0205	-0.212	0.272	0.157	0.051	0.484	0.429
		-0.185	0.515	0.117	NA	0.700	0.632
		-0.223	0.204	-0.009	0.192	0.427	0.213
		0.014	0.452	0.158	0.022	0.466	0.610
IVT 54, 120-grit finish	0.0305	-0.183	0.339	0.165	0.141	0.522	0.174
		0.008	0.326	0.195	0.180	0.334	0.131

[1] potentiodynamic polarization. NA = not available

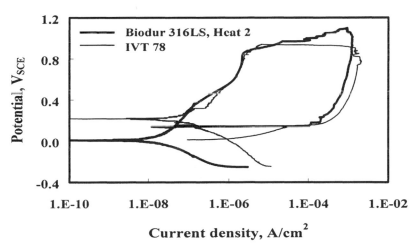

Figure 4 - *Potentiodynamic polarization results for Biodur 316LS, Heat 2, and IVT 78*

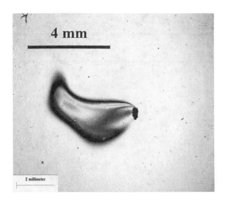
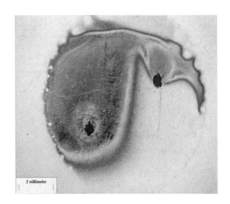

Biodur 316LS. Heat 2. annealed and electropolished.

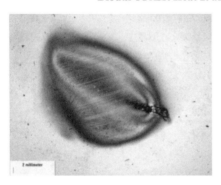
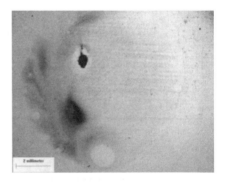

F2129   potentiodynamic polarization

IVT 78, vacuum annealed and electropolished.

Figure 5 - *Alloy surface following polarization tests in Ringers solution showing pits that formed following breakdown of the passive film (staining inconsequential to test).*

Effect of Alloy Oxygen Content on Localized Corrosion of IVT 50-series PERSS alloys
In general, local imperfections in passive films, such as inclusions, increase the susceptibility of an alloy to localized corrosion [14]. Oxygen incorporated into an alloy during melting and fabrication can result in the formation of oxide inclusions. Oxide inclusions at the surface of stainless steels can affect the stability of the passive film formed on stainless steels when evaluated by F2129. Inclusions can become sites for pit initiation, thereby reducing the alloy resistance to pitting corrosion. The IVT 50-series alloys were made with different oxygen contents and had second phases present in their microstructure. Results for the alloys are plotted in Figure 7 and show that E_{corr}, E_b, or E_{prot} were not a function of oxygen content in the range 0.01 to 0.03 wt % oxygen. However, IVT 50-series alloys were more susceptible to pitting corrosion than IVT 78.

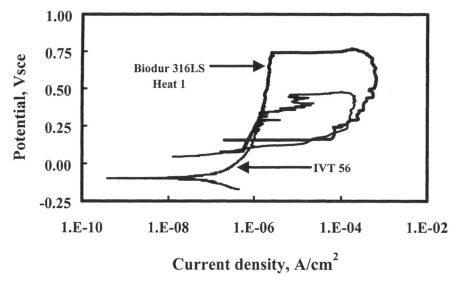

Figure 6 - *Cyclic potentiodynamic polarization curves for Biodur 316LS, Heat 1, and IVT 56 conducted according to ASTM F2129*

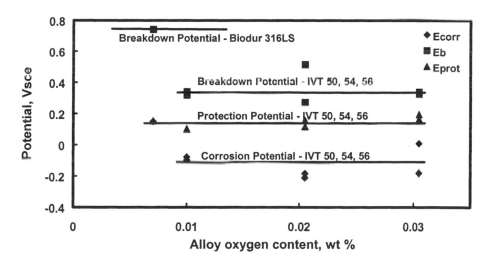

Figure 7 - *Effect of alloy oxygen content on electrochemical parameters for Biodur 316LS, Heat 1, and IVT 50-series alloys*

A262E   The behavior of alloys IVT 37 and IVT 38 was identical to that of BioDur 316LS, Heat 1, in the A262E test. Figure 8 shows the surface of the BioDur 316LS, Heat 1, and IVT 37 alloys after 24 hour immersion in the copper sulfate solution and then bending through a 180° arc. None of the samples exhibited cracks or fissures on the bend radius. This indicates the alloys were not susceptible to intergranular corrosion attack. As a consequence of these results it can be surmised that annealing did not precipitate chromium-rich carbides and the alloys were not susceptible to sensitization at the annealing conditions. While not tested by A262E, metallographic examination of BioDur 316LS, Heat 2, and IVT 78 alloy microstructures showed them to be single-phase austenitic materials with no evidence of inclusions or precipitates.

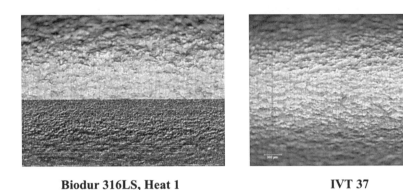

Biodur 316LS, Heat 1   **IVT 37**

Figure 8. Alloy surface after ASTM A262E test followed by bending through a 180° arc (20X).

ASTM F746

The results of F746 are shown in Table 6 for BioDur 316LS, Heat 1, and IVT 38. The critical potential for pit repassivation, E_{prot}, of the alloy in the saline solution for BioDur 316LS, 0.200 to 0.250 V_{SCE}, was slightly more noble than that for IVT 38, 0.100 to 0.150 V_{SCE}. In terms of ability to repassivate, BioDur 316LS, Heat 1, had greater resistance to pitting and crevice attack than IVT 38. Examination of the samples following the F746 test revealed no evidence of localized corrosion attack, either crevice corrosion attack around the tapered collar or pitting corrosion attack on the sample face.

Table 6 – *Results of ASTM F746 Experiments*

Sample	Exposed Area cm^2	Area Under Collar cm^2	Initial E_{corr} V_{SCE}	Final E_{corr} V_{SCE}	E_{prot} V_{SCE}
BioDur 316LS Heat 1	3.62	0.61	-0.177	-0.133	0.200
	3.62	0.61	-0.163	-0.124	0.250
	3.62	0.61	-0.177	-0.117	0.200
IVT 38	3.62	0.61	-0.171	-0.093	0.150
	3.62	0.61	-0.164	-0.102	0.100
	3.62	0.61	-0.221	-0.164	0.150

Discussion

Composition of alloys

The PERSS alloy IVT 78 exhibited substantially greater resistance to pitting corrosion than the IVT 50-series alloys. The value of E_{corr} was substantially more noble and more clearly in the passive region than that for the IVT 50-series alloys. The value of E_b for IVT 78 was more noble than that for the IVT 50-series alloys and comparable to that of BioDur 316LS. The value of I_{corr} for IVT 78 was more than a factor of 5 lower than that of the IVT 50-series alloys and comparable to that of BioDur 316LS. The value of (E_b-E_{corr}) for IVT 78 was substantially higher than most values for the IVT 50-series alloys and comparable to that for BioDur 316LS.

Results in Table 5 show that E_b values for IVT 78 were similar to those for BioDur 316LS. Values for the IVT 50-series alloys were less noble than those for BioDur 316LS. A reduction in E_b, similar to that seen for the IVT 50-series alloys was suggested in McGill's review [5-6] of the literature for two ferritic stainless steels, although no data were reported for austenitic stainless steels such as UNS S31673. Leclerc [10] has reported E_b values of 0.160-0.650 V_{SCE} for 316 stainless steel in Ringers solution. E_b values slightly more noble to these are reported in Table 5 for BioDur 316LS and for IVT 78. Values comparable to them are reported in Table 5 for the IVT series-50 alloys.

Another way to assess pitting corrosion susceptibility is to consider the derived parameters given in the last two columns of Table 5. A well-defined hysteresis loop indicates susceptibility to localized corrosion, and the width of the hysteresis loop (E_b-E_{prot}) characterizes that susceptibility (see for example Figure 4). A larger E_b-E_{prot} value generally indicates greater susceptibility to localized corrosion [17]. (E_b-E_{prot}) values in Table 5 for both BioDur 316LS and the PERSS alloys are similar in magnitude, indicating they have a similar susceptibility to localized corrosion. However, susceptibility to localized corrosion does not mean pitting corrosion will initiate.

Susceptibility to pit initiation is indicated by the second parameter, (E_b-E_{corr}). The greater the value of (E_b-E_{corr}), the lower the probability that pitting corrosion will initiate on an alloy surface [17]. Values of (E_b-E_{corr}) given in Table 5 are large (0.334 to 0.852 V) for all of the alloys, indicating low susceptibility to pit initiation. Furthermore, both BioDur 316LS and IVT 78 had values on the high end of this range, indicating even greater resistance to pit initiation.

None of the measured corrosion parameters for the PERSS alloys in deaerated Ringers solution were a function of alloy oxygen content between 0.01 and 0.03 wt %. Results in other environments may be different. However, the fabrication practice for the PERSS alloys is to keep the oxygen content as low as possible.

Surface finish and possible effects

Surface preparation of the BioDur 316LS alloy and the IVT 30-series and 50-series alloys was a 120-grit finish, which is much rougher than that of finished stents. Surface preparation of the BioDur 316LS, Heat 2, and IVT 78 was similar to that of electropolished (finished) stents. Surface finish can greatly affect the resistance of an alloy to localized corrosion. For example, the F2129 results for BioDur 316LS were quite different for Heat 1 ground to a 120-grit surface finish and Heat 2 polished to a 1 μm finish and then electropolished. A surface that is more homogeneous, both chemically and physically, will have a more noble value for E_b and a better resistance to localized corrosion [16]. Physical homogeneity of an alloy surface refers to roughness caused by the surface preparation process. E_b has been shown to be more noble as peak-to-peak surface roughness decreased from 100 to 0.02 μm [16]. While chemical homogeneity of an alloy surface can mean many things, one of the most critical factors is the amount of Cr in the passive surface film. Studies have shown that the amount of Cr in the passive film, and value of E_{corr} and E_b, increased as follows: dry polishing < wet polishing < HF etching < 10% HNO_3 etching < 30% HNO_3 passivation [16]. Clearly surface finish is an important factor and should be considered when evaluating alloy resistance to localized corrosion. The optimum surface finish is that of the finished stent, as was done with the BioDur 316LS, Heat 2, and the PERSS alloy IVT 78, and is reflected in the higher E_b values for these two materials, Table 5.

Potentiodynamic polarization scan rate

Scan rate can affect measured values of E_b and E_{prot} [17]. Faster scan rates tend to produce more noble values of E_b and E_{prot}. Scan rate also can affect different alloys differently. The scan rate used in the present tests was 10 mV/min, well within the range where E_b for 18Cr-9Ni stainless steels is reported to be unaffected by scan rate [17].

Potentiodynamic polarization scan versus F2129 scan

The potentiodynamic polarization and F2129 scans for BioDur 316LS, Heat 2, are given in Figure 9. The F2129 scan is seen to be identical to that of the potentiodynamic polarization scan over the potential range covered by the F2129 test criteria (the lower value of current after the scan direction was reversed is not considered to be significant). However, for materials like BioDur 316LS, Heat 2, and IVT 78 with an electropolished surface finish, the F2129 test did not permit a determination of E_{corr}, I_{corr}, or E_{prot}. The difficulty lies in the way E_{corr} and the scan start potential are determined in the test for a material that is strongly passive, as both BioDur 316LS and the IVT 78 alloys were. With a strongly passive material the "last measured E_{corr}" can vary widely over the passive region. The F2129 test limits the cyclic potential scan from a point 100 mV more negative than "the last measured E_{corr}" to E_b and back. Clearly from the results in Figure 8, this range is insufficient to measure some of the important parameters used to rate the performance of alloys in body fluids.

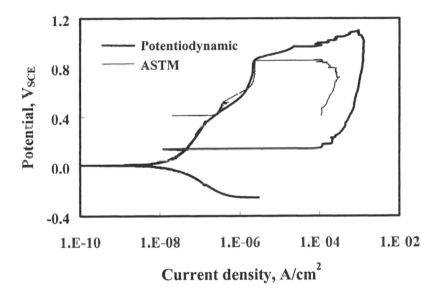

Figure 9 - *Comparison of F2129 and potentiodynamic polarization results for Biodur 316LS, Heat 2*

Conclusions

- The PERSS alloy IVT 78 alloy had a resistance to pitting corrosion in deaerated Ringers solution that was similar to that of the BioDur 316LS base (UNS S31673).

- Metallographic examination showed annealed IVT 78 and annealed BioDur 316LS to be single-phase alloys with no evidence of inclusions or precipitates.
- Values of (E_b-E_{corr}), which characterize the probability that localized corrosion will initiate, were fairly large and were similar for both BioDur 316LS and IVT 78, suggesting the probability was low that pits would initiate in deaerated Ringers solution.
- The IVT 78 alloy was more resistant to pitting corrosion in deaerated Ringers solution than were the IVT 50-series alloys.
- The corrosion performance of the IVT 50-series alloys, as measured in deaerated Ringers solution by the F2129 test procedure, was not a function of alloy oxygen contents between 0.01 and 0.03 wt %.
- There was no evidence of intergranular attack due to sensitization of either BioDur 316LS or the IVT 30-series alloys as measured by the A262E test procedure.
- There was no evidence of pitting or crevice attack on the BioDur 316LS and IVT 38 alloys as measured by the F746 test procedure. The IVT 38 results were similar to those obtained by F2129 for IVT 50-series alloys.
- Potentiodynamic polarization scans provide more information on the corrosion performance of alloys that are strongly passive in body fluids than does F2129. This arises primarily because of the way E_{corr} and the scan start potential is established in F2129. Potentiodynamic polarization measurements provided values for E_{corr}, I_{corr}, and E_{prot} for electropolished BioDur 316LS and IVT 78. These values were not available from F2129.

References

[1]   Pepine, C.J. and Holmes, D.R, "Coronary Artery Stents," Journal of the American College of Cardiology, Vol. 28, No. 3, 1996, pp. 782-94.

[2]   Sahagian, R., "Critical Insight: Marking Devices with Radiopaque Coatings," Medical Device and Diagnostic Industry, May, 1999, 6 pp.

[3]   Craig, C. H., Radisch, H. R., Jr., Trozera, T. A., Turner, P. C., Govier, R. D., Vesely, E. J., Jr., Gokcen, N. A., Friend, C. M., and Edwards, M. R., "Development of a Platinum-Enhanced Radiopaque Stainless Steel (PERSS®)," Stainless Steels for Medical and Surgical Applications, ASTM STP 1438, G. L. Winters and M. J. Nutt, Eds., ASTM International, West Conshohocken PA, 2003.

[4]   Dennis, J. Z., Craig, C. H., Radisch, H. R., Jr., Pannek, E. J., Turner, P. C., Hicks, A. G., Jenusaitis, M., Gokcen, N. A., Friend, C. M., and Edwards, M. R., "Processing Platinum Enhanced Radiopaque Stainless Steel (PERSS®) for Use as Ballon-Expandable Coronary Stents," Stainless Steels for Medical and Surgical Applications, ASTM STP 1438, G. L. Winters and M. J. Nutt, Eds., ASTM International, West Conshohocken PA, 2003.

[5]   McGill, I. R., "Platinum Metals in Stainless Steels – A Review of Corrosion and Mechanical Properties," Platinum Metals Review, Vol. 34, No. 2, 1990, pp. 85-97.

[6]   McGill, I. R., "Platinum Metals in Stainless Steels – Part II: Further Corrosion and Mechanical Properties," Platinum Metals Review, Vol. 34, No. 3, 1990, pp. 144-154.

[7]   Andersson, Ö.H. and Kangasniemi, I., "Calcium Phosphate Formation at the Surface of Bioactive glass *In Vitro*," *Journal of Biomedical Materials Research*, Vol. 25, 1991, pp. 1019-1030.

[8]   Canham, L.T., Reeves, C.L., Newey, J,P., Houlton, M.R., Cox, T.I., Buriak, J.M., and Stewart, M.P., "Derivatized Mesoporous Silicon with Dramatically Improved Stability in Simulated Human Blood Plasma," *Advanced Materials*, Vol. 11, No. 18, 1999, pp. 1505-1507.

[9]   Sella, C., Martin, J.C., Lecoeur, J., Bellier, J.P., and Davidas, J.P, "Corrosion and Protection of Surgical and Dental Metallic Implants," *Biomaterials and Clinical Applications*, Elsevier Science Publishers, Amsterdam, The Netherlands, pp. 119-124, 1986.

[10]   Leclerc, M.F., "Surgical Implants," *Corrosion – Volume 1: Metal/Environment Interactions*, Shreir, L.L., Jarman, R.A., and Burstein, G.T., eds., 3rd edition, Butterworth-Heinemann Ltd., Oxford, UK, 1994, pp. 2:164-2:180.

[11]   Szklarska-Smialowska, Z., Pitting Corrosion of Metals, National Association of Corrosion Engineers, Houston, TX, 1986, pp. 39-40.

[12]   Qvarfort R., "New Electrochemical Cell for Pitting Corrosion Testing," *Corrosion Science*, vol. 28, No. 2, 1988, pp 135-140.

[13]   Szklarska-Smialowska, Z., op.cit., pp. 3-4.

[14]   ibid., p. 69

[15]   Baboian, R. and Haynes, G.S., "Cyclic Polarization Measurements – Experimental Procedure and Evaluation of Test Data," *Electrochemical Corrosion Testing*, ASTM STP 727, American Society for Testing and Materials, West Conshohocken, PA, 1981, pp. 274-282.

[16]   Szklarska-Smialowska, Z., op.cit., pp. 240-246.

[17]   ibid., pp. 50-57.

Lyle D. Zardiackas,[1] Michael Roach,[1] Scott Williamson,[1] and Jay-Anthony Bogan[1]

Comparison of Corrosion Fatigue of BioDur® 108 to 316L S.S. And 22Cr-13Ni-5Mn S.S.

Reference: Zardiackas, L. D., Roach, M., Williamson, S., and Bogan, J. -A., "Comparison of Corrosion Fatigue of BioDur® 108 to 316L S.S. And 22Cr-13Ni-5Mn S.S.," *Stainless Steels for Medical and Surgical Applications, ASTM STP 1438*, G.L. Winters and M.J. Nutt, Eds., ASTM International, West Conshohocken, PA 2003.

Abstract: Fatigue testing was performed on three austenitic stainless steels in tension-tension in distilled water and in Ringer's solution at 37°C using an MTS servo-hydraulic testing system following the guidelines of ASTM F1801. The materials chosen were BioDur® 108, BioDur® 316LS and BioDur® 22Cr-13Ni-5Mn stainless steel. Samples with a 2.5 mm diameter in the gauge length of 10 mm were prepared from 8 mm diameter bar stock using low stress grinding techniques. A minimum of three samples at each of five load levels were cycled to failure or to a maximum of 10^6 cycles. S/N curves for each material under each condition were plotted and fracture surfaces were examined using scanning electron microscopy (SEM). Comparison between the fatigue response of each material in distilled water and Ringer's solution as well as between alloys was evaluated. Results showed typical S/N curve response comparison of stainless steels in distilled water vs. salt solutions with curves slightly shifted in a positive direction (higher numbers of cycles to failure at equal stress values) in distilled water as compared to Ringer's solution. Additionally, although not statistically evaluated, the fatigue curves were shifted toward higher numbers of cycles to failure for the two nitrogen strengthened alloys with the number of cycles to fracture for 22Cr-13Ni-5Mn being slightly higher in distilled water at lower stress values and the fatigue curves for 22Cr-13Ni-5Mn and BioDur® 108 in Ringer's solution were essentially equivalent. Evaluation of fracture surfaces by SEM showed variations in fatigue striation spacing as a function of loading in all alloys. A difference in fracture morphology of the BioDur® 108 was noted near the area of crack initiation as compared to the other two alloys. Flutes and terraces, not normally seen in fatigue of austenitic stainless steels at in vivo temperature, were seen.

Keywords: Stainless steel, fatigue, corrosion fatigue, implant materials

---

[1]Professor and Coordinator of Biomaterials and Professor of Orthopaedic Surgery, materials engineer, senior materials engineer and senior materials engineer, respectively, University of Mississippi Medical Center, 2500 North State Street, Jackson, MS, 39216.

Introduction

Austenitic stainless steels have enjoyed a wide variety of applications as biomedical implants. A spectrum of mechanical properties achieved by annealing, cold working and forging, good corrosion resistance and biocompatibility have contributed to their long term use. Retrieval studies [1-8] and fundamental research [9-11] conducted on orthopaedic implants as well as stainless steel alloys in the1960s and 1970s, indicated the need for compositional and processing changes to produce an implant quality 316L stainless steel with greater corrosion resistance and a lower concentration of inclusions. Since that time, significant changes in the composition requirements of 316L stainless steel, as reflected in the ASTM standards for "Wrought 18 Chromium-14 Nickel-2.5 Molybdenum Stainless Steel Bar and Wire for Surgical Implants (UNS S31673)[1]" (F138-00) and "Wrought-18 Chromium-14 Nickel-2.5 Molybdenum Stainless Sheet and Strip for Surgical Implants (UNS S31673)[1]" (F139-00), have occurred. The most significant of these changes include increases in the lower and upper limits of Ni, a decrease in the upper limit of Cr and a decrease in the upper limit of Mo. In order to meet the PRE requirement of 26 or greater and to reduce the possibility of δ-ferrite formation, alloy manufacturers raised the Mo concentration to near the maximum (3.0) and kept the Cr concentration near the middle of the allowed range. These changes have resulted in superior mechanical and corrosion properties as compared to their predecessors. Additionally, 22Cr-13Ni-5Mn stainless steel which is covered by ASTM standard for "Wrought Nitrogen Strengthened-22 Chromium-12.5 Nickel-5 Manganese-2.5 Molybdenum Stainless Steel Bar and Wire for Surgical Implants[1]" (F1314-95), which is a nitrogen strengthened austenitic stainless steel, has been added as another implant quality stainless steel for use especially in the area of orthopaedic fracture fixation.

As changes in composition and properties of 316L stainless steel have occurred, additional studies have reported on the results of implant retrieval [12-17]. These studies have shown that there continues to be some crevice and fretting corrosion which occurs in retrieved implanted devices of 316L stainless steel but that fracture of these devices, in essentially all cases, is due to fatigue. Basic research studies on the fatigue and corrosion fatigue of 316L stainless steel have shown that the fatigue resistance of this alloy is reduced when subjected to fatigue in NaCl solutions [11, 18-20] as compared to air or distilled water. Results of fatigue in air, generally using rotating beam samples or samples fatigued under bending loads, have indicated that the fatigue strength of 316L and 22Cr-13Ni-5Mn stainless steel is proportional to the yield strength and that higher fatigue endurance limits are achieved by increased cold working [21-22]. Studies have also shown that the percentage of increase in fatigue resistance of 22Cr-13Ni-5Mn stainless steel as a function of cold working is not linear but drops off as the percentage of cold working increases. Failure analysis of both retrieved implants and in vitro fatigue fractures have shown no difference in failure mechanism or fracture surface morphology as a function of test media in these alloys [17-18].

While providing excellent properties, implant quality austenitic stainless steels such as 316L and 22Cr-13Ni-5Mn stainless steel have been questioned by some as relates to their biocompatibility. Research has shown that the release of elements in vivo, particularly nickel and chromium, may lead to inflamation, toxicity or hypersensitivity over time [23-

27]. Questions related to biocompatibility have been one of the primary factors initiating research on the development of low Ni containing austenitic stainless steels.

The purpose of this research was to characterize and compare the corrosion fatigue of a new low Ni, austenitic stainless steel (BioDur® 108) to implant quality 316L stainless steel and implant quality 22Cr-13Ni-5Mn stainless steel using a tension-tension fatigue model as described by ASTM standard for "Corrosion Fatigue Testing of Metallic Implant Materials[1]" (F1801-97) [28]. Comparison was performed by the generation of S/N curves and through analysis of fracture surface morphology by scanning electron microscopy.

Materials and Methods

The low nickel stainless steel chosen for the study was BioDur® 108 (alloy A) supplied by Carpenter Specialty Alloys. The materials chosen for comparison were BioDur® 316LS (alloy B) and BioDur® 22Cr-13Ni-5Mn (alloy C) since they were available from the same source and represented the other two commonly used austenitic stainless steel alloys in compliance with ASTM F138 and ASTM F1314, respectively. Alloys were supplied as 8mm diameter centerless ground bar in the cold worked condition. In order to verify information supplied on primary certification documents and to establish baseline mechanical properties for fatigue testing, each alloy was characterized for composition, microstructure and tensile properties. Quantitative compositional evaluation of the major alloying elements of each alloy was determined using an inductively coupled plasma spectrometer (ICP) with a spark attachment for analysis of solid samples (SPECTRO[2] ICP with LISA). The microstructure of each alloy material was evaluated according to ASTM standard for "Determining Average Grain Size[1]" (E112-96) with all samples prepared in duplicate. The inclusion content was determined according to ASTM standard for "Determining the Inclusion Content of Steel[1]" (E45-97) Method A using Plate I-r. Prior to fatigue testing, smooth tensile samples with a gauge length of 36 mm, a diameter in the gauge length of 6 mm and a maximum surface roughness of 16 micro-inches (Ra=16) in the gauge were prepared by Low Stress Grind[3]. Testing was performed using an MTS[4] servo-hydraulic test system operating at 0.3 mm/min to yield and 3.0 mm/min from yield to fracture according to ASTM standard for "Tension Testing of Metallic Materials[1]" (E8-00b). Ultimate tensile strength, yield strength, elastic modulus, % elongation to fracture, and reduction of area were determined in order to establish baseline data for fatigue testing.

Corrosion fatigue was performed in tension-tension in aerated distilled/de-ionized water and in aerated Ringer's solution at 37°C using an MTS servo-hydraulic testing system. Testing followed the guidelines of ASTM F1801. Samples were prepared in an identical manner to the smooth tensile samples previously described except that the diameter in the gauge length of 10 mm was 2.5 mm (Figure 1). Samples were mounted vertically to facilitate complete submersion of the sample through the gauge section, and all fixturing in contact with the solution was either teflon or the same alloy as the samples to eliminate any corrosion couples. A tension-tension load was applied as a sinusoidal

---

[2]SPECTRO Analytical Instruments, Fitchburg, MA, USA
[3]Low Stress Grind, Cincinnati, OH USA
[4]MTS, Eden Prairie, MN, USA

wave function in load control at 1 Hz. A minimum of three samples was tested at each of five stress levels to failure or to a maximum of 10^6 cycles. Data was plotted as stress v. number of cycles to fracture to generate typical S/N curves for each alloy under each of the two test conditions.

Ra = 16 µin Gauge

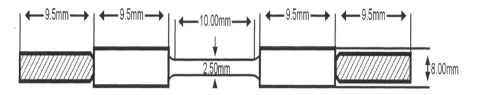

Figure 1 - *Sample drawing for corrosion fatigue samples*

After fatigue testing was completed, analysis of the fracture surfaces from at least one sample of each alloy in each test solution which fractured at less than 10^5 cycles and one sample of each alloy in each test solution that fractured at greater than 10^5 cycles was examined by scanning electron microscopy (SEM). Comparison was made between alloys to determine the area of crack initiation, fracture morphology during Stage II fatigue crack propagation, and the final fracture mode (Stage III fatigue). Additionally, comparison was made to identify differences in fracture surface morphology between fatigue in distilled/de-ionized water and Ringer's solution for each alloy.

Results

Results of the baseline evaluation of each of the three alloys including composition, microstructure and mechanical testing are reported elsewhere [29-30] and given for informational purposes in Table 1. S/N plots of the results of the fatigue testing to compare the fatigue behavior of each of the three stainless steel alloys evaluated in each of the two test media are seen in Figures 2 and 3. It must be remembered that the endurance limit for these alloys has not been statistically determined, and therefore, the values interpreted from the S/N curves are not statistically precise. As seen in Figures 2 and 3, the results indicate that in distilled/de-ionized water the fatigue curves cross with alloy A showing the greatest number of cycles to failure at the higher loads and alloy C showing the greatest number of cycles to failure at the lower loads. However, in Ringer's solution the curves are essentially superimposed. The fatigue strength of both alloy A and alloy C are greater than alloy B regardless of the solution used during testing. These results are essentially consistent with the data reported for fatigue testing in air regardless of testing methodology, although the actual fatigue strength numbers are not as great as those reported in most of the literature where testing has been performed in reverse bending [21,22].

Table I - *Mechanical Testing Results (n=5)*

Alloy	Alloy A	Alloy B	Alloy C
Elastic Modulus (GPa)	188±3	167±5	186±2
UTS* (MPa)	1344±7	1014±0	1351±13
0.2% YS** (MPa)	1179±21	793±7	1082±13
% ROA***	68±0	71±0	60±1
% Elongation	35±1	25±1	19±1

* UTS = ultimate tensile strength
** YS = 0.2% yield strength
*** ROA = reduction of area

Fracture analysis revealed a classical macroscopic fatigue pattern for samples fatigued in tension-tension with no stress concentration [31]. This pattern was consistent regardless of the alloy and the percentage of the fractured sample which experienced Stage II fatigue increased with decreasing load (Figure 4). The remainder of each fracture surface showed a Stage III fatigue fracture pattern (ductile overload). SEM fracture analysis of alloy B and alloy C showed crack initiation at the surface of the samples with the fracture morphology being typically fatigue striations with secondary cracking (Figures 5a and 5b). The striations were less clearly defined in some areas of the fracture surfaces in the samples tested in Ringer's solution presumably due to corrosion effects. This type of morphology is similar to that seen in retrieved fracture fixation devices [14, 17]. Final fracture of each sample was due to tensile overload as exhibited by ductile dimples (Figure 5c). While this type of morphology is typically seen in test samples, dimpling, due to ductile tensile or shear overloading, is very often not seen in retrieved devices where there has been some degree of bone healing which results in load sharing.

SEM fracture analysis of the fatigued samples of alloy A showed a more complex pattern with the morphology deviating from that typically seen in the other two FCC austenitic stainless steels evaluated. While fatigue striations were noted over much of the fracture surfaces regardless of testing media or stress level (Figure 6a), fluting, terraces with feather marks, and furrowing (Figures 6b and 6c) were noted especially in the areas near crack initiation.

Discussion and Conclusions

ASTM F1801 requires that a minimum of three samples be tested at each of five load levels to describe the fatigue curves. This same specification recommends that a minimum of six samples be tested at each load level to evaluate statistical significance. It has been our experience that ten samples are often required to perform statistical tests.

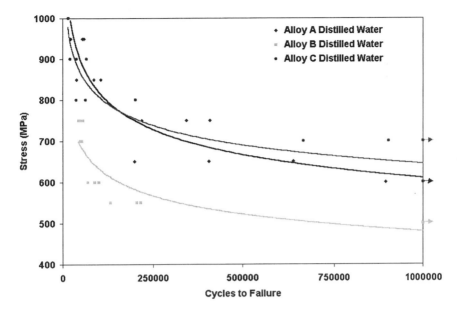

Figure 2 - *S/N curves of alloys A, B, and C in distilled/de-ionized water*

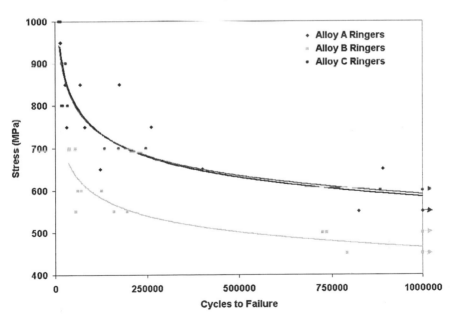

Figure 3 - *S/N curves of alloys A, B, and C in Ringer's solution*

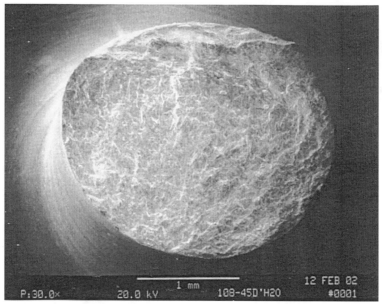

Figure 4 - *SEM micrograph showing the fracture surface of alloy A in distilled/de-ionized water (30X, 713,015 cycles)*

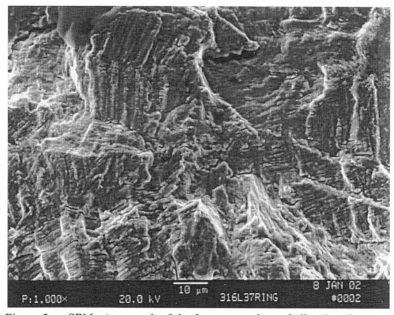

Figure 5a - *SEM micrograph of the fracture surface of alloy B in Ringer's solution showing fatigue striations with secondary cracking.*

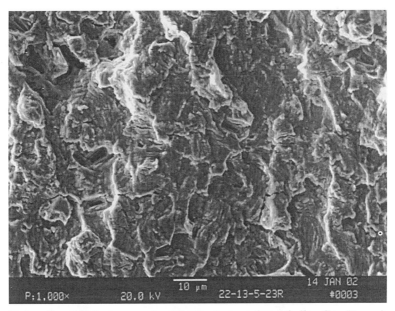

Figure 5b - *SEM micrograph of the fracture surface of alloy C in Ringer's solution showing fatigue striations with secondary cracking.*

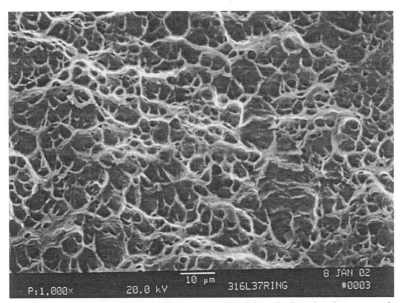

Figure 5c - *Representative SEM micrograph of ductile dimples due to tensile overload in the final fracture region of alloy B in Ringer's solution.*

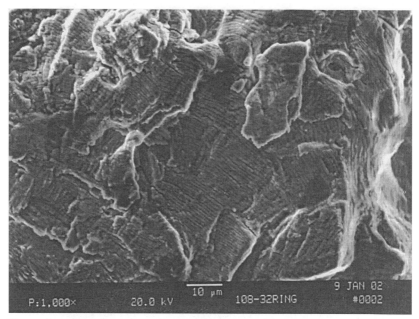

Figure 6a - *SEM micrograph showing the fatigue striations on alloy A in Ringer's solution.*

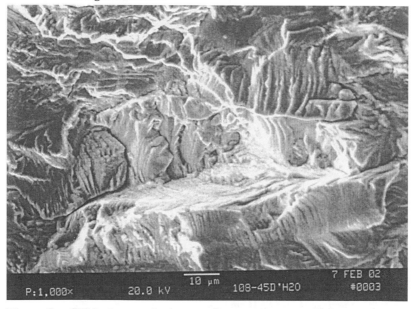

Figure 6b - *SEM micrograph showing fluting, terraces, and furrowing on the fracture surface of alloy A near crack initiation (Fatigue in distilled/de-ionized water).*

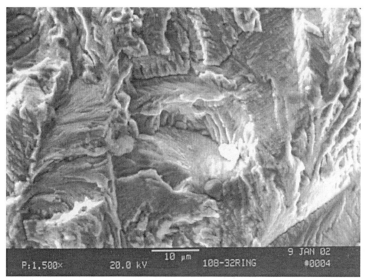

Figure 6c - *SEM micrograph showing terraces with feather marks on the fracture surface of alloy A near crack initiation (Fatigue in Ringer's solution).*

Due to the large number of samples required and thus the overwhelming machine time to statistically compare the fatigue of the three alloys, especially when testing at the recommended 1 hz, the initial testing regimen using three samples at each load level as described by ASTM F1801 was followed. Of significant interest is the comparison of the S/N curves between alloys in each of the two test solutions (Figures 2 and 3). These results show that in both Ringer's solution and distilled/de-ionized water the number of cycles to fracture at a given stress value are greater for the two nitrogen strengthened alloys as compared to alloy B. However, whilethere is a difference, it is not as great as anticipated in light of the much greater yield strength of alloy A (1179 MPa) and alloy C (1082 MPa) as compared to that of alloy B (793 MPa) and results reported elsewhere [21,22]. Because the differences seen between the fatigue curves of alloy A and alloy C are slight, they may or may not be seen if the testing were repeated using the same alloys from different lots with essentially identical properties. Information taken from the Carpenter data sheets as well as other sources indicates that an increase in fatigue strength is not necessarily proportional to the increase in tensile and yield strength especially in these nitrogen strengthened stainless steels which have been cold worked to achieve even higher strength values. It has been our observation that even though alloy A has high elongation to fracture, especially for material that has been highly cold worked to achieve high strength, the work hardening rate during deformation is very high and the amount of work hardening to fracture is also high. The work hardening rate and increase in tensile strength properties for the same percentage of cold working, including both yield strength and ultimate tensile strength, of the two nitrogen strengthened alloys is significantly greater than that of alloy B [32]. Through discussions with LSG and machinists' fabricating fixtures, as well as Carpenter, we have learned that alloy A cold works even more rapidly than does alloy C and much more rapidly than does alloy B. This phenomenon significantly increases the care required during machining of the material. However, these observations are even more significant in explaining the results of the fatigue data. Since fatigue cracks initiate and propagate due to applied or resolved tensile stresses, and the tensile stress is additive to any residual tensile stresses, any test regimen that continues to apply tensile stress and cold work the material in tension should result in increased fatigue damage (crack initiation and propagation). Because the nitrogen strengthened alloys are especially susceptible to cold working, cycling in a tension-tension mode could accelerate fatigue as compared to alternating tension and compression. If the material were not so highly cold worked, the relative fatigue strength to the yield strength might be increased. Even though the samples that were evaluated during the research reported here were prepared using low stress grinding procedures, the susceptibility of alloy A to very rapid cold working could, at least in part, contribute to the slightly lower than anticipated fatigue strength. If the surfaces were prepared with compressive residual stresses, the addition of applied tensile stresses should not result in as great a total tensile stress during loading. Previous unreported research in our laboratories comparing the bending fatigue of 316LS and 22Cr-13Ni-5Mn hip screw plates with a variety of surface finishes including shot peening and electro-polishing indicates improved fatigue properties of plates that are shot peened. Additionally, preliminary results of ongoing research related to fatigue testing of fracture fixation devices of alloy A indicates that surface treatment such as shot peening, which increases compressive residual stress, results in significantly greater fatigue strengths than expected from the results obtained during this study. Further research is also underway to examine the fatigue behavior and endurance limit of alloy A which has only been cold worked to achieve strength values in the range of those of alloy B evaluated during this project.

The results, comparing the fatigue of all three alloys in the two media (Figures 2 and 3), corroborate the results reported by others concerning the effect of NaCl containing solutions on the reduction of the number of cycles to fracture at a given stress value. The effect of NaCl containing solutions on the fatigue of the two nitrogen strengthened alloys might be even more clearly delineated if the endurance limits were statistically evaluated using the 'two point method' [33]. The use of NaCl solutions results in a negative displacement of the entire fatigue curve of austenitic stainless steels [11,22]. The consistency of the trend in the affect on the fatigue performance in the two different test solutions on each of the alloys is to be expected because the crystalline structure and mechanism of resistance to corrosion (passivation by Cr-O production) is the same for all three alloys. Additionally, little difference in the corrosion characteristics of the three alloys but especially the two nitrogen strengthened alloys (alloys A and C) occurs within the testing parameters of this experiment and as documented by other research [29].

It is well understood that fatigue is a brittle rather than ductile fracture mode, and that Stage II fatigue crack propagation of austenitic stainless steels generally exhibits a striation type of morphology when fatigue occurs at strain rates and temperatures in the range of those imposed here. Deformation that includes terraces, flutes and furrowing is often attributed to a more brittle fracture or fatigue of nitrogen strengthened austenitic stainless steels [34] at low temperatures or fracture of metals with far fewer slip systems such as titanium, especially when a complex state of stress is present [17]. Because this type of morphology is only present in the samples of alloy A and not present in the fatigued samples of alloy C, which is also nitrogen strengthened, it is hypothesized that this type of fatigue fracture morphology may be as a result of the cold working behavior of alloy A as previously described. Cold working during manufacturing as well as during the testing could lead to pinning of dislocations, especially due to the presence of a high concentration of nitrogen interstitials in the FCC lattice. This phenomenon could lead to a more brittle type of fracture, especially in areas where the material has experienced significant cold working creating localized high intensity stress fields or where the tensile stresses have been built up prior to crack initiation. These observations on the fracture surfaces reinforce the previous conclusions made concerning the trends observed in the S/N curves.

In conclusion, the results reported here indicate that based upon the fatigue performance, alloy A is a candidate for applications where 316LS or 22Cr-13Ni-5Mn stainless steel have been used previously. This alloy could be especially useful as an implant material for devices subjected to higher loading, especially if the hypothesis concerning the effects of compressive residual stress and the ability of altering the surface to increase the fatigue strength are accurate. The effects of surface treatments such as shot peening and electro-polishing, which removes areas of high surface tensile stress concentration, should serve to improve the fatigue characteristics of devices produced from this alloy.

Acknowledgment

This research supported by a grant from Carpenter Technology Corporation.

References

[1]   Cahoon, J.R., Paxton, H.W., "Metallurgical Analyses of Failed Orthopedic Implants," *Journal Of Biomedical Materials Research*, Vol. 2, 1968, pp.1-22.

[2]   Colangelo, V.J., "Corrosion Fatigue in Surgical Implants," *Journal of Basic Engineering*, December 1969, pp. 581-586.

[3]   Dumbleton, John H., Miller, Edward H., "Failures of Metallic Orthopaedic Implants," *Metals Handbook 8th Edition*, Howard E. Boyer, Ed., American Society for Metals, Vol. 10, 1975.

[4]   Gray, R.J. "Metallographic Examinations of Retrieved Intramedullary Bone Pins and Bone Screws from the Human Body," *Journal of Biomedical Materials Research Symposium*, No. 5, John Wiley & Sons, Inc., New York, 1974, pp. 27-38.

[5]   Gray, R.J., "Metallographic Examinations of Retrieved Intramedullary Bone Pins and Bone Screws from the Human Body," Report No. ORNLTM4068, Oak Ridge National Laboratory, Tennessee, U.S. Department of Commerce, National Technical Information Service, February 1973.

[6]   Hughes, A.N., Jordan, B.A., "Metallurgical Observations on Some Metallic Surgical Implants Which Failed in Vivo," *Journal of Biomedical Materials*, Vol. 6, 1972, pp. 33-48.

[7]   Sloter, L.E., Piehler, H.R., "Corrosion-Fatigue Performance of Stainless Steel Hip
      Nails - Jewett Type," *Corrosion and Degradation of Implant Materials, ASTM STP
      684*, B.C. Syrett and A. Acharya, Eds., American Society for Testing and Materials,
      1979, pp. 173-195.
[8]   Weinstein, A., Amstutz, H., Pavon, G., Franceschini, V., "Orthopedic Implants - A
      Clinical and Metallurgical Analysis," *Journal of Biomedical Materials Research
      Symposium*, No. 4, John Wiley & Sons, Inc., 1973, pp. 297-325.
[9]   Cahoon, J.R., Paxton, H.W., "A Metallurgical Survey of Current Orthopedic
      Implants," *Journal Of Biomedical Materials Research*, Vol. 4, 1970, pp. 223-244.
[10] Imam, M.A., Fraker, A.C., Gilmore, C.M., "Corrosion Fatigue of 316L Stainless Steel,
      Co-Cr-Mo Alloy, and ELI Ti-6AI-4V," *Corrosion and Degradation of Implant
      Materials, ASTM STP 684*, B.C. Syrett and A. Acharya, Eds., American Society for
      Testing and Materials, 1979, pp. 128-143.
[11] Pohler, O.E.M., Straumann, F., "Fatigue and Corrosion Fatigue Studies on Stainless-
      Steel Implant Material," *Evaluation of Biomaterials*, G.D. Winter, J.L. Leray, K. de
      Groot, Eds., John Wiley & Sons, Inc., 1980, pp. 89-113.
[12] Brantina, W.J., Young, S.B., Yue, S., Morgan, M.J., Pilliar, R.M., Wallace, A.C.,
      "Fatigue Deformation and Fractographic Analysis of Surgical Implants and Implant
      Materials," *Proceedings of the International Conference and Exhibits on Failure
      Analysis*, Montreal, Quebec, Canada, July 8-11, 1991, pp. 299-310.
[13] Brunner, H., Simpson, J.P., "Fatigue Fracture of Bone Plates," *Injury: the British
      Journal of Accident Surgery* Vol.11, No.3, pp. 203-207.
[14] Pohler, O.E.M, Straumann, I., "Failures of Metallic Orthopedic Implants,"*Metals
      Handbook 9th Edition*, American Society for Metals, Vol. 11, 1986.
[15] Sivakumar, M., Dhanadurai,K., Rajeswari, S., Thulasiraman, V., "Failures in Stainless
      Steel Orthopaedic Implant Devices: A Survey," *Journal of Materials Science Letters*,
      Vol. 4, Chapman & Hall, 1995, pp. 351-354.
[16] Zardiackas, Lyle D., Black, R. John, Hughes, James L., Reeves, R. Bradley, Jun, J.N.,
      "Metallurgical Evaluation of Retrieved Implants and Correlation of Failures to Patient
      Record Data," *Orthopedics*, Vol. 12, No. 1, January 1989, pp. 85-92.
[17] Zardiackas, Lyle D., Dillon, Lance D., "Failure Analysis of Metallic Orthopedic
      Devices," *Encyclopedic Handbook of Biomaterials and Bioengineering*, Part B:
      Applications, Vol. 1, Donald L. Wise, Debra J. Trantolo, David E. Altobelli, Michael
      J. Yaszemski, Joseph D. Gresser, Edith R. Schwartz, Eds., 1995, pp. 123-170.
[18] Nakajima, M., Akatsuka, Y., Tokaji, K., "Fatigue Crack Initiation and Growth of
      Stainless Steels in 3% NACL Solution," *Advances in Fracture Research*, Vols. 1-6,
      1997, pp. 1621-1628.
[19] Nakajima, M., Shimizu, T., Kanamori, T., Tokaji, K., "Fatigue Crack Growth
      Behaviour of Metallic Biomaterials in a Physiological Environment," *Fatigue &
      Fracture of Engineering Materials & Structures*, Vol. 21, Blackwell Science Ltd.,
      1998, pp. 35-45.
[20] Yu, J., Zhao, Z.J., Li, L.X., "Corrosion Fatigue Resistance of Surgical Implant
      Stainless Steels and Titanium Alloy," *Corrosion Science*, Vol, 35, Pergamon Press
      Ltd., Great Britain, 1993, pp. 587-597.
[21] Black, Jonathan, *Orthopaedic Biomaterials In Research and Practice*, 1988.

[22] Shetty, Ravi H. and Ottersberg, Walter H., "Metals in Orthopedic Surgery," *Encyclopedic Handbook of Biomaterials and Bioengineering*, Part B: Applications, Vol. 1, Donald L. Wise, Debra J. Trantolo, David E. Altobelli, Michael J. Yaszemski, Joseph D. Gresser, Edith R. Schwartz, Eds., 1995, pp. 509-540.

[23] Vieweg U., van Roost D., Wolf H.K., Schyma, C.A., Schramm, J. "Corrosion On Internal Spinal Fixator System," *Spine*, Vol. 24, 1999, pp. 946-951.

[24] Mofid M.N., Thompson, R.C., Pardo. C.A., Manson, P.N., Wander-Kolk, C.A., "Biocompatibility of Fixation Materials In the Brain," *Plastic Reconstruction Surgery*, Vol. 100, 1997, pp.14-21.

[25] Savarino, L., Stea, S., Granchi, D., Visentin, M., Ciapetti, G., Donati, M.E., Rollo, G., Zinghi, G., Pissoferrato, A., Montanaro, L., Toni, A., "Sister Chromatid Exchanges And Ion Release In Patients Wearing Fracture Fixation Devices," *Journal of Biomedical Material Research*, Vol. 50, 2000, pp. 21-26.

[26] Hensten-Pettersen, A., "Replacement of Restorations Based on Material Allergies," Quality Evaluation of Dental Restorations: Criteria for Placement and Replacement, Anusavice K.J., Ed., Quintessence Pub. Co., 1989, pp. 357-372.

[27] Kerosuo, H., Kullaa, A., Kerosuo, E., Kanerva, L., Hensten-Pettersen A., "Nickel Allergy In Adolescents In Relation To Orthodontic Treatment And Piercing Of Ears," *American Journal of Orthodontics and Dentofacial Orthopedic*, Vol. 109, 1996, pp. 148-154.

[28] Dobbs, H.S., Scales, J.T., "Corrosion Fatigue Testing of Metallic Implant Materials," *Medical Devices and Services, ASTM Vol. 13.01*, B.C. Syrett and A. Acharya, Eds., American Society for Testing and Materials, 1999, pp. 1289-1294.

[29] Zardiackas, L.D., Roach, M.D., Williamson, S., Bogan, J.A., "Comparison of Anodic Polarization And Galvanic Corrosion of a Low-Nickel Stainless Steel to 316L S.S. and 22Cr-13Ni-5Mn S.S.," *Stainless Steels for Medical and Surgical Applications, ASTM STP 1438*, G.L. Winters and M.J. Nutt, Eds., ASTM International, West Conshohocken, PA 2003.

[30] Zardiackas, L.D. Roach, M.D., Williamson, S., Bogan, J.A., "Comparison of Notch Sensitivity and SCC of a Low-Nickel Stainless Steel to 316L S.S. and 22Cr-13Ni-5Mn S.S.," *Stainless Steels for Medical and Surgical Applications, ASTM STP 1438*, G.L. Winters and M.J. Nutt, Eds., ASTM International, West Conshohocken, PA 2003.

[31] Powell, G.W., "Identification of Types of Failures," *Failure Analysis an Prevention*, ASM Handbook, Formerly 9th Edition, Metals Handbook, G.W. Powell and S.E. Mahmoud, Coordinators, 1986, pp. 75-81.

[32] Carpenter Technology "BioDur® and Other Specialty Alloys for Medical Applications," Reading, PA.

[33] Little, R.E., "Manual on Statistical Planning And Analysis For Fatigue Experiments," *ASTM STP 588*, American Society for Testing and Materials, Philadelphia, PA, 1975.

[34] Vogt, J.B., "Fatigue Properties of High Nitrogen Steels," *Journal of Materials Processing Technology*, Vol. 117, 2001, pp. 364-369.

Wear and Corrosion-Related Wear

Markus Windler,[1] Julie E. MacDougall,[2] and Rolf Schenk[2]

Investigation Into Wear-Induced Corrosion of Orthopaedic Implant Materials

---

Reference: Windler, M., MacDougall J. E., and Schenk, R., **"Investigation Into Wear-Induced Corrosion of Orthopaedic Implant Materials,"** *Stainless Steels for Medical and Surgical Applications, ASTM STP 1438*, G. L. Winters and M. J. Nutt, Eds., ASTM International, West Conshohocken, PA, 2003.

Abstract: The purpose of this study was to compare the corrosion behaviour under sliding wear of four materials commonly used for surgical implants: Ti-6Al-7Nb, Co-28Cr-6Mo, and two stainless steels, high-nitrogen stainless steel (Fe22Cr10NiN) and AISI 316L. A machine was constructed to simulate sliding wear, and the current density was measured to compare the response of each material to wear and to study the effect of pH (varied from 1 to 6). The results indicate that titanium exhibits higher current densities during wear than other materials tested over the pH range of 2.5 to 6. Additionally, pH has a greater effect on the corrosion behaviour of the two stainless steels than on the titanium or cobalt alloys.

Keywords: high nitrogen stainless steel, stainless steel, CoCr alloy, titanium alloy, corrosion behaviour, sliding wear, repassivation

Introduction

Currently, a major issue in orthopaedic implant design (e.g. hip or knee prosthesis) is wear of metallic components. Primarily, wear occurs on articulating surfaces, such as on the femoral head of total hip implant. In modular designs, the combination of different materials and components can promote micromotion between parts, which can result in

---

[1] Director materials research , Material Research Department, Sulzer Orthopedics Ltd., P.O. Box 65, 8404 Winterthur, Switzerland.

[2] Corrosion scientist and material engineer, respectively, Sulzer Innotec, Sulzer Markets and Technology AG, P.O. Box 414, 8401 Winterthur, Switzerland.

fretting wear and lead to crevice corrosion [1-4]. With cemented hip prostheses, loosening may occur at the cement/implant interface and can lead to wear of the stem component [5-7]. In addition, in total hip replacements, wear between articulating components causes scratching and polishing of the metal surfaces [8]. This phenomenon is well-known in hip prostheses especially in metal-on-metal articulations where both components are made of CoCr alloys [9]. Fretting corrosion can also take place in the connection between plates and screws [10].

In all such situations, the passive layer of the metal component is subject to degradation. If the passive layer is destroyed and bare metal exposed, leading to a rise in current density, the metal surface must repassivate to prevent corrosion of the material. If repassivation is inhibited in any way, severe corrosion can result, which can lead to the failure of the implant. Therefore, due to the importance of maintaining corrosion resistance in the body, characterizing wear of implant materials or, more specifically, testing for *wear-induced* corrosion of such materials is crucial. This is an area of implant material characterisation that has not been extensively researched to date.

The purpose of this study was to compare the corrosion behaviour *under sliding wear conditions* of four materials commonly used for surgical applications: Ti6Al7Nb, Co28Cr6Mo, and two stainless steels, Fe22Cr10NiN and 316L stainless steel. The corrosion behaviour was evaluated at different pH valued from ~1.0 to ~6.0 as low pH levels are present during crevice corrosion.

Materials and Procedures

Potentiodynamic testing (without wear) and potentiostatic testing (with wear) were used to characterize the corrosion behaviour of four implant materials: 316L stainless steel (ISO 5832-1E), Fe22Cr10NiN high-nitrogen stainless steel (ISO 5832-9), Co28Cr6Mo (ISO 5832-12), and Ti6Al7Nb (ISO 5832-11). All bar materials were in wrought and annealed conditions and had diameters from 20 to 22 mm. Each material was cut into cylindrical coupons. Each coupon was connected to an insulated copper wire and encased in a cold-curing resin (Technovit 4071, Kulzer GmbH, Wehrheim, Germany). Its surface was ground to 1200 grit specification. The reference electrode used in all experiments was the Standard Calomel Electrode (SCE) and all testing was conducted with N_2 gas bubbling.

Potentiodynamic Corrosion Tests (no wear)
In order to characterize the general corrosion behaviour of each material initially (breakthrough potential, passive current density, etc.), potentiodynamic testing was performed in the absence of wear (scan rate: 0.167 mV/s). A standard potentiodynamic corrosion cell (ASTM-G5) was used to measure the effects of pH and temperature (Potentiostat: Schmitzo AG, Switzerland, Software: CMS 100, Version 2.40a, Gamry Instruments Inc., Warminster, PA, USA). Electrolyte pH was varied from 1.2 to 6 at a constant temperature of 24°C: 0.15mol/L HCl at pH 1.2; 0.9% NaCl at pH 4 (pH adjusted with diluted HCl); and 0.9% NaCl at pH 6. The temperature was varied from 24°C to

60°C (Julabo HC5/2 water bath, Julabo Inc., Allentown, PA, USA) at a constant pH of 4. All the potentiodynamic corrosion experiments were performed using one specimen. The materials were also analyzed for correct chemical composition, physical properties, and microstructure before they were tested.

Potentiostatic Tests under Sliding Wear Condition

Potentiostatic testing was used to measure the passive current density produced during sliding wear. The samples were fixed in a PVC frame and placed in a basin filled with the same electrolytic solutions used in the potentiodynamic tests (Figure 1). A 1.5mm diameter alumina ceramic head was lowered onto the flat sample surface and the downward stress adjusted to 2.78 MPa using a specially designed spring-controlled loading system. The counter electrode was platinum wire. Potentiostatic scans were taken for each sample over the potential range of the passive region. Initially, the material was allowed to reach a constant passive current density (steady state). Sliding wear was then simulated by running the flat ceramic head back and forth over the material surface for an interval, allowing for repassivation between trials. Current density data was recorded every 10 seconds during the whole experiment. The horizontal movement and vertical position of the ceramic head were controlled by a motor-driven precision cross-table (Jacob AG, Switzerland). The length of the scratch was fixed at 7.5mm with linear potentiometers (LP-200F-5K, Midori Precisions, Japan) and the scratching speed set to 1.5 mm/s (DC-motor GNM 2145, Engel GmbH, Germany). The current-time data were recorded using CMS-100 software (Gamry Instruments Inc., USA).

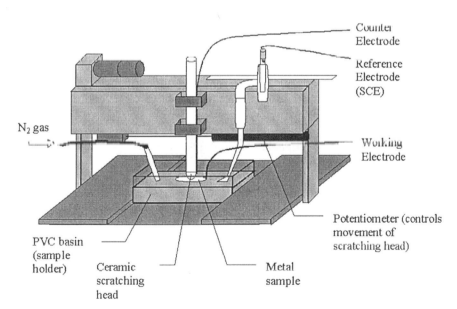

Figure 1 – *Custom made construction to study the corrosion behaviour during sliding wear condition*

The following tests were performed under sliding wear conditions:

Influence of Scratching Time

Only Ti6Al7Nb was tested at an applied potential of +100 mV and pH 4. Six different scratch times were introduced: 10 s, 30 s, 60 s, 300 s, 600 s, 1800 s. All tests were repeated twice.

Influence of Speed

All materials were tested at an applied potential of 0 mV, pH 4 for a scratch time of 2 minutes. Three different speed levels were used: 1.1 mm/s, 1.9 mm/s and 2.5 mm/s. All test were repeated twice.

Influence of pH

All materials were tested at three applied potentials of −100, 0 and +100 mV, each for a scratch time of 2 minutes. Four different pH levels: 0.15mol/L HCl at pH 1 and 0.9% NaCl at pH 2.5, pH 4, and pH 6 were tested, all tests were repeated twice. NOTE: In living tissue, at pH~7.4, the typical redox potential is ~0 mV$_{[SCE]}$ [11].

Results

Potentiodynamic Corrosion Tests (no wear)

From the potentiodynamic testing, it was found that Ti6Al7Nb exhibited the best overall corrosion resistance in terms of the breakdown potential (>1.5 V) at any pH level or temperature, followed by Fe22Cr10NiN, Co28Cr6Mo, and finally 316L stainless steel (Table 1 and 2). The values of passive current density showed a trend of increasing with a decreasing pH value. This trend was especially pronounced when the pH varied from 4.0 to 1.2 (the only exception was for Fe22Cr10NiN at pH 1.2).

It was found that all materials, particularly 316L stainless steel, were more sensitive to changes in pH than to changes in temperature. In fact, temperature had no significant effect on the corrosion behaviour of any material over the tested range (24°C-60°C). It has therefore been proposed that data collected from experiments carried out at room temperature are reasonable approximations of data generated at slightly higher temperatures (e.g. at 37°C – the average human body temperature).

The effect of pH was only predominant at very low pH values and the corrosion behaviour of the test materials did not vary significantly over the pH range of 4 to 6.

Table 1 – *Influence of Temperature on the Breakdown Potential (Eb) and Passive Current Density (PCD), measured at pH 4*

	Temperature [°C]	Eb [mV$_{(SCE)}$]	PCD [μA/cm^2]
316L	24°C	100	0.63
(ISO 5832-1E)	40°C	-40	0.44
	60°C	-100	0.63
Fe22Cr10NiN	24°C	1000	0.40
(ISO 5832-9)	40°C	1050	0.79
	60°C	1050	0.89
Co28Cr6Mo	24°C	620	0.63
(ISO 5832-12)	40°C	600	0.63
	60°C	550	0.67
Ti6Al7Nb	24°C	1500	0.79
(ISO 5832-11)	40°C	1700	0.84
	60°C	1650	0.99

Table 2 – *Influence of pH on the Breakdown Potential (Eb) and Passive Current Density (PCD), measured at 24°C*

	pH	Eb [mV$_{(SCE)}$]	PCD [μA/cm^2]
316L	1.2	-60	19.95
(ISO 5832-1E)	4.0	100	0.40
	6.3	160	0.38
Fe22Cr10NiN	1.2	840	0.45
(ISO 5832-9)	4.0	1000	0.63
	6.3	1000	0.56
Co28Cr6Mo	1.2	820	0.79
(ISO 5832-12)	4.0	620	0.63
	6.3	600	0.56
Ti6Al7Nb	1.2	2000	1.26
(ISO 5832-11)	4.0	1500	0.79
	6.3	1700	0.79

Potentiostatic Tests under Sliding Wear Condition

Figure 2 shows a typical potentiostatic scan taken of the material Fe22Cr10NiN (superimposed) at pH 4 and –200 mV. From this figure three different current densities can be identified: (1) the passive current density (PCD), which was the current density before the material was scratched, (2) I $_{peak}$, which was the maximum average current density, and (3) delta current density (Δ CD), which was the difference between I $_{peak}$ and passive current density. In this study the focus was on the delta current density (Δ CD), which was normalized on the total scratched area (T.S.A.) 7.5 mm x 1.5 mm.

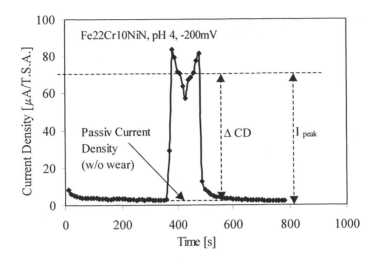

Figure 2 – *Typical potentiostatic scan of Fe22Cr10NiN at pH 4 and +100mV.*
NOTE: The current density is normalized to the total scratched area (T.S.A.) which is
7.5mm x 1.5mm = 11.25mm^2

Influence of Scratching Time

Figure 3 shows the influence of scratching time on Ti6Al7Nb. No difference could be demonstrated when varying the scratching time in steps from 10 seconds up to 30 minutes (1800 s). Only the standard deviation increased slightly from 14% (10 s) to 39% (1800 s).

Influence of Speed

Increased scratch speed resulted in an increase of delta current density (Table 3). This phenomenon could be observed with all materials except 316L stainless steel. It is hypothesized that, as the scratching speed increases, a larger amount of surface area of bare material is exposed at any given time. The data collected for 316L stainless steel did not follow the trend observed with the other materials. Other factors (e.g., pitting corrosion) might have influenced this result.

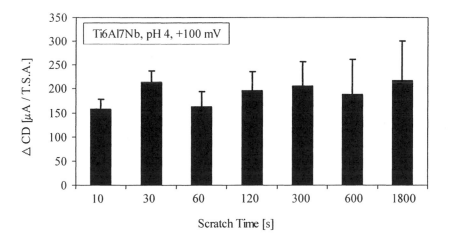

Figure 3 – *Influence of the scratching time on Ti6Al7Nb at pH 4 and applied potential of +100 mV*

Table 3 – *Influence of speed on the delta current density of all tested materials at pH 4 and applied potential of 0 mV*

Materials	Speed [mm/s]	Δ CD [μA / T.S.A.]
316L	1.1	194.4 ± 50.7
(ISO 5832-1E)	1.9	143.6 ± 22.3
	2.5	158.1 ± 19.9
Fe22Cr10NiN	1.1	54.6 ± 15.0
(ISO 5832-9)	1.9	84.0 ± 19.2
	2.5	132.4 ± 33.6
Co28Cr6Mo	1.1	77.9 ± 15.1
(ISO 5832-12)	1.9	143.6 ± 15.7
	2.5	164.8 ± 24.6
Ti6Al7Nb	1.1	111.6 ± 36.5
(ISO 5832-11)	1.9	184.2 ± 48.2
	2.5	217.3 ± 106.1

Influence of pH

Figure 4 shows the average change (Δ CD) in current density measured during sliding wear as a function of pH for all materials tested. The plotted values were calculated by averaging the current densities found over the potential range of –100mV to +100mV as listed in Table 4.

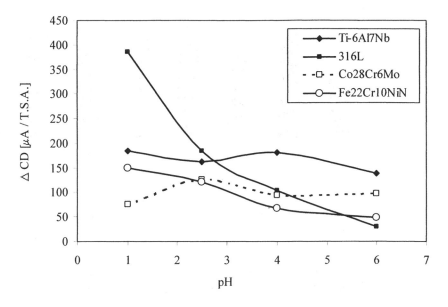

Figure 4 – *Delta current density (Δ CD) as a function of pH for all materials tested*

Potentiostatic testing under sliding wear demonstrated that, as in the potentiodynamic testing, 316L stainless steel was the most sensitive material to changes in pH. The most significant difference between non-wear (potentiodynamic) and sliding wear testing (potentiostatic) lies in the corrosion behaviour of Ti6Al7Nb. In the absence of wear, Ti6Al7Nb showed excellent corrosion behaviour, as quantified by a high breakdown potential and a passive current density on the same order as those of other materials tested. However, Ti6Al7Nb showed extremely high values of current density when placed under wear, indicating that the material requires more energy to repassivate and will corrode faster if subjected to wear. Although, in the absence of wear, Ti6Al7Nb showed slightly higher relative passive current densities (25% more than Fe22Cr10NiN and Co28Cr6Mo, see Table 1), the current density recorded for Ti6Al7Nb during wear was *200% to 300%* (see Table 4) larger than those found for the other materials tested.

From Figure 4, it is evident that the corrosion resistant behaviour of 316L stainless steel is highly dependent on pH. At pH 6, the material exhibits excellent corrosion resistance under wear; the average ΔCD measured at pH 6 for 316L stainless steel (30 μA/T.S.A.) was well below those measured for the other materials. However, as pH is decreased to 1, the average current density gradually increases and eventually surpasses those of other materials, with an increase of more than 12 times in ΔCD. This indicates that, at low pH, 316L stainless steel performs very poorly against wear-induced corrosion.

Contrarily, the cobalt and titanium alloys showed very little dependence on pH. Although there is some fluctuation in the results, no definite trend is seen to suggest that pH has a large effect on the potentiostatic behaviour of these materials under sliding wear conditions.

Table 4 – *Delta current density (Δ CD) as a function of pH for all tested materials*

Materials	[mV$_{(SCE)}$]	Δ CD @ pH 6	Δ CD @ pH 4	Δ CD @ pH 2.5	Δ CD @ pH 1
	-100	174.6 ± 83.7	153.1 ± 33.5	157.2 ± 62.3	152.5 ± 47.5
	0	139.4 ± 41.0	205.6 ± 65.3	177.6 ± 42.2	168.6 ± 49.3
	100	133.9 ± 29.2	185.5 ± 46.3	151.7 ± 69.2	232.1 ± 138.8
Ti6Al7Nb	Mean	**139.0 ± 45.2**	**181.4 ± 53.9**	**161.8 ± 60.0**	**184.2 ± 94.7**
	-100	78.0 ± 11.2	92.6 ± 13.5	137.4 ± 15.5	39.2 ± 7.3
	0	102.0 ± 14.8	95.1 ± 9.4	112.3 ± 17.4	66.0 ± 20.5
	100	112.1 ± 8.7	96.7 ± 13.0	128.0 ± 12.5	119.6 ± 8.9
Co28Cr6Mo	Mean	**97.9 ± 18.3**	**94.9 ± 12.1**	**125.7 ± 18.2**	**76.2 ± 36.5**
	-100	46.8 ± 5.7	65.1 ± 11.2	101.3 ± 6.2	168.2 ± 13.3
	0	44.3 ± 13.7	67.6 ± 12.5	141.7 ± 9.6	147.6 ± 9.1
	100	55.4 ± 9.6	69.1 ± 13.5	121.6 ± 10.3	135.3 ± 6.2
Fe22Cr10NiN	Mean	**49.0 ± 11.0**	**67.3 ± 12.3**	**121.5 ± 21.9**	**150.0 ± 16.7**
	-100	27.6 ± 5.1	98.8 ± 13.8	190.1 ± 6.9	378.25 ± 49.7
	0	33.1 ± 7.1	100.6 ± 5.5	177.8 ± 15.1	391.9 ± 17.8
	100	31.3 ± 6.2	120.7 + 16.4	n.m.	n.m.
316L	Mean	**30.6 ± 6.6**	**103.9 ± 14.5**	**183.7 ± 13.3**	**384.8 ± 38.3**

NOTE: n.m. = not possible to be measured because pitting corrosion stated

As the pH is lowered from 6 to 1, Fe22Cr10NiN shows a slight, but steady, increase in the values found for the average ΔCD (300%); still, the increases are much smaller than those found for 316L stainless steel. More important, however, is the fact that Fe22Cr10NiN shows the best overall resistance to wear-induced corrosion over the pH range of 2.5 to 6. Therefore, even though it is more sensitive to changes in pH than the cobalt or titanium alloys, Fe22Cr10NiN produces the lowest values of current density over the pH range of 2.5 to 6 and is surpassed only by the cobalt alloy at low pH.

Thus, as seen from Figure 4, the titanium alloy generally showed the highest change and Fe22Cr10NiN generally showed the smallest change in current density during wear of all materials tested at any pH. The two exceptions to this statement occured at low pH where (1) the ΔCD of 316L stainless steel surpassed that of Ti6Al7Nb and (2) the cobalt alloy behaved slightly better than Fe22Cr10NiN.

Discussion and Conclusion

The primary aim of this study was to damage mechanically the passive oxide layer of four materials by sliding wear and to measure the repassivation current transients generated during the redevelopment of the passive film. A secondary goal was to investigate the effects of scratch time, scratch speed, and pH on the current density generated during sliding wear.

Initially, potentiodynamic testing and material characterization were performed on all implant metals in order to obtain a reference set of corrosion data, which could be compared with data collected during sliding wear. From the results outlined in this report, one of the most important results to note is that the titanium alloy (Ti6Al7Nb), on average, corrodes at a significantly higher rate during wear than all other materials tested over the potential range of −100mV to +100 mV, despite its excellent corrosion resistance in the absence of wear. Secondly, pH does not greatly affect the wear-induced corrosion behaviour of Co28Cr6Mo or Ti6Al7Nb, but does significantly affect that of 316L stainless steel and, to a lesser extent, that of Fe22Cr10NiN.

The current generated during repassivation of any metal is due to at least three factors: the disruption and rebuilding of the double layer, the passive oxide film regeneration, and the ionic dissolution of soluble ionic species [12]. However, Gilbert et al. proposed that approximately 80% of the total current generated is due solely to the oxide film regeneration [12]. Therefore, it can be assumed that the current densities measured in this study are largely associated with the regeneration of the oxide film. Gilbert et al. [12] reported values of I_{peak} of 13 to 27 A/cm^2 for titanium using a similar testing method to the one employed in our series or testing, except with high speed scratching (90μm scratches in 0.5 to 1.0 ms). It should be noted that, in our study, the entire scratched surface (7.5mm x 1.5mm) was used to calculate the current densities; this is an incorrect assumption, for the actual activated area at any given time is considerably smaller. This explains the discrepancy between the two sets of results; Gilbert et al. used an extremely small area to calculate the current densities, which more closely approximate the actual activated surface area at any given time.

It is proposed that the poor performance of Ti6Al7Nb during wear is due to two factors: (1) The freshly formed titanium oxide layer is relatively softer than those of the other materials tested and is more easily destroyed by mechanical wear; and (2) higher current densities are generated during wear because of the four valence electrons needed to reform the titanium oxide passive layer (mostly made up of TiO$_2$). Titanium is known for its high corrosion resistance, due to relatively fast regeneration of the passive layer and its subsequent thickening over time. However, if the passive oxide is fractured or abraded at a frequency that is greater than its ability to repassivate fully, severe corrosion of titanium is a definite possibility. Thus, the results presented in this paper indicate that Ti6Al7Nb has the potential to corrode severely if placed under conditions of continual wear, particularly in the case where oxygen transport is inhibited.

One final point to note is that, at any given current density, the rate of titanium material loss is less than that of other materials studied, due to its low density and four valence electrons count. Therefore, although the current densities recorded for titanium during wear are significantly higher than those found for other materials, the impact on the corresponding wear rate is not as great as the measured current densities would suggest. However, the difference in current densities measured is large enough that the material loss of Ti6Al7Nb is still greater than both Fe22Cr10NiN and Co28Cr6Mo at any pH.

References

[1]   Willert, H.-G., Brobäck, L.-G., Buchhorn, G.H., Jensen, P.H., Köster, G., Lang, I., Ochsner, P., and Schenk, R., "Crevice Corrosion of Cemented Titanium Alloy Stems in Total Hip Replacements," *Clinical Orthopaedics and Related Research*, No. 333, 1996, pp. 51-75.

[2]   Gilbert, J.L., Buckley, C.A., and Jacobs J.J., "In Vivo Corrosion of Modular Hip Prosthesis Components in Mixed and Similar Metal Combinations. The Effect of Crevice, Stress, Motion, and Alloy Coupling," *J. Biomedical Materials Research*, Vol. 27, 1993, pp.1533-1544.

[3]   Brown, S.A., Flemming, C.A.C., Kawalec, J.S., Placko, H.E., Vassaux, C., Merritt, K., Payer, J.H., and Kraay, M.J., "Fretting Corrosion Accelerates Crevice Corrosion of Modular Hip Tapers," *J. Applied Biomate*rials, Vol. 6, 1995, pp. 19-26.

[4]   McKellop, H.A., Sarmiento, A., Brien, W., Park, S.H., "Interface Corrosion of a Modular Head Total Hip Prosthesis," *J. Arthroplasty*, Vol. 7, 1992, pp. 291-294.

[5]   Verdonschot, N., and Huiskes, R., "Mechanical Effects of Stem Cement Interface Characteristics in Total Hip Replacement," *Clinical Orthopaedics and Related Research*, No. 329, 1996, pp. 326-336.

[6]   Wimmer, M.A., Bluhm, A., Kunze, J., Heckel, L., Morlock, M.M., and Schneider, E., "Fretting Wear of Titanium and Cobalt-Chromium Alloys against Bone-Cement," *Proceedings of 44th Annual Meeting of the Orthopaedic Research Society*, New Orleans, March 1998, p. 353.

[7]   Rabbe, L.M., Rieu, J., Lopez, A., and Combrade, P., "Fretting Deterioration of Orthopaedic Implant Materials: Search for solutions," *Clinical Materials*, 15, 1994, pp. 221-226.

[8]   Hirakawa, K., Bauer, T.W., Stulberg, B.N., Wilde, A.H., and Secic, M, "Characterisation and Comparison of Wear Debris from Failed Total Hip Implants of Different Types," *J. Bone and Joint Surg*ery, Vol. 78A, 1996, pp. 1235-1243.

[9]   Rieker, C., Shen, M., and Köttig, P., "In-Vivo Tribological Performance of 177 Metal-on-Metal Hip Articulations," *World Tribology Forum in Arthroplasty*, C. Rieker, S. Oberholzer and U. Wyss, Eds., Huber Verlag, Bern, 2001, pp. 137-142.

[10]   Brown, S.A., and Merritt, K., "Fretting Corrosion of Plates and Screws: An In Vitro Test Method," *Corrosion and Degradation of Implant Materials*, ASTM STP 859, A.C. Fraker and C.D. Griffin, Eds., ASTM International, West Conshohocken, PA, 1985, pp. 117–135.

[11]   Steinemann, S.G., "Corrosion of Implant Alloys," *Technical Principles, Design and Safety of Joint Implants,* G.H. Buchhorn and H.G. Willert, Eds., Hogrefe & Huber Publishers, 1994, pp. 168-179.

[12]   Gilbert, J.L., Buckley, C.A., and Lautenschlager, E.P., "Titanium Oxide Film Fracture and Repassivation: The Effect of Potential, pH and Aeration," *Medical Applications of Titanium and Its Alloys: The Material and Biological Issues*, ASTM STP 1272, S.A. Brown and J.E. Lemons, Eds., Philadelphia, 1996, pp. 199–215.

Dieter Wirz[1], Bruno Zurfluh[2], Beat Göpfert[3], Feng Li[4], Willi Frick[5] and Erwin W. Morscher[6]

Results of in Vitro Studies about the Mechanism of Wear in the Stem-Cement Interface of THR

Reference: Wirz, D., Zurfluh, B., Göpfert, B., Li, F., Frick, W. and Morscher, E. W., " Results of in Vitro Studies about the Mechanism of Wear in the Stem-Cement Interface of THR," *Stainless Steels for Medical and Surgical Applications, ASTM STP 1438*, G. L. Winters and M. J. Nutt, Eds., ASTM International, West Conshohocken, PA, 2003.

Abstract: Experiments were performed in a wear machine especially constructed to simulate the natural in vivo process of wear in a de-bonded metal-cement interface. Four different bone cements were fretted against S-30 stainless steel with mat surface finish. The validation of the metal surfaces of the in vitro experiments revealed excellent correspondence to examined retrieved hip stems. No scratches or fretting orientation was noted on the polished surfaces. ZrO_2 particles did not play a decisive role in the wear mechanism. PMMA as a softer material than S-30 steel did not mechanically abrade the metallic surface. Further no steel particles could be found within the wear debris. Metal is removed by dissolution in a process of fretting and crevice corrosion. Fretting corrosion causes the formation of debris in the form of a mixture of particles of metallic oxides (but not metallic particles!), polymer and serum.

Keywords: Arthroplasty; Biomechanics; Bone Resorption; Corrosion, Crevice; Corrosion, Fretting; Foreign-Body Reaction; Hip Prosthesis; Macrophages; Metals; Microscopy, Electron; Middle Age; Particle Size; Polymethylmethacrylate; Steel, Stainless

---

[1] MD, Laboratory of Orthopaedic Biomechanics, University of Basel, Burgfelderstr. 101, CH-4012 Basel, Switzerland.

[2] PhD, Laboratory of Orthopaedic Biomechanics, University of Basel, Burgfelderstr. 101, CH-4012 Basel, Switzerland.

[3] BS Eng., Laboratory of Orthopaedic Biomechanics, University of Basel, Burgfelderstr. 101, CH-4012 Basel, Switzerland.

[4] MS Eng., Laboratory of Orthopaedic Biomechanics, University of Basel, Burgfelderstr. 101, CH-4012 Basel, Switzerland.

[5] PhD, Laboratory of Orthopaedic Biomechanics, University of Basel, Burgfelderstr. 101, CH-4012 Basel, Switzerland.

[6] Professor em., MD, Laboratory of Orthopaedic Biomechanics, University of Basel, Burgfelderstr. 101, CH-4012 Basel, Switzerland.

Introduction

The main problem of total hip replacement (THR) remains aseptic implant loosening due to osteolysis. The main mechanism of osteolysis appears to be enzymatic induced resorption of wear particles by macrophages. Wear particles are generated first in the articulation itself, especially through wear of polyethylene. However, wear particles can be generated at any interface of a THR, such as the implant-bone interface in non-cemented endoprostheses or the stem-cement interface in cemented ones. Wherever particles are generated they may be distributed in the "effective joint space" [1], thus leading to osteolysis.

Various clinical observations showed the importance of the stem-cement interface as a place where osteolysis has its source.

The tapered Exeter stem, an Fe-alloy (FeCrNiMnMo) device was introduced into clinical practice in 1970 with a smooth surface. Between 1976 and 1980 this stem was provided with a mat surface. As a consequence of the change of the surface an increased rate of aseptic loosening of this stem was observed. Since 1986, the Exeter has a smooth polished surface [2,3].The superiority of the polished version of the Exeter stem over the mat one has been confirmed by Howie et al.[4] and the Swedish Implant Register [5].

The Müller Straight Stem, introduced in clinical practice in 1977, originally was made of Protasul 10 (CoCr alloy) and stainless steel (AISI 316-L). From 1985 until 1994, it was manufactured of a titanium alloys including Ti6Al4V and Ti6Al7Nb. In the early nineties, several Swiss orthopedic institutions reported a high rate of early development of osteolysis with the cemented Müller Straight Stem manufactured from titanium alloy with mat surface, which led to early revisions [6]. The early development of osteolysis was unexpected, since several cemented titanium femoral stems were - and still are - on the market with excellent mid-term results: Céraver [7], Perfecta [8], Bicontact [9] etc. The poor results of the cemented Müller Titanium Straight Stem, however, could not be confirmed at our institution [10]. There are currently contrasting clinical results with the same type of cemented stem. While there was a high rate of aseptic loosening with revision rates of 12 % and 8 % in clinics A and B, the clinics C (our own institution) and D had revision rates of only 1.6 % and 1.5 %, respectively. These different results were achieved with exactly the same endoprosthesis and after about the same time interval of 6 - 8 years! In light of these results, it is obvious that when a significantly different number of osteolyses and revisions is observed in different institutions using the same endoprosthesis identical in design, surface, material, - some other variables must be considered as likely causes for the differences in osteolysis and revision rates. These variables, i.e., the reason for the above-mentioned, different results, may stem from a difference in bone cement, cementing technique, operative technique and/or surgeon. It is to be noted that all four clinics used modern cementing techniques, but clinics A and B, the ones with the poor results, used a different cement than clinics C and D. The logical conclusion, therefore, would be that bone cement does not equal bone cement! This statement was also convincingly made by the Swedish and the Norwegian Implant Registers [5,11-13]. From the Norwegian Implant Register of the year 2000, it became obvious that the bone cements Palacos and Simplex are superior to Sulfix 6 or Boneloc. The latter two have been withdrawn from the market in the meantime. The risk ratio with 95 % confidence interval are shown in the Swedish National Hip Register of the year 2000 [5] for all revisions, in all diagnoses, and aseptic loosening in osteoarthritis. The risk ratio, Sulfix 6 being the nominator (equals one) is 0.49 for Palacos- Gentamicin, 0.51 for Palacos, 0.60 for Simplex and 0.73 for CMW. An equally good outcome for the Palacos cement is given by the Norwegian Implant Register [11-13]. This register also indicated that bone cement has a greater influence on the outcome of a THR than the prosthesis itself!

From these clinical observations, we conclude that a verdict on a total hip replacement component should never be made in an uni-dimensional way, in other words, not without assessment of the whole system. In any case, the design, the surface characteristics, the material, the quality, and the operative the cementing technique, must be considered.

The significant difference in clinical outcomes of THRs with different bone cements was also unexpected, because the results of the preclinical test methods of bone cements did not reveal such important differences [14]. The question, therefore, arises: Are current testing methods adequate to assess bone cements? Mechanical testing of different brands of bone cement in compression, tension or bending alone did not reveal any significant differences. There is no evidence that bone cement with higher compressive and tensile strengths improves the clinical longevity of the cement mantle. In contrast to static test methods, dynamic fatigue testing has proven to be a more relevant test method in the laboratory. Significant differences with regard to the quality of bone cements in terms of survival rates, in accordance with the results of the Swedish and the Norwegian Implant Register, were found by Harper and Bonfield [15] with a dynamic fatigue testing method. On the other hand, Hopf and Fritsch/Germany [16,17] demonstrated convincingly that the application of the Wöhler method [17] for testing the fatigue strength of PMMA is inadequate and misleading as polymers - such as PMMA - behave differently than metals. With the Wöhler method to measure fatigue strength of metals, a sample has to undergo a certain number of cycles at a defined bending moment without breaking. According to Wöhler, 3 - 5 million cycles are appropriate for the testing of metals. Hopf and Fritsch performed their fatigue tests up to a minimum of 20 million loading cycles if breakage of the polymer specimens did not occur [17]. They found a correspondence between the maximum number of loading cycles and the clinical results of bone cements. These tests convincingly show that failures of the cement mantle, i.e., breakage, may even occur a long time after implantation in contrary to failures of the (metallic) hip stem.

Wear particles - as mentioned earlier - are thought to be the cause of osteolysis and subsequent aseptic loosening of implants [18]. However, very little is known about the interaction of different bone cements with different prosthetic surface finishes when fretted, simulating a debonded stem/cement interface. Nothing is known about possible differences of bone cements under fretting. Different combinations of bone cement types and surfaces might hypothetically lead to different quantities of wear particles (bone cement and metal), thus explaining the variant clinical outcome with one type of prosthesis.

In order to learn more about the basic mechanisms of the generation of wear debris originating from the cement-stem interface, it was decided to perform wear studies in collaboration with the Research Department of Sulzer Orthopedics Ltd.

It was hypothesized that the amount of wear particles, their geometry and size after debonding in the cement-stem interface depends mainly on three factors:

1. ZrO_2 particles as x-ray additives in PMMA break off and then act as third body particles under wear conditions
2.   Bone cements with proven good clinical outcomes (for example Palacos) "generate" less wear debris(particles)
3.   The rougher the surface of the stem, the more cement is abraded and the more particles are generated.

The wear studies were focused first - as mentioned above - on the basic mechanism of the development of wear particles at the metal/cement interface. Secondly, it was attempted to examine why different cements behave differently under wear conditions. Thirdly, the role of the radio-opaque additives, i.e. ZrO_2 was assessed, and, finally, it was aimed at getting more insight into the impact of the surface finish of the implants. A basic hypothesis was that, the more wear debris are generated, i.e. abraded - both, from the metallic the cement surface - the more particles are produced.

In order to elucidate experimentally the wear mechanism at the metal/cement interface, the laboratory set-up has to be able to replicate the in vivo mechanisms of wear generation. The respective surfaces and the particles generated must then be studied and compared to the findings from retrieved loosened stems and bone cements fragments.

Material and Methods

In Vitro Simulation of the Wear Mechanism

For this purpose, a wear machine had to be designed and constructed. Simulating the natural fretting mechanisms at the stem/cement interface must take into account the materials fretting against each other, the conditions of the fretting surfaces, the pressure between the two surfaces facing each other, the amplitude of the two surfaces' movement and, last but not least, the direction of the (respective) movements. Movement can only occur when the two surfaces are physically separated from each other, i.e., when they are debonded. Once debonded, the direction of the wear motion depends on the direction of the forces and the geometry of the implants surface, i.e., the stress distribution from the stem to the cement mantle and vice versa. These forces (which are eventually also responsible for the loosening of the endoprosthesis stem) become effective in three dimensions during gait: in the horizontal plane as rotational forces, "moving" the stem into retroversion (1) and in the axial direction, as demonstrated by subsidence of the femoral stem (2). On the other hand, axial loading increases the stability of collarless tapered stems in the cement mantle. Finally, in the frontal plane, the forces are transmitted to the calcar and the stem is "moved" into varus (3). The stress distribution in a total hip replacement, therefore, is a complex combination of forces acting in all three dimensions. From the burnishing pattern on retrieved hip stems it is known that the interface micromotion is not uni-dimensional but rather consists of translational and rotational components. A potential migration and movement of the metal/cement surfaces against each other occurs in two dimensions, the rotation of the stem within the cement mantle being the most important one [19-21]. Simulating the "natural" loosening process in vitro, movements of the two surfaces fretting against each other must be multidimensional, respecting the alternating direction of forces between the prosthesis stem and the cement/bone complex.

The fretting machine, therefore, has to fulfill the following requirements: 1. two-dimensional movements, 2. simulation of subsidence by the superposition of a slow linear component to the cyclic loading, 3. variable amplitudes between 20 and 200 μm, 4. normal pressures up to 4 MPa, 5. fretting frequencies of about 1 Hz (the cyclical frequency is comparable to the average walking frequency of the human body), 6. a physiological environment using lubrication with calf serum, 7. body temperature of 37°C.

The fretting samples have a contact area of 10 x 10 mm. Frequency, temperature, amplitudes and pressure have to be measured and acquired by a computer over all the experiment.

Tests Performed

1.   Evaluation of the in vivo process of wear in the cement-stem interface: Surfaces of retrieved MS-30 stems with mat surface were compared with the surfaces of test specimens after fretting, both manufactured both manufactured of S-30 steel, a high nitrogen stainless steel (FeCrNiMnMo, ASTM F1586, ISO 5832-9). In addition, one sample was fretted with 1 Hz, over 1 million cycles in one direction (uni-dimensional). This test was performed in order to show the differences in polishing by uni- and multi-directional.
2.   The impact of ZrO2 particles on the fretting mechanism: PMMA samples either with or without ZrO_2 were fretted against S-30 stainless steel samples with a mat surface (Table 1).

Table 1 - *Fretting tests with PMMA alone (no ZrO_2) and Duracem 3 with ZrO_2 and Gentamicin (currently not on the market)against S-30 steel*

Components	Parameters	number of Tests (2 samples each)	total number of Samples
Pure PMMA without ZrO_2 / S-30 mat	100 μm, 1Hz, 1Million cycl., bi-dimensional	3	6
Duracem 3 with ZrO_2 and Gentamicin / S-30 mat	100 μm, 1Hz, 1Million cycl., bi-dimensional	3	6

3.   Differences of the outcome of wear experiments with different bone cements against S-30 mat surface: Three different bone cements were fretted against a mat S-30 surface (Table 2).
4.   The impact of longer fretting: 1 sample of S-30 with mat surface was fretted against Duracem 3 with Gentamicin and ZrO_2 for 5 million cycles.

Table 2 - *Fretting tests: 3 different bone cements against S-30 stainless steel*

Components	Parameters of movement	number of Tests (2 samples each)	total number of Samples
Duracem 3 with Gentamicin and ZrO₂ / S-30 mat	100 µm, 1Hz, 1Million cycl., bi-dimensional	3	6
Palacos R with Gentamicin and ZrO₂ / S-30 mat	100 µm, 1Hz, 1Million cycl., bi-dimensional	3	6
CMW 2000 and BaSO₄ / S-30 mat	100 µm, 1Hz, 1Million cycl., bi-dimensional	2	4

5.   The impact of high speed fretting at 5 Hz, over 0.5 million cycles, in order to account for the impact of heat to wear.

All tests where performed with sinusoid movements with a path of 0.1mm, either uni-directional or bi-directional with slightly different frequency, all mat specimen have a Ra value of 1.4 µm.

Evaluation of the Specimens

1.   Photo documentation of the surfaces before and after fretting.

2.   Scanning Electron Microscopy (Philips XL30 ESEM and Philips XL20, Philips Inc, Eindhoven NL) of the surfaces before and after fretting.

3.   Laserprofilometry with UBM Laser Surface Profilometer (UBM Corporation, Sunnyvale CA). The shape, the roughness and the reflecting power were examined before and after fretting. Mean, standard-deviation and graphs of the stainless steel sample's surface were performed.

4.   Measurement of weight loss because of fretting. The amount of debris worn off as determined by measuring the loss of weight of the samples using a Mettler AT 261 Delta Range scale (Mettler-Toledo Inc., Greifensee, Switzerland) with a precision of ± 0.01mg.

Results:

The photographs and the SEM pictures of fretted, mat S-30 stainless steel surfaces correspond well with the appearance of in vivo retrieved stems with the same original surface. They both revealed no distinct direction of scratches, indicating that the polishing of a mat metal surface is caused rather by multi- than by uni-directional movements (Figure 1).

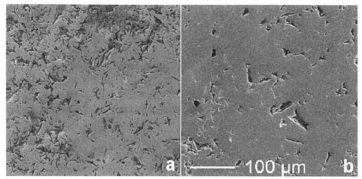

Figure 1 - *Comparison of the surface of a mat S-30 sample after 5 million wear cycles in laboratory simulation (a) and a femoral MS-30 stem retrieved for aseptic loosening 50 months postop. (b). During wear against bone cement, the S-30 surface lost its roughness resulting in a surface with polished areas and isolated 'valleys'.*

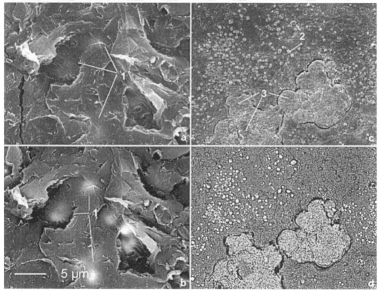

Figure 2 - *Surface of PMMA-bone cement samples before (left) and after fretting (right). a: ZrO₂ particles totally embedded in PMMA, b: in Back Scattering Electron technique (BSE) shining through. c: Surface of PMMA bone cement sample after fretting of 1 million cycles against sand blasted surface of S-30 steel in SEM technique and d: in BSE technique. 1: Clusters of ZrO₂ particles, in (a, b) wholly embedded in PMMA visible on the surface and partially abraded in (c, d). 2: Debris consists in a mixture of PMMA debris, 3: ZrO₂ particles and bovine serum building a sludge covering the surface partially.*

At the end of the fretting tests, very small particles (< 0.5 µm) which could be identified as Zr-oxide were detected within the sludge on the abraided cement surface (Figure 2).

ZrO$_2$ in the pre-polymerized stage is found in clusters of 5 to 30 µm. Apparently, the larger Zr-oxide conglomerates are broken up into very small particles.

Laser profilometry showed non significant differences only in the polishing effect of bone cement with or without the X-ray additive ZrO$_2$. The Ra-values of the S-30 samples fretted against pure PMMA without ZrO$_2$ are reduced by 7.7 ± 12%, the ones fretted against Duracem 3 with Gentamicin (with ZrO$_2$) by 15 ± 21% compared to the original surface before fretting.

Figure 3 shows the number of measured points with a reflection of more than 60% on the surface of the matte S-30 steel samples. Surprisingly - and in contrast to our hypothesis that a "good cement" reveals less wear - Palacos R (clinically proven as bone cement with the best performance[5,11-13]) produced even more reflection and, therefore, revealed a higher polishing effect on the mat stem surface than other bone cements as determined by laser profilometry. This finding is significant (Figure 3). The percentage of light reflection can be taken as a measure of polish. Ra measurements revealed the highest roughness reduction by Palacos too.

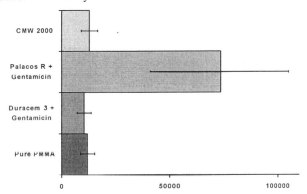

Figure 3 – *Number of measured Points with a reflection of more than 60% on the surface of the matte S-30 steel samples after fretting against four different bone cements (1 million cycles, 4 MPa pressure, two-dimensional fretting 100µm). No significant difference can be found for Duracem 3 (with Gentamicin and ZrO$_2$) and pure PMMA (without ZrO$_2$). ZrO$_2$ has no special polishing effect to a S-30 steel surface.*
Note the significantly higher polishing of S-30 steel after fretting against Palacos R (with Gentamicin and ZrO$_2$)!

The weight loss of bone cement when fretting CMW 2000 (-19.78 ± 12.59 mg) against mat S-30 (-0.40 ± 0.24 mg) is about 50 times larger than the metal loss. In the case of pure PMMA (-5.02 ± 2.41 mg), Duracem 3 with ZrO$_2$ and Gentamicin (-0.56 ± 2.02 mg) and Palacos R with Gentamicin (-4.87 ± 4.15 mg), this ratio is much smaller.

Palacos apparently removed less S-30-material from the mat S-30 surface than pure PMMA or Duracem 3, and the same amount as CMW 2000. The difference, however, is not significant. (Figure 4)

Furthermore, the only fretting particles detected in the sludge were identified as ZrO_2 particles. No steel particles from the S-30 alloy could be found! The ZrO_2 particles, however , were smaller than 0.2 μm, and, therefore much smaller than the original particles seen in the PMMA before fretting. In other words Zr-Oxide particles were mechanically broken up by the fretting process.

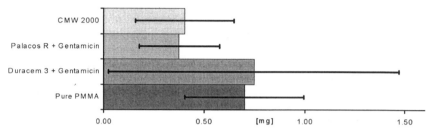

Figure 4 – *Weight loss of the mat S-30 steel samples after fretting against four different bone cements (1 million cycles, 4 MPa pressure, two-dimensional fretting 100μm).*

Discussion

The presented experiments are the first published data about the mechanism of wear in the metal-cement interface of cemented total hip replacements based on in vitro with multi-directional, i.e. relevant movements. The experiments were performed in a wear machine designed to replicate the natural in vivo process of wear at a debonded metal-cement interface. The validation of the metal surfaces of the in vitro experiments revealed excellent correspondence with examined retrieved hip stems. No scratches or fretting orientation on the polished surfaces does occur, in contrast to uni-directional wear experiments with larger fretting paths done by others [22-26].

Fretting a S-30 mat surface against bone cement results: 1. In a loss of weight and decrease of roughness through "removal" of the tops of the asperities. 2. In a more polished and more reflecting surface. This increase of reflection is not due to "valleys" filled with PMMA debris but due to an increase amount of polished surface by the fretting process and polishing the "peaks" of the rough surface. 3. In a progressive filling of the "valleys" between the asperities with PMMA debris as the wear process is going on. The abraded metal cannot be identified as particles within the wear debris, apparently it is dissolved.

The respective measurement of the Ra-value of the S-30 stainless steel surface with Laserprofilometry revealed only a slightly higher reduction of the roughness after fretting against PMMA with ZrO_2 than against PMMA without ZrO_2. Thus it must be concluded that the X-ray additive ZrO_2 does not play a significant role in the process of wear generation and for the development of osteolyses. This is in contrast to the tests performed by Cooper et al. showing an increased abrasion due to ZrO_2 [27]. In pin on disk fretting experiments, neither fretting- nor crevice- corrosion takes place. Further, ZrO_2 conglomerates of a size of 5 to 30 µm are pulverized into very small particles with a size of less than 0.2µm and particles of this size are supposed to be too small to induce enzymatic bone resorption [28].

Palacos - a clinically proven, good bone cement - has a significantly higher polishing effect. A more extensively polished surface is supposed to generate less wear debris by abrasion. On the other hand, Palacos produced the smallest loss of metal weight with fretting. This, however, was not significant.

By wearing S-30 stainless steel against pure PMMA the rough surface of the S-30 stainless steel is polished by removing material though pure PMMA contains no hard materials like ZrO2 that might abrade and polish the surface mechanically. Further, no S-30 particles could be found neither within the wear debris nor in the bovine serum. A different process than mechanical abraison of metal particles alone thus must be brought into consideration. This might be described as chemical dissolution of oxide layers in the process of fretting corrosion, or, under very specific conditions, even crevice corrosion in a strongly acidic, oxygen depleted medium [29].

Fretting corrosion causes the formation of debris in the form of a mixture of polymer, serum and metallic oxides (but not metallic particles!). Serum is rich in chlorides, promoting the process of corrosion. [29]. The metal dissolves, forms complexes with peptides or proteins or forms insoluble salt deposits as is the case on titanium surfaces [30]. Furthermore, oxygen depletion in confined pockets of serum enhances crevice corrosion.

According to these observations, we conclude that the differences in the quality of bone cements consist first of all in their capability to induce a process of fretting corrosion, which also greatly depends on the surface characteristics of the metal (roughness, nature of the oxide surface, material etc) [2].

CoCr alloys show a lower de-passivation pH-value, and thus show less corrosion in crevice conditions than alloys of austenitic stainless steel as e.g. S-30. It, therefore must be assumed that endoprosthetic femoral stems manufactured from CoCr-alloys reveal different fretting behaviour in the cement-stem interface than steel prostheses. On the other hand, clinical experience with polished steel prostheses has shown excellent long term results with extremely low incidence of osteolyses.

A complete cement mantle covering the tip of the stem, modern cementing technique used together with a clinically proven good bone cement avoid debonding of hip prosthesis stem with a mat surface. Such implants obtain good results, at least in the midterm [31]. Nevertheless, for tapered collarless femoral stems, the use of polished surfaces is recommended and the use of a mat surface should definitively be abandoned as subsidence within the cement mantle is no more considered with aseptic loosening of a prosthesis. If the stem is implanted in combination with an "open" centralizer, i.e. a centralizer designed in order to allow subsidence, the use of a mat surface has to be avoided.

Further wear studies fretting polished steel surfaces and CoCr alloys will have to show whether there is a potential for further improvement of results of cemented THR by improving implant surfaces and improving bone cements. For a specific endoprosthesis system the design, the implants surface, the materials and the operative, i.e., cementing technique must be considered as an entity. Most failures in endoprosthetics are the result of "improvements" based on conclusions from a mono-causal approach!

Progress in THR will continue, though we find ourselves already in the upper area of the asymptotic curve of the "margin revenue". Despite that, we can get even better results of THRs with better implant designs, better surfaces, better materials, including better bone cements, better operative, i.e., cementing techniques, and corrosion resistant metals. However, we must not forget that the surgeon still is the greatest variable.

Industry should keep in mind that better clinical results at lower costs are not achieved with ever new implant designs, but with continuous improvements of existing systems and, even more importantly, with measures to improve the operating surgeon's knowledge and skills.

Acknowledgments

The authors would like to thank Dieter Stoll and Scott Wilson (Sulzer INNOTEC, Winterthur, Switzerland) for performing the Laserprofilometry, Ralf Klabunde (Sulzer Orthopedics, Winterthur, Switzerland) for supplying the samples and the scientific support, Richard Guggenheim, Marcel Düggelin (REM-Lab., University of Basel) and Udo M. Spornitz (Institute of Anatomy, University of Basel) for their support in electron microscopy. This work was supported by the Hardy and Otto Frey-Zünd Foundation, Basel, Switzerland and Sulzer Orthopedics, Winterthur, Switzerland.

References

[1]   Schmalzried, T.P., Jasty, M. and Harris, W.H. "Periprosthetic Bone Loss in Total Hip Arthroplasty. Polyethylene Wear Debris and the Concept of the Effective Joint Space," Journal of Bone Joint Surgery Am. Vol. 74, No. 6, 1992, pp. 849-863.

[2]   Ling, R.S. "Observations on the Fixation of Implants to the Bony Skeleton," Clinical Orthopedics and Related Research Vol. 210, 1986, pp. 80-96.

[3]   Fowler, J.L., Gie, G.A., Lee, A.J. and Ling, R.S. "Experience with the Exeter Total Hip Replacement since 1970," The Orthopedic clinics of North America. Vol. 19, No. 3, 1988, pp. 477-489.

[4]   Howie, D.W., Middleton, R.G. and Costi, K. "Loosening of Matt and Polished Cemented Femoral Stems," Journal of Bone Joint Surgery Br. Vol. 80, No. 4, 1998, pp. 573-576.

[5]   Malchau, H., Sodermann, P. and Herberts, P. "Swedish Hip Registry: Results with 20-Year Follow Up with Validation Clinically and Radiographically," Orlando, 67th Annual Meeting of the American Academy of Orthopaedic Surgeons, 2000.

[6]   Maurer, T.B. and Ochsner, P. "Results and Guidelines after 78 Revisions of Cemented Titanium Stems," Beaune, European Hip Society meeting, 1998.

[7]   LeMouel, S., Allain, J. and Goutallier, D. "Analyse actuarielle à 10 ans d'une cohorte de 156 prothèses totales de hanche cimentées à couple de frottement alu-

mine/poly-ethylène," Revue de chirurgie orthopédique et reparatrice de l'appareil
moteur. Vol. 8, 1998, p. 345.

[8]   Van der Straeten, C., Goossens, M. and Gruen, T. "Cemented and Non-Cemented
        Hip Arthroplasty with a Proximal Plasma Sprayed Titanium Stem," Journal of
        Bone Joint Surgery Br. Vol. 81, Supplementum II, 1999, p. 173

[9]   Eingartner, C., Volkmann, R., Kummel, K. and Weller, S. "Niedrige Lockerungs-
        rate einer zementierten Titan-Geradschaftprothese im langerfristigen Verlauf,"
        Swiss Surgery Vol. 3, No. 2, 1997, pp. 49-54.

[10]   Acklin, Y.P., Berli, B.J., Frick, W., Elke, R. and Morscher, E.W. "Nine-Year Re-
        sults of Muller Cemented Titanium Straight Stems in Total Hip Replacement,"
        Archives of Orthopaedic and Trauma Surgery. Vol. 121, No. 7, 2001, pp. 391-
        398.

[11]   Havelin, L.I., Espehaug, B., Vollset, S.E. and Engesaeter, L.B. "Early Aseptic
        Loosening of Uncemented Femoral Components in Primary Total Hip Replace-
        ment. A Review Based on the Norwegian Arthroplasty Register," Journal of Bone
        Joint Surgery Br. Vol. 77, No. 1, 1995, pp. 11-17.

[12]   Havelin, L.I., Espehaug, B., Vollset, S.E. and Engesaeter, L.B. "The Effect of the
        Type of Cement on Early Revision of Charnley Total Hip Prostheses. A Review
        of Eight Thousand Five Hundred and Seventy-Nine Primary Arthroplasties from
        the Norwegian Arthroplasty Register," Journal of Bone Joint Surgery Am. Vol.
        77, No. 10, 1995, pp. 1543-1550.

[13]   Havelin, L.I., Engesaeter, L.B., Espehaug, B., Furnes, O., Lie, S.A. and Vollset,
        S.E. "The Norwegian Arthroplasty Register: 11 years and 73,000 Arthroplasties,"
        Acta orthopaedica Scandinavica. Vol. 71, No. 4, 2000, pp. 337-353.

[14]   Kühn, K.D. "Up-to-Date Comparisons of Physical and Chemical Properties of
        Commercial Materials," Berlin, Heidelberg, New York: Springer, 2000.

[15]   Harper, E.J. and Bonfield, W. "Tensile Characteristics of Ten Commercial Acrylic
        Bone Cements," Journal of biomedical materials research. Vol. 53, No. 5, 2000,
        pp. 605-616.

[16]   Hopf, T., Zell, J. and Hanser, U. "Methods of Fatigue Testing of PMMA Bone
        Cement," Medizinisch Orthopädische Technik. Vol. 105, 1985, pp. 20-25.

[17]   Hopf, T. and Fritsch, E.W. "Fatigue Strength of Vacuum-Mixed Polymethyl
        Methacrylate Bone Cement," Orthopedics International Vol. 5, 1997, pp. 98-104.

[18]   Wilson-MacDonald, J., Morscher, E. and Masar, Z. "Cementless Uncoated
        Polyethylene Acetabular Components in Total Hip Replacement. Review of Five-
        to 10-Year Results," Journal of Bone Joint Surgery Am. Vol. 72, No. 3, 1990, pp.
        423-430.

[19]   Alfaro-Adrian, J., Gill, H.S. and Murray, D.W. "Cement Migration after THR. A
        Comparison of Charnley Elite and Exeter Femoral Stems using RSA," Journal of
        Bone Joint Surgery Am. Vol. 81, No. 1, 1999, pp. 130-134.

[20]   Alfaro-Adrian, J., Gill, H.S. and Murray, D.W. "Should Total Hip Arthroplasty
        Femoral Components be Designed to Subside?: A Radiostereometric Analysis
        Study of the Charnley Elite and Exeter stems," Journal of Arthroplasty. Vol. 16,
        No. 5, 2001, pp. 598-606.

[21]   Bergmann, G. "In vivo Messung der Belastung von Hüftimplantaten," Berlin,
        Verlag Dr. Köster, 1997.

[22]   Stoll, D. "Knochenzementversuche, Interner Bericht Sulzer Innotec," 1998.

[23]   Charrière, E. "Projet de diplôme en ingénierie biomédicale, EPFL Lausanne," 1998.

[24]   Wimmer MA, Nassutt R, Lersner A, Kunze J, Schneider E. "Schwingverschleiss von Titan gegen Knochen verursacht Abriebpartikel kleiner als Zellgrösse", *in: Zuin Gohr, Reibung und Verschleiss,* DGM Verlag, 1996.

[25]   Wimmer MA, Schneider E, "Fretting Wear of Titanium and Cobalt-Chromium Alloys Against Bone Cement", *Annual Meeting of the Orthopedic Research Society.* 353, New Orleans, 16.-22.3.1998.

[26]   Wimmer MA, Bluhm A, Hansen I, Heckel L, Schneider E, "Fretting Wear of Titanium against Bone-Cement depends on the Surface Finish of Titanium", *Annual Meeting of the European Orthopedic Research Society,* Amsterdam (NL), 1998.

[27]   Cooper, J. R, Dowson, D. Fisher, J. and Jobbins, B. "Ceramic Bearing Surfaces in Total Artificial Joints: Resistance to Third Body Wear Damage from Bone Cement Particles," Journal of Medical Engineering and Technology., Vol. 15, No. 2, 1991, pp. 63-67.

[28]   Ingham, E. and Fisher, J. "Biological Reactions to Wear Debris in Total Joint Replacement," Proceedings of the Institution of Mechanical Engineering, Vol. 214, No. 1, 2000, pp. 21-37.

[29]   Tritschler, B., Forest, B. and Rieu, J. "Fretting corrosion of materials for orthopaedic implants: a study of a metal/polymer contact in an artificial physiological medium," Tribology International, Vol. 32, 1999, pp. 587-596.

[30]   Willert, H.G., Broback, L.G., Buchhorn, G.H., Jensen, P.H., Koster, G., Lang, I., Ochsner, P. and Schenk, R. "Crevice corrosion of cemented titanium alloy stems in total hip replacements," Clinical Orthopedics and Related Research. Vol. 333, 1996, pp. 51-75.

[31]   Berli, B., Elke, R. and Morscher, E.W. "MS-30 stems - matte versus polished surfaces; clinical and radiological results of a 5 year follow-up," *Annual Meeting of the European Federation of Orthopaedic Research and Traumatology*, Rhodos, Greece 6. 4. 2001.

Mengke Zhu[1] and Markus Windler[2]

Fretting and Anodic Current of the Taper Interface of Stainless Steel Hip Stems/Cobalt-Chromium Femoral Heads

Reference: Zhu, M. and Windler M., **"Fretting and Anodic Current of the Taper Interface of Stainless Steel Hip Stems/Cobalt-Chromium Femoral Heads,"** *Stainless Steels for Medical and Surgical Applications, ASTM STP 1438*, G. L. Winters and M. J. Nutt, Eds., ASTM International, West Conshohocken, PA, 2003.

Abstract: Three types of hip stems, MS-30^{TM} high-nitrogen stainless steel, Natural Hip^{TM} cobalt-chromium, and APR$^{®}$ II porous titanium were interfaced with cobalt-chromium femoral heads. They were tested according to ASTM F 1875-98. In the initial 1 Hz cyclic loading up to 480 cycles, the average fretting current generated from the taper interface was 0.4, 0.6, and 1 μA, respectively for the stainless steel, cobalt-chromium, and titanium stems. In the following 2 Hz cyclic loading up to 3600 cycles, the average fretting current was 1.3, 0.6, and 2.25 μA, accordingly. In the potentiodynamic polarization, the titanium stems showed relatively high anodic current in the range of -100 to 500 mV. The cobalt-chromium stems had the highest anodic current in the range of 500 to 1200 mV. The stainless steel stems exhibited the best corrosion resistance in the whole potential range of polarization.

Keywords: stainless steel, cobalt-chromium, titanium, fretting corrosion, orthopedic hip stems, femoral head, taper interface

Introduction

Modular orthopedic hip prostheses are widely used in total hip arthroplasty due to their clinical flexibility. However, clinically retrieved modular hip prostheses have manifested corrosion related problems particularly at the taper interfaces [1, 2]. The taper interfaces of hip stems and femoral heads are subjected to micro-motion that might lead to fretting corrosion. The modular connection of the hip stem and head of different materials is susceptible to galvanic corrosion. Moreover, stainless steel hip implants have

---

[1]Senior Research Engineer, Research and Analysis Department, Sulzer Orthopedics Inc., 9900 Spectrum Dr., Austin, TX 78717, USA.
[2]Manager of Materials, Research and Analysis Department, Sulzer Orthopedics Ltd., P. O. Box 65, CH-8404, Winterthur, Switzerland.

been also used clinically, which requires special attention to their corrosion behavior as a less frequently used type of material. *In vivo* corrosion of Charnley and Müller 316L stainless steel hip implants was reported occurring around the one piece design stems [3]. However, little is reported on the corrosion behavior of modular stainless steel hip implants. The purpose of this study was to evaluate the *in vitro* fretting corrosion behavior of a high-nitrogen stainless steel stem/cobalt-chromium (CoCr) head taper interface and compare it to that of CoCr stem/CoCr head and titanium stem/CoCr head taper interfaces.

Materials

The following number of hip stems and femoral heads (Figure 1) were used in this study.

   6   MS-30™ high-nitrogen stainless steel hip stems, size 12
                                       (Protasul S-30, ASTM F 1586, stainless steel stems)
   5   Natural-Hip™ CoCr stems, size 4 (ASTM F 1537, CoCr stems)
   5   APR® II Porous Ti-6Al-4V hip stems, size 15 mm
                                       (ASTM F 136, titanium stems)
 16   Sulzer CoCr femoral heads, size 28 mm, neutral (ASTM F 1537, CoCr heads)

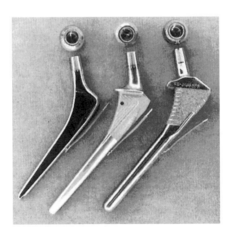

Figure 1– *Parts tested*
From left to right: MS-30 stainless steel, Natural-Hip CoCr, APR II Porous titanium

All parts had a 12/14 mm taper with threads on the stem cone.
Lactated Ringer's Injection USP, Baxter Healthcare Corp., Deerfield, IL 60015

Methods

This study was conducted per the ASTM Standard Practice for Fretting Corrosion Testing of Modular Implant Interfaces: Hip Femoral Head-Bore and Cone Taper Interface (F1875-98). Fretting corrosion tests were conducted in two configurations corresponding to Procedure B and Procedure A of Test Method II of the standard. A total of five tests described in Test Method II were conducted; two tests were performed in Configuration I and three tests were in Configuration II. Each of the 16 stem and head assemblies was set up and went through the five tests in the sequence described as follows, with the most destructive test executed at the end.

Setup of the Hip Stem and the Femoral Head

Each set of a hip stem and a femoral head was assembled on an Instron material test machine in a dry condition. The stem was fixed with the neck aligned with the load axis. The femoral head was pushed onto the stem cone by applying a static load to 2000 N. The fretting corrosion tests were conducted on a servo-hydraulic MTS material test machine. The stem and head assembly was set up in an inverted position as per ASTM Cyclic Fatigue Testing of Metallic Stemmed Hip Arthroplasty Femoral Components without Torsion (F1440). The femoral head articulated against an acetabular insert that was fixed in a fluid chamber mounted on the lower platen of the MTS test machine. The distal portion of the stem was fixed on the upper platen of the machine (Figures 2 and 3). The stem and head were either unloaded or cyclically loaded according to the requirements of individual fretting corrosion tests. If required, cyclic loads of 2000 N in a sinusoidal waveform, with a minimum of 40 N and a maximum of 2040 N, were applied to the stem and head assembly at either 1 or 2 Hz.

Fretting Corrosion Testing

Configuration I Fretting Current at Open Circuit Potential – The stem and head assembly was the working electrode (A in Figure 2), while an identical hip stem as the test stem (B in Figure 2) was employed as the counter electrode. Both working and counter electrodes were immersed in 500 mL lactated Ringer's solution in the fluid chamber. The current generated at the taper interface was measured using a galvanic corrosion program of an EG&G 273A Potentiostat/Galvanostat, which served as a zero resistance ammeter.

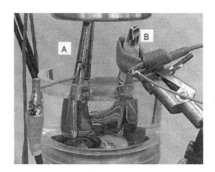

Figure 2 – *Setup in Configuration I*

The current was measured while the stem was cyclically loaded in the following two loading periods.

Test 1 Cyclic loading at 1 Hz Current was measured for a total of 600 seconds (s), including 120 s while the stem was not loaded and 480 s while it was cyclically loaded (current increase due to fretting was recorded in this period).

Test 2 Cyclic loading at 2 Hz Current was measured for 120 s at 360, 1000, 1800, and 3600 cycles periodically.

Configuration II Corrosion potential (Rest Potential) and Anodic Current at Applied Potentials – In this test configuration, the working electrode was the stem and head assembly (A in Figure 3). A platinum wire counter electrode (B in Figure 3) was placed close to the CoCr head and the lugging probe of a saturated calomel reference electrode (SCE, C in Figure 3) was positioned near the taper interface. To reduce the effect of size and geometry differences between the three types of stems, the stem and head assembly was immersed in 160 mL Ringer's solution such that only the CoCr head and the stem neck portion was exposed to the solution. The following three tests were conducted using the EG&G 273A Potentiostat/Galvanostat.

Test 3 Corrosion potential measurement Corrosion potential of the working electrode was measured for one hour while the stem was cyclically loaded at 1 Hz. To display the effect of fretting, measurement was first performed without applying the loads for 5 minutes.

Test 4 Potentiostatic polarization Potentiostatic polarization was conducted at 50 mV/5 minutes for five steps from -150 mV through 50 mV. The current was measured for five minutes at each applied potential. Cyclic loads at 1 Hz were applied in this test.

Test 5 Potentiodynamic polarization Potentiodynamic polarization was conducted at 0.667 mV/s from the then open circuit potential to 1200 mV. No cyclic loads were applied in this test.

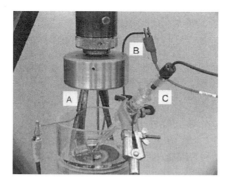

Figure 3 – *Setup in Configuration II*

The taper interfaces of the stems were examined using an SEM before and after the tests. The stem and head couples were disassembled by using a head extractor.

Results

Fretting Current at Open Circuit Potential (Configuration I)
Test 1– Figure 4 shows the initial response of current to fretting of the modular interface. Current jumped in response to the commencement of the cyclic loads at 120 s. In the initial 8 minutes of cyclic loading at 1 Hz, several stems showed unstable current variation, and the titanium stems scattered most in the current output. When the curves of the stems in each type were averaged, the fretting current was approximately 0.4 μA, 0.6 μA, and 1.3 μA, respectively for the stainless steel, CoCr, and titanium stems (Figure 5).

Test 2– In the following periodical current measurements with cyclic loading at 2 Hz, no consistent variation was observed between the current of each stem and the cycle number. In view of that, all measurements (started at 360, 1000, 1800, and 3600 cycles) of the stems in each group were averaged (Figure 6). The averaged fretting current values corresponding to the three types of stems were approximately 1.3 μA, 0.6 μA, and 2.25 μA. In the cyclic loading at 2 Hz, the current of the individual stems appeared relatively stable. In comparison to the values in the initial 1 Hz cyclic loading, the averaged fretting current of the stainless steel and titanium stems rose by approximately 225% and 73%, respectively. In contrast, no apparent change was observed for the CoCr stems.

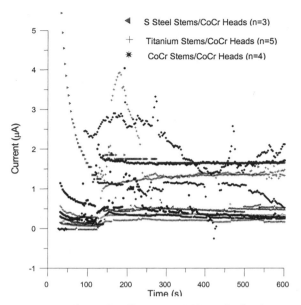

Figure 4 – *Current in 1 Hz cyclic loading*
Cyclic loads started at 120 s

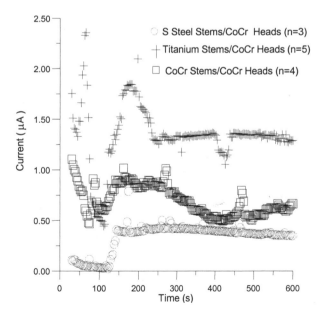

Figure 5 – *Average current in 1 Hz cyclic*
loading Cyclic loads started at 120 s

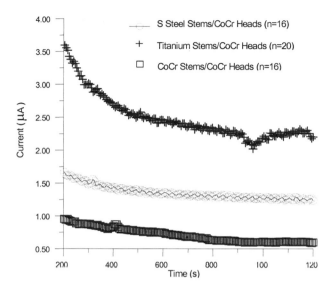

Figure 6 – *Current in 2 Hz cyclic loading*
Average of results measured at 360, 1000, 1800, and 3600 cycles
and the stems from the same group

Corrosion Ppotential (Rest Potential) and Anodic Current at Applied Potentials
(Configuration II)

Test 3– Corrosion potential dropped when the modular interface was subjected to the cyclic loads at 1 Hz at 300 s (Figure 7). The titanium stems showed the highest (noblest) corrosion potential, while the stainless steel and CoCr stems appeared to be comparable.

Test 4– In the potentiostatic measurement with the 1 Hz cyclic loading, current increased with increased applied potential for all stems, as represented by an stainless steel stem (Figure 8). At an applied potential of - 100 mV, the three types of stems showed similar levels of anodic current (Figure 9). When the applied potential reached 50 mV, titanium stems showed the highest anodic current, while the stainless steel stems the lowest (Figure 10).

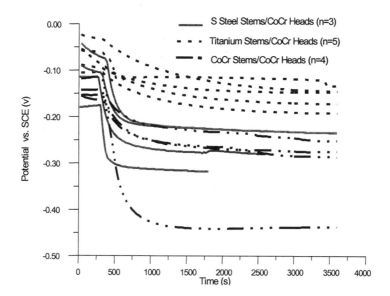

Figure 7 – *Corrosion potential measured in 1 Hz cyclic loading Cyclic loads started at 300 s*

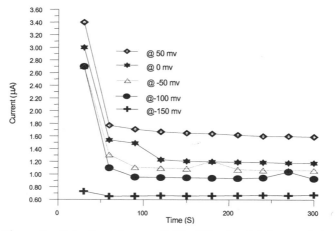

Figure 8 – *Potentiostatic scan @50 mV/5 min, stainless steel stem*

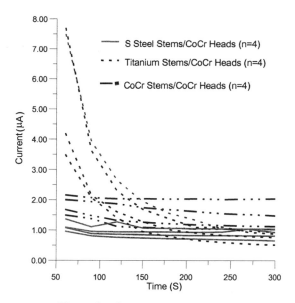

Figure 9   *Potentiostatic measurement*
@ - 100 mV vs. SCE
cyclic loads @ 1 Hz

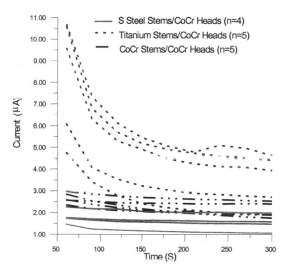

Figure 10 – *Potentiostatic measurement*
@ 50 mV vs. SCE
cyclic loads @ 1 Hz

Test 5– In the potentiodynamic measurement without cyclic loading (Figure 11), starting at 550 mV, the CoCr stems showed much higher anodic current than the other two types of stems. The severity of corrosion of the CoCr stems was indicated

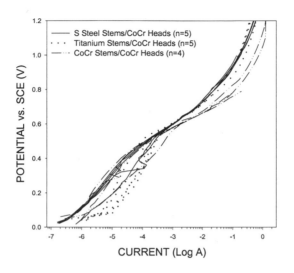

Figure 11 – *Potentiodynamic scan @ 0.67 mV/S*

by the size of the corroded area and its extent of discoloring on the CoCr head and neck (Figure 12), and by the thick and dark electrolyte left after the test. The titanium stems showed relatively higher anodic current in the potential range up to 500 mV. The stainless steel stems exhibited the least anodic current in the whole polarization range.

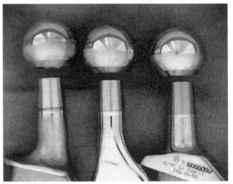

Figure 12 - *Corrosion damage after*
the potentiodynamic polarization
From left to right: Natural Hip CoCr, MS-30, APR II Titanium

SEM Examination of the Stem Taper Sections

The threaded taper appeared similar on the three types of stems. Typical for all stems, no detectable corrosion damage was found in the threaded taper sections covered by the femoral heads. Corrosion damage due to the potentiodynamic polarization was primarily present on the area close to the taper and neck junction (Figure 13) and the stem neck section below the taper as shown in Figure 12.

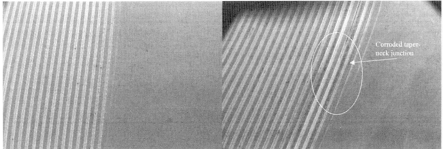

(a) before corrosion test   *(b) after potentiodynamic polarization*
Figure 13 *SEM pictures of the threaded taper section (MS-30)*

Discussion

Corrosion at the femoral stem/head taper interface may result from fretting due to micro motion, crevice at the taper mismatch, and galvanic coupling of dissimilar materials or a combination of these three. This study investigated the fretting current due to cyclic loading and galvanic corrosion behavior of the tree types of modular interfaces. Since all parts had the same taper design, a large variation in the crevice of the tapers can be dismissed.

The effect of cyclic loading was demonstrated in both the initial fretting current and the corrosion potential measurements. Fretting at the taper interface creates fresh surface areas that contribute to an increased current. The variation of the fretting current may indicate how stem cones of different materials fit in the CoCr head bore. The fretting current varied greatly in the initial cyclic loading due probably to the irregular micro motion at the taper interface in the "sit-in" phase. The titanium stems appeared to have most initial micro motion, while the stainless steel stems seemed to have the best initial match with the CoCr head. As the cyclic load frequency increased to 2 Hz, both the stainless steel and titanium stems revealed to be sensitive to the increased frequency. The CoCr stems appeared to have the best fit with the CoCr head by showing the very low fretting current and insensitivity to the frequency change. Since fretting current results from changes of the surface state, its magnitude should mainly depend upon the materials of the components and has little to do with the galvanic effect of mixed materials. The generally higher fretting current of the titanium group appears to be characteristic of titanium that reacts and repassivates sensitively to surface changes.

The CoCr head was a universal component of the modular taper interface. However, the degree of corrosion of the modular portion as a whole was greatly affected by the stem cones and necks of different materials. The coupling of the titanium stems had the noblest corrosion potential, resulting probably from the sintering process of the stem. As demonstrated by both potentiostatic and potentiodynamic polarization measurements, titanium stems showed the highest anodic current in the lower range of applied potential (- 50 mV to 500 mV). Although made of the same material, the coupling of the CoCr stems and heads exhibited the highest anodic current or corrosion in the upper scan range of 550 mV to 1200 mV. Noticeably, the coupling of the stainless steel stems had the best corrosion resistance in the whole range of polarization. These results demonstrate that the anodic current of a hip stem/head assembly is less dependent on the galvanic coupling of dissimilar materials than on the polarization behavior of a particular material. In fact, the polarization behavior of the three groups shown in Figure 11 reflected that of the CoCr head, which dominated the polarization process because of its higher anodic current than components of the other two materials [4].

Although only short-term testing was performed, this *in-vitro* study covered several conditions that a hip stem may encounter *in-vivo,* including cyclic loading and a wide range of applied potential. A limitation of this study was that the proximal bodies of the stems were partially immersed in the electrolyte in the fretting current measurement, which had different surface areas and shapes. Whether the additional surface area would affect the fretting current was not examined. Under such a circumstance of testing and with the said design features, the stainless steel stems behaved well, if not superior to the titanium and the CoCr stems.

References

[1] Collier, J. P., Surprenant V. A., Jensen, R., Mayor, M. B., and Surprenant, H., "Corrosion Between the Components of Modular Femoral Hip Prostheses," *Journal of Bone and Joint Surgery [Br]*, Vol. 74-B, No. 4, 1992, pp. 511-517.

[2] Gilbert, J. L., Buckley, C. A., and Jacobs, J. J., "In vivo Corrosion of Modular Hip Prosthesis Components in Mixed and Similar Metal Combinations. The Effect of Crevice, Stress, Motion, and Alloy Coupling," *Journal of Biomedical Materials Research*, Vol. 27, 1993, pp. 1533-1544.

[3] Walczak, J., Shahgaldi, F. and Heatley, F., "In vivo Corrosion of 316L Stainless Steel Hip Implants: Morphology and Elemental compositions of Corrosion Products," *Biomaterials*, Vol. 19, 1998, pp. 229-237.

[4] Zhu, M., "Fretting Corrosion Testing of the Taper Interface of Four SOAG Hip Femoral Stem/Head Combinations," Technical Report 00026G, Department of Research and Analysis, Sulzer Orthopedics Inc., 2000.

Clinical Experience

Bernhard Berli[1], Reinhard Elke[2], Erwin W. Morscher[3]

The Cemented MS-30 Stem in Total Hip Replacement, Matte versus Polished Surface: Minimum of Five Years of Clinical and Radiographic Results of a Prospective Study

Reference: Berli, B., Elke, R., and Morscher, E. W., "The Cemented MS-30 Stem in Total Hip Replacement, Matte versus Polished Surface: Minimum of Five Years of Clinical and Radiographic Results of a Prospective Study," *Stainless Steels for Medical and Surgical Applications*, ASTM STP 1438, G. L. Winters and M. J. Nutt, Eds., ASTM International, West Conshohocken, PA, 2003.

Abstract: The MS-30 femoral stem is a three-dimensionally tapered, collarless implant for cement fixation in THR, manufactured from an FeCrNiMnMoNb-alloy with either a matte or polished surface. One hundred twenty-seven MS-30 stems with matte surface and 128 stems with polished surface, respectively, were implanted in an alternated manner.

The mean observation period was 5.6 years. No patients were lost to the follow-up. In both groups 88 patients with 108 stems were included in the clinical and radiographic follow-up examinations. Only one stem with a matte surface was revised for aseptic loosening. There was no death related to surgery and no infection.

Conclusion: Both, the clinical and radiographic evaluation (radiolucencies, osteolyses and subsidence) did not show any statistically significant difference between the two groups.

The main reason for the equally excellent performance of both the matte and the polished version of the MS-30 stem may be the design of the centralizer which resists both debonding of the stem, and subsequent subsidence as a precondition for fretting in the metal/cement interface.

Clinical relevance: Since, on the one hand, debonding of the stem/cement interface cannot entirely be excluded, we recommend the discontinuation of tapered stems with a matte surface - especially if they do not have a centralizer which resists the stem to subside.

Keywords: Total Hip Replacement, Cement Fixation, Tapered Stem, Implant Surface

[1] MD, Orthopaedic Department, University of Basel, Burgfelderstr. 101, CH-4012 Basel, Switzerland
[2] Private Dozent, MD, Orthopaedic Department, University of Basel, Burgfelderstr. 101, CH-4012 Basel, Switzerland
[3] Professor em., MD, Laboratory of Orthopaedic Biomechanics, University of Basel, Burgfelderstr. 101, CH-4012 Basel, Switzerland

Introduction:

The MS-30 femoral stem (SULZER Orthopedics, Baar/Switzerland, Figure 1), manufactured in stainless steel (FeCrNiMnMo ISO 5832-9) and designed for cemented fixation in Total Hip Replacement, was developed by the senior author (EWM) and L. Spotorno/ Italy. The primary goal for the development of this stem was to generate an optimal cement mantle, which is known to be the most important factor for the longevity of a cemented femoral stem.

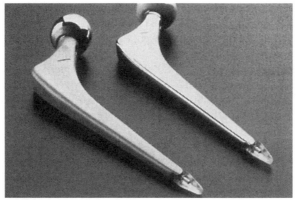

Figure 1 - *MS-30 femoral stem with centralizer and modular head. Left: Matte surface, metallic head, Right: Polished surface, ceramic head.*

The quality of the cement mantle itself depends on the implant design, its surface conditions, the material characteristics (both, of the implant and the cement) and, last but not least, on the operative, i.e. the cementing technique. In contrast, inadequate cementing techniques were the main cause of the high rates of aseptic loosening and, thus,of the increase in revision rates in the past. Main causes of failure of cemented femoral stems are an insufficient medial support [1], an insufficient cement mantle with metal/bone contact [2], an insufficient cement/bone interdigitation [3] and an inadequate positioning of the stem [4 - 6]. Therefore, a series of various factors, which are closely related to each other, play a decisive role for the outcome of a THR .

The design of the implant determines the amount and the direction of the forces transmitted from the bone to the prosthesis and vice versa. Furthermore, the design and size of the implant determine the thickness of the cement mantle. Preoperative planning, therefore, is vital for the success of a THR. According to experimental and clinical experiences, the optimum thickness of the cement mantle can be defined as asymmetric and non-uniform. It is thicker in the region where the main forces are transmitted, i.e. in Gruen zones 7, 3 and 5. Overall, the thickness of the cement mantle around the stem should be not less than 2 mm [1, 7].

The MS-30 stem is three-dimensionally tapered. Thus, if the cement debonds from the stem, the system functions according to a press-fit concept. The selected stem is - compared to the medullary canal prepared by reamers – undersized, in order to provide the necessary space for the bone cement between implant and bone. This is already taken into account in the preoperative planning. The edges of the stem are rounded off, in order to minimize stresses within the cement mantle. The flanges on the proximo-lateral part of the prosthesis increase its rotational stability. Furthermore, rotational stability is improved by a high neck resection of 30° to the horizontal plane.

An integral part of the system is the centralizer to position the component distally, hence avoiding metal/bone contact and - in combination with excessive lateral reaming of the proximal end of the femur – avoiding malalignment [8].

The cemented MS-30 stem was introduced in clinical practice with a matte surface in 1990. From March 1990 until December 31, 2001, 1,465 stems were inserted at the Orthopaedic Department of the University of Basel/Switzerland.

Aseptic loosening caused by osteolysis through wear particles [9] is still the most limiting factor for the longevity of a hip arthroplasty. Wear particles are generated predominantly in the articulating surface of a THR. However, fretting corrosion at the cement/implant interface has been identified as an additional cause of osteolysis of cemented femoral stems [10 - 12]. For both, the generation of wear particles and for fretting corrosion, the implant surface and the quality of the bone cement play a decisive role.

Only when the interface between the cement mantle and the endoprosthetic stem is debonded and relative movements allow friction, both wear particles are produced and corrosion at the cement/stem interface can take place. As the literature documents that the tapered collarless Exeter stem yielded better results with a polished rather than a matte surface [13 - 16], SULZER Orthopedics Ltd, Switzerland, also offered the MS-30 stem in a polished version. Our own results with this stem with a matte surface revealed excellent results with no revision and no osteolysis during a four-year period from 1990 to 1994.

In order to compare the outcome of the MS-30 stem in relation to the surface characteristics, we decided to perform a prospective study including a total number of 255 stems: 127 with a matte, 128 with a polished surface. The first MS-30 stem of this series was inserted on November 15, 1994, the last one on March 20, 1997. A prospective study with the careful use of criteria for inclusion and exclusion allowed the investigators to minimize the number of variables [17]. The only variable of the study was the characteristic of the surface.

The main goals of the study were to elucidate whether there is a significant difference with regard to radiolucencies, osteolyses and stem subsidence on the X-rays, and the clinical survival rate between stems with matte and polished surface.

Patients and Methods:

The study included 127 stems with a matte and 128 stems with a polished surface. All but one of these stems were combined with the Morscher Press-Fit Cup and a 28 mm head (metal or ceramic). In 21 patients, the MS-30 stem was inserted bilaterally during the index period, in 16 cases in one operation, and in 5 cases in two stages. All the implants were assigned by the head nurse of the operating theater in a randomized, blinded manner. In cases where a patient was to receive a total hip replacement in both hips in one stage surgery, one prosthesis had a matte, the other one a polished surface. There was one exception, where a polished stem was inserted in both hip joints. The operative procedures were performed by 15 different surgeons of the Orthopaedic Department of the University of Basel/Switzerland, including the senior author EWM, with different lengths of training and experience levels.

Forty patients (19 women, 21 men)already had undergone a total hip replacement on the opposite side prior to the index surgery period, and 17 patients (10 women, 7 men), were treated on the opposite side after the index surgery period. Five patients had a bilateral total hip replacement done in two stages during the index surgery period (2 with a matte surface and 1 with a polished surface in both hips: 2 patients received a matte in one and a polished stem in the opposite hip). Sixteen Patients had a bilateral THR done in one stage (15 with a mat on one and a polished on the opposite side, 1 patient got a polished stem on both sides). In the first group with a matte surface, there are 61 men with a mean age at surgery of 65 years, and 66 women with a mean age of 73 years. In the second group with a polished stem surface, there are 63 men with a mean age of 64 years, and 65 women with a mean age of 70 years. The right hip was treated in 53 cases with a matte, in 73 hips with a polished stem; 71 stems with a matte and 58 stems with a polished surface were inserted on the left hip. Sixteen patients in the first group with a matte surface and 14 patients with a polished MS-30 surface in the second group, i.e., a total number of 30 patients (14 men and 16 women), died during the observation period. Six patients with 7 hips (2 with a matte, 5 with a polished surface) were not able or not willing to come to the last, 5-year, follow-up. They were, however, interviewed by telephone. All had their endoprosthesis stem in situ. One hundred and eight hips with a MS-30 stem with a matte surface and 108 hips with a polished surface had a minimum 5-year clinical and radiological check. No patient was lost to follow-up (Table 1).

Table 1- *Patients Data: N = 234 Patients / 255 Hips, 127 mat, 128 polished surface*

| | Total | Uni-lateral THR | | Bi-lateral THR | | |
| | | mat | polished | mat-mat | mat-polished | polished - polished |
					mat polished	
Patients male	111	47	55	1	6	2
Patients female	123	59	52	1	11	0
Age at surgery male		65 Y	66 Y	76 Y	60 Y	52 Y
		(41–86)	(35-88)		(52-72)	(44-60)
Age at surgery female		72 Y	70 Y	54 Y	65 Y	-
		(54-89)	(40-91)		(56-73)	
Hips male	120	47	55	2	6 6	4
Hips female	135	59	52	2	11 11	0
Stem revisions	1	1	0	0	0	0
Deceased (until Dec. 2001)	30/31	15	14	0	1	0
Lost for FU	0	0	0	0	0	0
Not able to come	6/7	1	4	0	1	0
Patients controlled	197	89	89	2	15	2
Hips controlled	2/6	89	89	4	15 15	4

Table 2 - *Preoperative Diagnosis:*

Surface	Total	matte	polished
Primary Osteoarthritis	198	105 (82.7%)	93 (72.7%)
Avascular Necrosis	24	9 (7.1%)	15 (11.7%)
Dysplasia	17	7 (5.5%)	10 (7.8%)
Posttraumatic OA	9	4 (3.1%)	5 (3.9%)
Rheumatoid Arthritis	7	2 (1.6%)	5 (3.9%)
Total N:	255	127 (100%)	128 (100%)

Out of the 255 hips, the preoperative diagnosis was osteoarthritis in 198 (77 %), avascular necrosis in 24 (9.5%), dysplasia in 17 (7%), rheumatoid arthritis in 7 (3 %) and post-traumatic osteoarthritis in 9 cases (3.5%) (Table 2).

Stem sizes were not different in the two groups (p > 0.05) (Fig. 2).

Figure 2 - *Sizes of the MS-30 Stem*

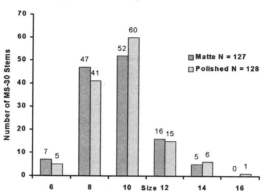

The only criterion for exclusion from the study was the surgeon's decision to use a non-cemented femoral stem. During the study period, this was the case in 52 hips.

As an acetabular component, the senior author's Press-Fit Cup (SULZER Orthopaedics, Baar/Switzerland) was used for all patients except in one with post-traumatic osteoarthritis, where a Ganz Reinforcement Ring was inserted. The articulation chosen was metal on conventional polyethylene in 7 cases of MS-stems with a matte, and in 4 cases with a polished stem, with ceramic on conventional polyethylene in 120 cases with a matte, and in 124 cases with a polished surface.

The patients were operated on in supine position and all THRs were inserted by a lateral approach. The rasp is oversized compared to the stem, in order to provide the necessary space for the cement. The medullary canal was irrigated and packed with sponges until immediately before introducing the bone cement. The cementing technique included the use of a cement gun, plugging of the distal femoral canal and pressurization. The centralizer designed to position the stem distally is an integral part of the MS-30 system. It serves to prevent contact between implant and bone and to avoid malalignment. The centralizer selected is in general 1 size larger than the respective stem size. The femoral component was fixed with Gentamicin-Palacos (Kulzer GmbH, Bad Homburg/Germany), according to the manufacturer's instructions. The mean duration of surgery was 1½ hours (range: 1 – 2¼ hours).

Because the MS-30 stem with distal centralizer was at first introduced in the matte version only, and because the controversy about the condition of the surface arose only after that time, the patients were not informed about the nature of the surface condition of their cemented stem. On the X-rays, it cannot be distinguished whether the stem surface is matte or polished. The evaluating authors were informed about the surface condition only after the clinical and radiological evaluation, i.e., the evaluation part of the study was performed in a double-blind fashion.

The perioperative regimen was the same for all patients. It included the use of antibiotics (Mandokef, 2 g preoperatively) as well as prophylaxis against venous thrombosis (Heparin 5000 U and Sintrom from the 2nd postoperative day). The postoperative treatment (rehabilitation) was uniform in the whole series. The patients were mobilized either the evening after the operation or the first postoperative morning.

Partial weight bearing was allowed up to half body weight for 6 weeks. Physiotherapy was prescribed for about 3 months if there was no specific indication for a prolonged aftertreatment.

The average observation time, i.e. the time between surgery and the last radiographic follow-up, was 67.3 (60 - 87) months. The minimum observation time, therefore, was 5 years.

Clinical assessment occurred according to the IDES forms of the Institute of Documentation of the M.E.Müller Foundation in Berne/Switzerland [18].

The clinical evaluation was done according to the Harris Hip Scores [19].

Radiographic evaluation

For the radiographic assessment, an X-ray of the pelvis including both hip joints was taken. The radiographic appearance of the initial cementing was graded on the 6-week check according to the classification of Barrack et al. [1992]: A: complete filling of the medullary cavity by cement, a so-called "white out" at the cement/bone interface, B: slight radiolucency of the cement/bone interface, C: radiolucency involving 50% to 99% of the cement/bone interface or a defective or incomplete cement mantle, D: radiolucency at the cement/bone interface of 100% in any projection, or a failure to fill the canal with cement to such an extent that the tip of the stem was not covered [20].

Fixation of the acetabular socket (Press-Fit Cup) was also assessed with regard to osteolyses and radiolucencies in zones I to III of DeLee & Charnley [21].

The radiograph of the latest follow-up was examined for radiolucent lines at the cement/bone interface which had not been present on the 6-week radiograph. The cortical bone was checked for the development of osteolyses, the stem for varus/valgus position, and the cement mantle for cement fractures. Subsidence of the stem within the cement mantle was measured as the difference of the distance between the upper circumference of the prosthesis shoulder and the sclerotic line above the shoulder [22, 23].

In the radiological evaluation, osteolysis was defined as a newly developed, cystic lesion with endosteal scalloping and/or migration, which had not been noticed on the immediate postoperative radiograph [24]. The sites of radiolucent lines (< 1 mm, 1-2 mm, >2mm) at the cement/bone interface) and osteolyses were recorded as being present in one or more of the 7 Gruen zones.

Ectopic ossification was assessed using the method of Brooker et al.[25].

The data were analyzed and the descriptive statistics (means and standard deviations) were calculated with the Excel 95 (Microsoft Corp., Redmont, CA) program. Survivorship was corrected according to Kaplan-Meyer [26].

Results:

Clinical Results

The mean preoperative Harris Hip Score improved from 67 points (range 44 - 84) to a postoperative score of 93 points (67 - 100). There was no significant difference between the hips with a matte or polished femoral stem with regard to the overall score (p > 0.05), the subscore for pain (p > 0.05) or the subscore for function (p > 0.05) The overall results were excellent in the group with stems with a matte surface in 79 patients (73%), and in 87 patients (81%) with a polished surface. Good results were observed in 21patients (19%) and 11 patients (10%), moderate results in 5 patients (5%) and 7 patients (6%), poor results in 3 patients (3%) with a matte surface, 3 patients (3%) with a polished surface.

None of the 21 patients with bilateral hip replacement, one with a matte MS-30, the other one with a polished surface, indicated a preference for either hip.

Complications

A preoperative fracture pf the great trochanter occurred in 6 cases, five of them were stabilized by cerclage wires. In two additional cases a crack of the proximal femur occurred that had to be cerclaged as well.

There was no death related to surgery and no infection has been observed.

Revisions

One revision had to be done for aseptic loosening of a stem with a matte surface 4 years after surgery. Two hips (acetabula) had to be revised for recurrent dislocation. The overall revision rate is, thus, three of 255 (1.2%), and one of 255 for aseptic loosening (0.4%).

Radiological Results

37 MS-30 stems out of the 216 stems (17%, 27 of the stems with matte and 12 stems with polished surface) showed a varus position between 3 and 6° (av. 4.2°).

Femoral cementing was classified on the postoperative radiographs in the 108 hips with a matte MS-30 stem as grade A in 72, grade B in 34 and grade C in 2 cases. There was no grade D. In the cohort of stems with a polished surface, the respective numbers are 78 grade A, 30 grade B and none with grade C and D.

Radiolucencies – all below 2 mm - in 1 to 3 zones were observed in 16 cases of the group with matte surface and in 15 cases in the group of the polished stems.

The number, the extension and distribution of osteolyses according to the seven Gruen zones is shown in Table 3.

Subsidence of less than 2 mm was found in 3 cases of the group with a matte surface and in 2 cases in the group with a polished one, subsidence of 2 - 5 mm in 6 stems with a matte and 7 stems with a polished surface (Table 4).

Table 3 - *Osteolyses (according to the Gruen zones)*

Gruen zones	Matte surface	Polished surface
1	1	0
2	0	0
3	0	0
4	0	0
5	0	2
6	0 } 2	1
7	1	2

Table 4 – *Subsidence*

Surface condition	Matte surface	Polished surface
< 2 mm	3	2
2 – 5 mm	6	7
> 5 mm	1	0

Subsidence was related significantly to the quality of the cement mantle: out of 150 stems with Barrack A cementing 15 (10%) subsided between 1 and 3 mm (av. 1.9mm), out of 64 stems with B cementing 10 (16%) subsided between 1 and 8 mm (av. 2.9 mm). The stem that subsided 8 mm has a matte surface and shows severe osteolysis in the proximal part of the femur. The patient is asymptomatic up to now. Nevertheless, revision surgery will be necessary in the not too distant future. On 12 radiographs no plug could be detected. Despite this, cementing was qualified A according to Barrack in 7, as B in 5 cases. Two stems only subsided within the cement mantle, one 2, the other one 4 mm. In both cases cementing had to be qualified as B.

Two cement fractures in zones 3/5 were observed.

Two periacetabular ossifications (PAO) III according to Brooker were identified in each group, but no PAO IV were seen.

Acetabular cup

There was no osteolysis and no revision for aseptic loosening, however, two revisions for dislocation for the Morscher Press-Fit Cup.

Discussion:

In contrast to the experience with the Exeter stem reported by Ling [13], Howie [14] and the Swedish Implant Register [16], no statistically significant difference in the outcome between the MS-30 stem with a matte or a polished surface was found in this prospective study over a 5-year observation period. There is, up to now, no difference between the MS-30 stem with a matte or a polished surface, not in relation to survivorship, subsidence or the incidence of osteolyses. However, there seems to be a tendency for a higher percentage of excellent clinical scores in the polished group vs. a higher percentage of good clinical scores in the matte group. Furthermore the only revision for aseptic loosening had to be performed with a stem with a matte surface and the only THR with severe osteolysis of the femur has a stem with matte surface as well.

A follow-up of 60 to 87 months, with an average time of 5.6 years, is, of course, too short to give a final verdict, at least concerning survivorship. There is still the theoretical possibility of a "type-II error", in other words, the probability of concluding that no difference between groups exists, when, in fact, there is a difference [27]. Type-II errors are to be expected especially in studies with a small sample size. In the present study, however, the sample size was 127 stems with a matte, and 128 stems with a polished surface. It was the aim of this study to compare the rate of *early* loosening of the MS-30 stem with respect to the surface conditions. Our findings should be considered sound, as it is known that debonding with subsidence of a stem within the cement mantle starts within the first 2 years after surgery. Furthermore, it is known that migration is more pronounced during the first year, then becomes slower and more continuous [28 - 32].

The main reason for the difference of the rate of osteolyses may be explained by the difference in the design of the centralizer of the Exeter and the MS-30 stem. Whereas the centralizer of the Exeter stem is directly put over the stem's tip and has a hollow space underneath to allow for the stem to subside, the centralizer of the MS-30 stem is made from PMMA and therefore bonds strongly with the surrounding bone cement and is as well fixed with a metallic pin into a hole at the tip of the stem. This provides resistance against debonding and subsidence.

The rationale to allow a tapered stem to subside (migrate) is the recognition of the fact that subsidence within the cement mantle has not only no correlation with regard to pain [13, 38], but allows the stem to restabilize as is also shown with the tapered Müller Straight Stem [37, 38].

According to the clinical experience with the Exeter stem [13, 14, 33, 34] it must be assumed that once debonded a MS-30 stem with a matte surface will produce more particles and/or corrosion compared to a polished surface. Despite the almost equally good results observed to date with the matte version, we, therefore, recommend the exclusive use of the MS-30 stems with polished surface. Furthermore, it has been shown that subsidence of a tapered polished stem is not harmful, but quite in contrast, is advantageous [13, 33].

On the other hand, according to studies of stem surface roughness and creep-induced subsidence of Norman et al.[35], it appears that stem subsidence is not important for the maintenance of a "taper-lock"; and creep-induced subsidence does not result in an increase of normal stress patterns at the stem/cement interface as previously proposed [36].

When designing the MS-30 stem, the main goal was to improve the quality of the cement mantle without abandoning the proven concept of a tapered design (press-fit principle), realized, i.e., in the Müller Straight Stem or the Exeter Stem. Thus, there is the possibility of a "second line of defense" in case of debonding of the metal/cement interface with migration (subsidence) [37].One has to bear in mind that, with a straight stem, the risk of a thin cement mantle in zones 8 and 9 increases [38]. In order to avoid this risk of metal/bone contact, Wroblewski et al. [6] and Breusch et al.[39] consider a low-neck osteotomy and aggressive removal of the posterior calcar femorale a necessity. However, with a low resection of the femoral neck, rotational stability is seriously compromised [40, 41]. Since loosening of a femoral stem rotates the stem into retroversion and a high neck resection secures the prosthesis stem effectively against migration into retroversion, we prefer the "high", i.e., 30° instead of 45° resection, as it is part of the "fixation philosophy" of the MS-30 stem.

In conclusion, no significant difference in the outcome of MS-30 stems with a matte or a polished surface could be found during a 5-year observation period. Neither did the incidence of radiolucencies, osteolyses or subsidence reveal a significant difference between the two surfaces. The main reason for the almost equally excellent performance of both the matte and polished version of the MS-30 in contrast to the matte Exeter stem may be the design of the centralizer of the MS-30 stem, which resists both, a debonding of the stem from the cement, and subsequent subsidence as a precondition for fretting between the two surfaces at the metal/cement interface. Another reason for the fact that no significant difference was found to date between the two implant surfaces, may be differences in the bone cement used in the different studies. However, this is a matter of ongoing research at the „Laboratory of Orthopaedic Biomechanic„ of the University of Basle/Switzerland. Furthermore, since it could be shown in our own experiments that the main mechanism for inducing osteolysis is fretting corrosion at the interface of bone cement (PMMA) and a matte stainless steel surface [12], only tapered stems with a polished surface must be used in combination with a hollow centralizer.

References:

[1]   Ebramzadeh, E., Sarmiento, A., McKellop, H.A., Llinas, A., Gogan, W. "The cement mantle in total hip arthroplasty" J Bone Joint Surg Am 76, 1994, pp.77-87.

[2]   Draenert, K. and Draenert, Y. "Die Adaptation des Knochens an die Deformation durch Implantate - Strain-Adaptive Bone Remodelling". Art & Science München, 1992

[3]   Miller, J. and Johnson, A. "Advances in cementing techniques in total hip arthroplasty". In: Stilwell, W.T. (ed.) The art of total hip arthroplasty, 1987, pp. 277-292, Grunde & Stratton.

[4]   Markolf, K.L. and Amstutz, H.C. "A comparative experimental study of stresses in femoral total hip replacement components: the effects of prosthesis orientation and acrylic fixation". J Biomech. 9, 1976, pp. 73-79.

[5]   Gruen, T.A., McNeice, G.M. and Amstutz, H.C. "Modes of failure of cemented stem-type femoral components. A radiographic analysis of loosening". Clin Orthop. 141, 1979, pp.17-27.

[6]   Wroblewski, B.M., Siney, P.D., Fleming, P.A. and Bobak, P. "The calcar femorale in cemented stem fixation in total hip arthroplasty". J Bone Joint Surg Br 82, 1979, pp. 842-845.

[7]   Estok, D.M., Orr, T.E. and Harris, W.H. "Factors affecting cement strains near the tip of a cemented femoral component". J Arthroplasty. 12, 1997, pp. 40-48

[8]   Morscher, E.W., Spotorno, L., Mumenthaler, A. and Frick, W. "The Cemented MS-30 Stem". In: Morscher, E.W.(Ed.) Endoprosthetics, 1995, pp.211-219, Springer Berlin, New York.

[9]   Willert, H.G. and Semlitsch, M. "Reactions of articular capsule to wear products of artificial joint prostheses". J Biomed Mater Res. 11, 1977, pp. 157-164.

[10]   Morscher, E.W., Wirz, D. "Current state of cement fixation in THR". Acta Orthop Belg. 2002 (in press).

[11]   Tritschler, B., Forest, B. and Rieu, J. "Fretting corrosion of materials for orthopaedic implants: a study of a metal/polymer contact in an artificial physiological medium. Tribol Int. 32, 1999, pp. 587-596.

[12]   Wirz, D., Zurfluh, B., Goepfert, B., Li, F., Frick, W., Klabunde, R., Stoll, D. and Morscher, E.W. "Results of in vitro studies about the mechanism of wear in the stem-cement interface of THR, ASTM, Symposium on Steels for Medical and Surgical Applications, Pittsburgh PA,USA, May 6-7, 2002.

[13]   Ling,R.S. "The use of a collar and precoating in cemented femoral stems is unnecessary and detrimental". Clin Orthop. 285, 1992, pp. 73-83.

[14]   Howie, D.W., Middleton, R.G. and Costi, K. "Loosening of matte and polished cemented femoral stems". J Bone Joint Surg. Br 80, 1998, pp. 573-576.

[15]   Rockborn, P. and Olsson, S.S. "Loosening and bone resorption in Exeter hip arthroplasties. Review at a minimum of five years". J Bone Joint Surg. Br 75, 1993, pp. 865-868.

[16]   Malchau, H. and Herberts, P. "Prognosis of total hip replacement. Revision and rerevision rate in THR: A revision risk study of 148, 359 primary operations". Scientific exhibition, 65th Annual Meeting AAOS, February 19-23, 1998, New Orleans/USA

[17]   Clark, C.R. "The prospective, randomized, double-blind clinical trial in orthopaedic surgery". J Bone Joint Surg. Am 79, 1997, pp. 1119-1120.

[18]   Johnston, R.C., Fitzgerald, R.H., Harris, W.H., Poss, R., Müller, M.E. and Sledge, C.B. "Clinical and radiographic evaluation of total hip replacement". J Bone Joint Surg. Am 72, 1990, pp. 161-168.

[19]   Harris, W.H. "Traumatic arthritis of the hip after dislocation and acetabular fracture: treatment by mold arthroplasty. J Bone Joint Surg. Am 51, 1969, pp. 737-755.

[20]   Barrack, R.L., Mulroy, R.D. Jr and Harris, W.H. "Improved cementing techniques and femoral component loosening in young patients with hip arthroplasty. A 12-year radiographic review". J Bone Joint Surg. Br 74, 1992, pp. 385-389.

[21]   DeLee, J.G. and Charnley, J. "Radiological demarcation of cemented sockets in hip replacement". Clin Orthop. 121, 1976, pp. 20-33.

[22]   Kelly, A.J., Lee, M.B., Wong, N.S., Smith, E.J. and Learmonth, I.D. "Poor reproducibility in radiographic grading of femoral cementing technique in total hip arthroplasty". J Arthroplasty. 11, 1996, pp. 525-528.

[23]   Acklin, Y.P., Berli, B.J., Frick, W., Elke, R. and Morscher, E.W. "Nine-year results of Müller cemented titanium straight stems in total hip replacement". Arch Orthop Trauma Surg. 121, 2001, pp. 391-398.

[24]   Joshi, R.P., Eftekhar, N.S., McMahon, D.J. and Nercessian, O.A. "Osteolysis after Charnley primary low-friction arthroplasty". J Bone Joint Surg. Br 80, 1998, pp. :585-590.

[25]   Brooker, A.F., Bowerman, J.W., Robinson, R.A. and Riley, L.H. Jr "Ectopic ossification following total hip replacement. Incidence and a method of classification". J Bone Joint Surg. Am 55, 1973, pp. 1629-1632.

[26]   Kaplan, E.L. and Meier, P. "Nonparametric estimation from incomplete observations". J Am Stat Assoc. 53, 1958, pp. 457-481.

[27]   Lochner, H.V., Bhandari. M. and Tornetta III, P. "Type-II error rates (Beta Errors) of randomized trials in orthopaedic trauma". J Bone Joint Surg. Am 83, 2001, pp. 1650-1655.

[28]   Alfaro-Adrián, J., Gill, H.S., Murray, D.W. "Should total hip arthroplasty femoral components be designed to subside? A radiostereometric analysis study of the Charnley elite and Exeter stems". J Arthroplasty. 16, 2001, pp. 598-606.

[29]   Harris, W.H., McCarthy, J.C. and O'Neill, D.A. "Femoral component loosening using contemporary techniques of femoral cement fixation". J Bone Joint Surg. Am 68, 1986, pp. 1064-1066.

[30]   Kiss, J., Murray, D.W., Turner-Smith, A.R., Bithell, J. and Bullstrode, C.J. "Migration of cemented femoral components after THR: Roentgen stereophotogrammetry analysis". J Bone Joint Surg. Br 78, 1996, pp. 796-801.

[31]   Kärrholm, J. and Snorrason, F. "Subsidence, tip and hump micromovement of noncoated ribbed femoral prostheses". Clin Orthop. 287, 1993, pp. 50-60.

[32]   Søballe, K., Toksvig-Larson, S. and Gelinek, J. "Migration of hydroxyapatite coated femoral prostheses: a roentgen stereophotogrammetric study". J Bone Joint Surg. Br 75, 1993, pp. 681-687.

[33]   Fowler, J.L., Gie, G.A., Lee, A.J.C. and Ling, R.S.M. "Experience with the Exeter total hip replacement since 1970". Orthop Clin North Am. 19, 1988, pp. 477-489.

[34]   Alfaro-Adrián, J., Gill, H.S. and Murray, D.W. "Cement migration after THR. A comparison of Charnley elite and Exeter femoral stems using RSA". J Bone Joint Surg. Br 81, 1999, pp. 130-134.

[35]   Normann, T.L., Thyagarajan, G., Saligrama, V.C., Gruen, T.A. and Blaha, J.D. "Stem surface roughness alters creep induced subsidence and "taper-lock" in a cemented femoral hip prosthesis". J Biomech. 34, 2001, pp. 1325-1333.

[36]   Lee, A.J.C., Perkins, R.D., Ling, R.S.M. "Time dependent properties of polymethylmethacrylate bone cement". In: John, O. (Ed) In implant bone interface. Springer New York, 1990, pp. 85-90.

[37]   Wilson-MacDonald, J. and Morscher, E. "Comparison between straight- and curved-stem Müller femoral prostheses; 5- to 10-year results of 545 total hip replacements". Arch Orthop Trauma Surg. 109, 1989, pp. 14-20.

[38]   Räber, D.A., Czaja, S. and Morscher, E.W. "Fifteen-year results of the Müller CoCrNiMo straight stem". Arch Orthop Trauma Surg. 121, 2001, pp. 38-42.

[39]   Breusch, S.J., Lukoschek, N., Kreutzer, J., Brocai, D. and Gruen, T.A. "Dependency of cement mantle thickness on femoral stem design and centralizer". J Arthroplasty. 16, 2001, pp. 648-657.

[40]   Freeman, M.A.R. "Why resect the neck?". J Bone Joint Surg. Br 68, 1986, pp. 346-349.

[41]   Nunn, D., Freeman, M.A.R., Tanner, K.E. and Bonfield, W. "Torsinal stability of the femoral component of hip arthroplasty. Response to an anteriorly applied load". J Bone Joint Surg. Br 71, 1989, pp. 452-455.

Robert M. Urban, [1] Joshua J. Jacobs, [1] Jeremy L. Gilbert, [2] Anastasia K. Skipor, [1] Nadim J. Hallab, [1] Katalin Mikecz, [1] Tibor T. Glant, [1] J. Lawrence Marsh, [3] and Jorge O. Galante [1]

Corrosion Products Generated from Mechanically Assisted Crevice Corrosion of Stainless Steel Orthopaedic Implants

Reference: Urban, R. M., Jacobs J. J., Gilbert, J. L., Skipor, A. K., Hallab, N. J., Mikecz, K., Glant, T. T., Marsh, J. L., and Galante, J. O., "**Corrosion Products Generated from Mechanically Assisted Crevice Corrosion of Stainless Steel Orthopaedic Implants,**" *Stainless Steels for Medical and Surgical Applications, ASTM STP 1438,* G. L. Winters and M. J. Nutt, Eds., ASTM International, West Conshohocken, PA, 2003.

Abstract: Accelerated corrosion of metallic implants *in vivo* can generate both soluble and insoluble products that can be detected locally and systemically. Retrieved stainless steel implants for trauma fixation or spinal instrumentation demonstrate iron and chromium-containing solid products of corrosion deposited around corroded modular junctions and as phagocytosable particles in the adjacent tissues. In some cases, the resulting adverse local tissue reaction has been associated with pain, inflammation and osteolysis, requiring removal of the implant. *In vitro* cell and organ culture studies confirm that corrosion products such as particles of chromium phosphate can elicit proinflammatory cytokine secretion from macrophages and promote macrophage-mediated bone resorption. Systemically, soluble corrosion products of chromium can be detected in the serum of selected patients with accelerated corrosion of chromium-containing implants. Metal-protein binding studies indicate that the high molecular weight serum proteins including immunoglobulins have the highest affinity for chromium. These findings stress the importance of the design of modular junctions to minimize corrosion of stainless steels used in orthopaedic appliances.

Keywords: Stainless steel, corrosion, crevice, fretting, modularity, chromium, particulate debris, metal ions, osteolysis, cytokines, serum proteins, systemic dissemination

[1]Director, Implant Pathology Laboratory, Professor and Director, Section of Biomaterials Research, Director, Metal Ion Laboratory, Assistant Professor and Director, Biomaterials Testing Laboratory, Associate Professor, Professor and Director, Section of Biochemistry and Molecular Biology, and Professor, respectively, Department of Orthopedic Surgery, Rush-Presbyterian-St. Luke's Medical Center, 1653 W. Congress Parkway, Chicago, IL 60612.
[2]Professor and Chairman, Department of Bioengineering and Neuroscience, Syracuse University, Syracuse, NY 13244.
[3]Professor, Department of Orthopaedic Surgery, the University of Iowa College of Medicine, Iowa City, IA 52242.

Introduction

Type AISI 316L (ASTM F138) stainless steel continues to be a dominant alloy for fabrication of internal fixation devices where biocompatibility, high strength and ductility are required. This paper summarizes the clinical, histopathological, micro-analytical and *in vitro* findings from previously reported and ongoing studies in our laboratories as they relate to the nature and significance of corrosion products generated by a variety of contemporary spinal instrumentation and trauma fixation devices made from stainless steel.

Corrosion of Stainless Steel Implants

Corrosion of single-part internal fixation devices is rare [1]. Retrieved stainless steel hardware generally demonstrates a bright, "as-implanted" finish indicative of the low rate of uniform dissolution of this alloy in its passivated state. The multi-part or modular design of many internal fixation devices consistently introduces the potential for crevice corrosion, to which all stainless steels are prone [2]. Screw and plate interfaces in fracture fixation devices and hook, screw and rod systems for spinal instrumentation provide environments for fretting and crevice corrosion, which can challenge even the most corrosion-resistant alloys. The elements of these interface corrosion processes have been well described and are the subject of current review articles [3,4].

As a result of the susceptibility of multi-component stainless steel implants to interface corrosion, the incidence of observed localized corrosion in retrieved implants is high. A study of 250 multi-part stainless steel fracture fixation devices removed in the late 1970s and early 1980s showed some degree of crevice corrosion in 89% of plates and 88% of screws [5].

In a previously unreported study conducted in our laboratory, 24 consecutively retrieved, contemporary, stainless steel spinal instrumentation devices (Table 1) removed after a mean of 68 months (range 4 to 277 months) were examined using a stereo light microscope (8 to 75 X) for evidence of interface corrosion. In selected cases, scanning electron microscopy with energy-dispersive X-ray analysis (model JSM-5900LV, JEOL) was used to determine the elemental composition of adherent corrosion products adjacent to the modular junctions. Ninety-two percent of the spinal devices demonstrated localized corrosion at the junctions between rods and connectors. Iron and chromium-containing degradation products were identified surrounding the sites of corrosion (Figure 1).

Despite the high incidence of interface corrosion with stainless steel implants, most often, the reaction is focal and usually not severe enough to require implant removal [1, 4, 6]. "Metal intolerance" manifested as late operative site pain is one reason for removal of stainless steel devices. In practice, however, the relationship among corrosion, local inflammation and pain is often difficult to demonstrate. Infection [7], mechanical irritation, or rarely metal allergy [8] plays a possible role in some cases. In plate and screw devices for fracture fixation, accelerated corrosion occurs at the very small area of screw/plate contact, limiting the amount of degradation products and the magnitude of the response in the surrounding tissues. Hence, the importance of corrosion as a clinical phenomenon is uncertain in this circumstance. However, oxide abrasion can induce large potential (electric field) transients that may play a role in pain generation [9].

Accelerated corrosion of larger modular junctions of different geometry provides

Table 1 – *Retrieved Stainless Steel Spinal Implants*

Implant	Instrumentation System[1]	Interface Corrosion (Yes / No)	Duration (Mos.)	Reason for Removal
1	Harrington	Yes	208	Flat back deformity
2	Rogozinski	Yes	103	Transition syndrome
3	ISOLA	Yes	13	Pain, flat back deformity
4	ISOLA	Yes	33	Flat back deformity
5	ISOLA	Yes	17	Transition syndrome
6	TRSH	Yes	47	Infection
7	Simmons	Yes	13	Fell, numbness
8	C-D	No	38	Pseudoarthrosis
9	C-D	Yes	60	Prominent hardware
10	Harrington	No	277	Flat back deformity
11	TRSH	Yes	41	Rod breakage
12	ISOLA	Yes	35	Flat back deformity
13	TRSH	Yes	175	Flat back deformity
14	C-D	Yes	103	Broken rod
15	C-D	Yes	145	Broken hardware
16	Simmons	Yes	44	Low back pain
17	ISOLA	Yes	33	Infection
18	ISOLA	Yes	25	Pain from iliac screws
19	C-D	Yes	86	Painful hardware
20	ISOLA	Yes	4	Flat back deformity
21	ISOLA	Yes	47	Transition syndrome.
22	ISOLA	Yes	10	Flat back deformity
23	Simmons	Yes	58	Pseudoarthrosis.
24	ISOLA	Yes	16	Extension of fusion

[1]Harrington (Zimmer, Warsaw, IN); Rogozinski (Surgical Dynamics, Norwalk CT); ISOLA (DePuy AcroMed, Warsaw, IN); TRSH, Texas Rite Scottish Hospital (Sofamor Danek, Memphis, TN); C-D, Cotrel-Dubousset (Sofamor Danek, Memphis, TN); Simmons (Smith & Nephew Richards, Memphis, TN).

increased contact area and does appear to generate a greater volume of degradation products that can result in local inflammation and pain, necessitating removal of an implant. A well-studied example of clinically significant local reactions to corrosion and metallic degradation products was described by Jones et al. [10], who reported interface corrosion of a three-piece modular 316L stainless steel intramedullary nail used to treat femoral diaphyseal fractures. Osteolysis, periosteal reaction or cortical thickening localized to one or both of the modular junctions were present in 23 of 27 femora at a mean of 21 months following fracture fixation (Figure 2). The level of thigh pain was significantly greater in patients with the modular nails compared to a similar group of patients whose femoral fractures had been treated with single-piece stainless steel nails. Fretting corrosion at the modular junctions and a granulomatous reaction to particulate corrosion products in the adjacent tissues was noted in retrieved specimens.

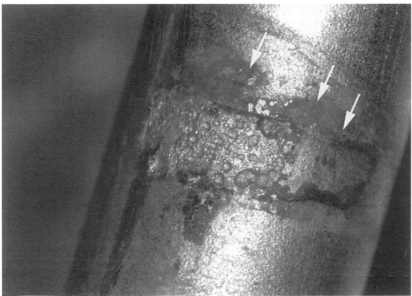

Figure 1 - *Spinal instrumentation rod removed after 33 months for infection demonstrated severe pitting at a rod/connector junction. Adherent corrosion products (arrows) surrounded the site of crevice corrosion.*

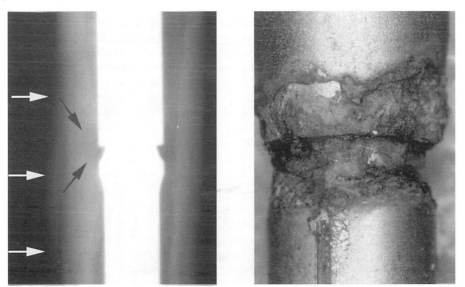

Figure 2 - *Radiograph (Left) shows periosteal reaction (white arrows) and focal osteolysis (black arrows) at the level of a junction of a modular stainless steel intramedullary nail. A retrieved nail (Right) shows adherent corrosion products surrounding a modular junction.*

Solid Corrosion Products and Local Tissue Effects

Generalized corrosion currently is not known to be of consequence in the tissues adjoining stainless steel implants, since in histological sections there is no evidence of a specific response to the slow release of metallic species that characterizes this process [4]. However, insoluble metallic degradation products are often found surrounding sites of accelerated corrosion. These products exist as deposits adherent to the implant and as particulate debris, which can provoke an inflammatory response in the peri-implant tissues. The adherent deposits may be recognized as black, dark green and rust-colored encrustations associated with interface corrosion at screw-plate junctions seen at routine removal of stainless steel internal fixation devices. Both the adherent deposits and the particulate debris within the tissue can be identified as metallic degradation products having similar compositions.

The nature of this particulate debris was first reported by Williams and Meachim [11], Sevitt [12] and Winter [13], who described two types of corrosion products in the tissues surrounding stainless steel implants retrieved in the 1970s. The first of these particles was a chromium compound containing iron and a substantial amount of phosphorus that appeared in histological sections as yellow or "apple-green" plate-like particles. These particles were termed, "microplates". The microplates ranged in size from as much as several hundred micrometers down to sub-micron dimensions. The second type of particles consisted of abundant, 1-3 micrometer, "yellow-brown", hemosiderin-like granules identified as oxides and hydrated oxides of iron.

More recent studies indicate that corrosion of contemporary stainless steel devices generates degradation products similar in morphology and elemental composition to those described above for implants retrieved in the 1970s. Our laboratory conducted supplementary analyses on the retrieved implants and peri-implant tissues from the study of Jones et al. [10] concerning corroded modular intramedullary nails. Correlated histological, energy-dispersive X-ray analysis (JSM-5900LV, JEOL) and selected area electron diffraction (JEM-4000FX, JEOL) revealed the existence of at least two types of microplates. No crystallinity was detected in either type of microplate particle. The microplates that appeared yellow by transmission light microscopy of the histological sections proved on microanalysis to be an iron phosphate hydroxide compound (Figure 3). The microplates appearing green in the light microscope were confirmed to be a hydrate-rich, chromium phosphate compound (Figure 4). The latter material has been described previously in association with corrosion of cobalt-chromium alloy head/neck junctions in hip replacement prostheses [14]. Nanometer size particles of chromium phosphate have been identified within macrophages in peri-implant tissue. The valance of chromium in this material has been determined to be 3+ using comparisons of parallel electron energy loss spectra [15]. Microplate-like particles have been reported in association with corroded junctions of spinal instrumentation devices as well [16, 17]. Energy-dispersive x-ray analysis of the yellow-brown, hemosiderin-like granules indicated high concentrations of oxygen and iron and traces of chromium (Figure 5).

Histopathological examination of the tissues adjacent to the modular junctions of the intramedullary nails demonstrated an inflammatory response to the various-size particles of the corrosion products. The cellular response to the two types of microplates, iron phosphate hydroxide and chromium phosphate, was similar (Figures 6 and 7). Multinucleated giant cells and macrophages surrounded large deposits of microplates;

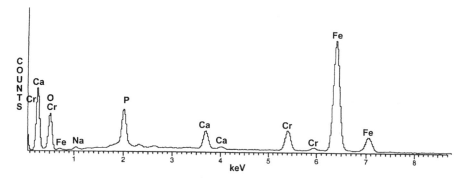

Figure 3 - *Energy-dispersive X-ray spectrum of a "yellow microplate" particle identified as an iron phosphate hydroxide corrosion product.*

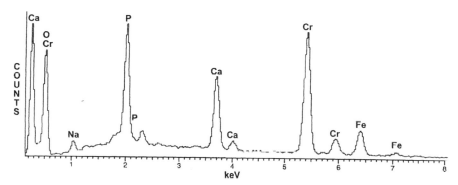

Figure 4 - *Energy-dispersive X-ray spectrum of a "green microplate" particle identified as a chromium phosphate hydrate-rich corrosion product.*

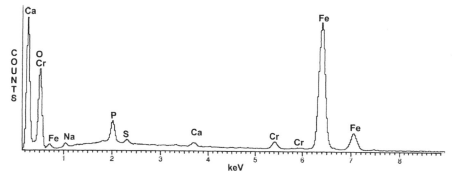

Figure 5 - *Energy-dispersive X-ray spectrum of a "yellow-brown", hemosiderin-like particle identified as an iron oxide corrosion product containing trace amounts of chromium.*

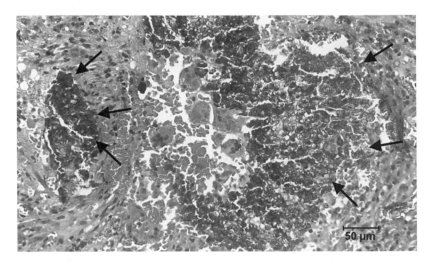

Figure 6 - *Multinucleated giant cells (center) adjacent to an accumulation of "yellow microplate" particles (arrows), identified as an iron phosphate hydroxide, in the peri-implant tissue from a corroded stainless steel modular intramedullary nail (H&E, X78).*

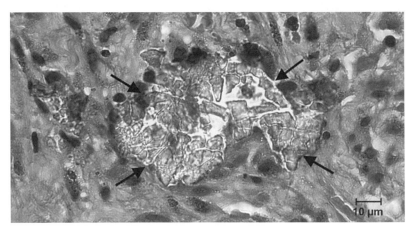

Figure 7 - *Macrophages surround a collection of "green microplate" particles (arrows), identified as chromium phosphate, in the tissue adjacent to a corroded modular stainless steel intramedullary nail removed after 20 months. (H&E, X234).*

while microplates of 5 micrometers and less were found within macrophages. Abundant iron oxide granules were present within macrophages and occasionally fibroblasts (Figure 8). The macrophages and multinucleated giant cells were accompanied by a mild infiltrate of lymphocytes and plasma cells. As would be expected, the magnitude of the cellular response was dependent on the size and concentration of the particles.

In vitro cell and organ culture studies have confirmed that phagocytosable chromium phosphate particles (1.42 ± 0.83 micrometers) can elicit proinflammatory cytokine (IL-1α, IL-1β and prostaglandin E$_2$) secretion from macrophages, promote macrophage-mediated bone resorption [18], and suppress osteoblast procollagen gene expression [19].

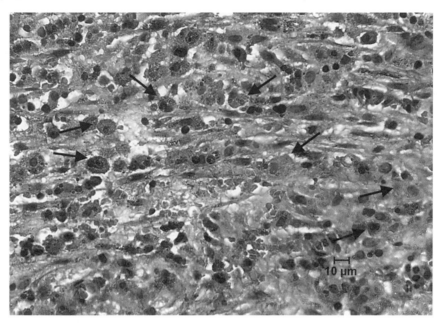

Figure 8 - *Hemosiderin-like "yellow-brown" 1 to 3 micrometer particles imparted a granular appearance to numerous macrophages (arrows) in this tissue adjacent to a corroded modular stainless steel intramedullary nail removed after 20 months. The particles were identified as iron oxides containing traces of chromium. (H&E, X156).*

Soluble Corrosion Products and Systemic Dissemination

Much of the metal released by corrosion of implants *in vivo* is transported systemically as minute particles and organometallic complexes via the lymphatic and blood circulatory systems. This is evident from post-mortem studies of implants and remote organs and from studies of metal ion concentrations in serum and urine of patients hosting metal implants. Case [20] studied specimens from 13 cadavers with implants, including 5 with stainless steel hip screws and 5 with stainless steel hip or knee replacement prostheses, using inductively coupled plasma-mass spectroscopy. Increased metal levels thought to be from the implants were found in lymph nodes, liver, spleen, and bone marrow. Post-mortem retrieval studies from our laboratories using electron microprobe analysis have shown that systemic distribution of metallic particles generated by total joint replacements to the liver, spleen and lymph nodes is common [21]. One case also demonstrated dissemination of corrosion products from the screw/plate interfaces of a stainless steel femoral fixation plate to the para-aortic lymph nodes where abundant particles of chromium phosphate were detected. Both of these post-mortem studies reported that the highest concentrations of disseminated metal were associated with mechanical failure of the implant.

Chromium can be released and disseminated systemically from stainless steel or cobalt-chromium alloys. Increased concentrations of metals in the serum and urine, particularly chromium, have been associated with interface corrosion of multi-part stainless steel as well as cobalt-chromium implants. In the study of Jones et al. [10], patients with corrosion at the modular junctions of a three-piece femoral intramedullary stainless steel nail had a 20-fold increase in the mean level of serum chromium compared to a control group of patients without metallic implants, and a fourfold increase compared to a group with one-piece stainless steel nails. Another study from our laboratories suggests that fretting corrosion at the modular head/neck coupling of otherwise well-functioning cobalt-chromium hip replacements was responsible for increases in serum and urine chromium levels of as much as fivefold and eightfold, respectively, over preoperative levels [22]. Serum protein-metal binding studies of patients with cobalt-chromium alloy hip prostheses indicate that chromium is bound to serum proteins within two specific molecular weight ranges at approximately 70 and 180 kilodaltons [23]. The higher molecular weight range, which includes the immunoglobulins, had the highest affinity for chromium.

Summary

Interface corrosion of multi-component stainless steel implants can generate both soluble and insoluble metallic degradation products that can be detected locally and systemically. The local tissue response to corrosion of screw/plate junctions is limited and not of clinical importance in most circumstances. However, accelerated corrosion of modular junctions with different geometries can generate a greater volume of degradation products, resulting in local inflammation, pain, and the need for removal of an implant. Spinal instrumentation systems employ connectors of various geometries. Neither the local tissue response, the potential effects on the proximate neural elements, nor the systemic metal levels have been studied comprehensively in patients with these devices.

Systemically, serum chromium levels can be substantially elevated in patients with accelerated corrosion at modular junctions of stainless steel devices and may be used as a marker for mechanical dysfunction. The long-term biological significance of these circulating organometallic complexes is currently unknown. These findings stress the importance of the design of modular junctions to minimize corrosion of stainless steels used in orthopaedic appliances.

Acknowledgment

This work was supported by grant AR39310 from the National Institute of Arthritis and Musculoskeletal and Skin Diseases.

References

[1]   Black, J., Biological Performance of Materials. *Fundamentals of Biocompatibility, Second Edition*, Marcel Decker, New York, 1992.

[2]   Rostoker, W., and Galante, J. O., "Materials for Human Implantation," *Journal of Biomechanical Engineering*, Vol. 101, 1979, pp. 2-14.

[3]   Gilbert, J. L., and Jacobs, J. J., "The Mechanical and Electrochemical Processes Associated with Taper Fretting Crevice Corrosion: A Review," *Modularity of Orthopedic Implants, ASTM 1301*, Donald E. Marlowe, Jack E. Parr and Michael B. Mayor, Eds., American Society for Testing and Materials, West Conshohocken, PA, 1997, pp. 45-59.

[4]   Jacobs, J. J., Gilbert J. L., and Urban, R. M., "Corrosion of Metallic Implants," *Journal of Bone and Joint Surgery,* Vol. 80-A, 1998, pp. 268-282.

[5]   Cook, S. D., Thomas, K.A., Harding, A. F., Collins, C.L., Haddad, R. J., Jr., Millicic, M., and Fischer, W. L., "The In Vivo Performance of 250 Internal Fixation Devices. A Follow-Up Study," *Biomaterials*, Vol. 8, 1987, pp. 177-184.

[6]   Sutow, E. J., and Pollack, S. R., "The Biocompatibility of Certain Stainless Steels," *Biocompatibility of Clinical Implant Materials, Vol. 1*, David F. Williams, Ed., CRC Press, Boca Raton, 1981, pp. 45-98.

[7]   Gaine, W. J., Andrew, S. M., Chadwick, P., Cooke, E., and Williamson, J. B., "Late Operative Site Pain With Isola Posterior Instrumentation Requiring Implant Removal. Infection or Metal Reaction?," *Spine*, Vol. 26, Number 5, 2001, pp. 583-587.

[8]   Hallab, N., Merritt, K., and Jacobs, J. J., "Metal Sensitivity in Patients with Orthopaedic Implants," *Journal of Bone and Joint Surgery*, Vol. 83-A, 2001, pp. 428-436.

[9]   Goldberg, S., Gilbert, J.L., "Transient Electric Fields Induced by Mechanically Assisted Corrosion of Ti-6Al-4V," *Journal of Biomedical Materials Research,* Vol. 56, 2001, pp. 184-194.

[10]   Jones, D. M., Marsh, J. L., Nepola, J. V., Jacobs, J. J., Skipor, A. S., Urban, R. M., Gilbert, J. L., and Buchwalter, J. A., "Focal Osteolysis at the Junctions of a Modular Stainless-Steel Femoral Intramedullary Nail," *Journal of Bone and Joint Surgery,* Vol. 83-A, 2001, pp. 537-548.

[11]   Williams, D. F., and Meachim, G., "A Combined Metallurgical and Histological Study of Tissue-Prosthesis Interactions in Orthopaedic Patients," *Journal of Biomedical Material Research Symposium 5 (part 1)*, 1974, pp. 1-9.

[12]   Sevitt, S., "Corrosion of Implants and Tissue Metallosis," *Bone Repair and Fracture Healing in Man*, Churchill and Livingstone, Edinburgh, 1981, pp. 281-295.

[13]   Winter, G.D., "Wear and Corrosion Products in Tissues and the Reactions They

Provoke," *Biocompatibility of Implant Materials*, David F. Williams, Ed., Sector Publishing, London, 1976, pp. 28-39.

[14]   Urban, R. M., Jacobs, J. J., Gilbert, J. L., and Galante, J. O., "Migration of Corrosion Products from Modular Hip Prostheses," *Journal of Bone and Joint Surgery*, Vol. 76-A, 1994, pp. 1345-1359.

[15]   Jacobs, J. J., Urban, R. M., Gilbert, J. L., Skipor, A. S., Black, J., Jasty, M., and Galante, J. O., "Local and Distant Products of Modularity," *Clinical Orthopaedics and Related Research*, Vol. 319, 1995, pp. 94-105.

[16]   Mody, D. R., Esses, S. I., and Heggeness, M. H., "A Histologic Study of Soft-Tissue Reactions to Spinal Implants," *Spine,* Vol. 19, Number 10, 1994, pp. 1153-1156.

[17]   Vieweg, U., van Roost, D., Wolf, H. K., Schyma, C.A., and Schramm, J., "Corrosion on an Internal Spinal Fixator System," *Spine*, Vol. 24. Number 10, 1999, pp. 946-951.

[18]   Lee, S. H., Brennan, F. R., Jacobs, J. J., Urban, R. M., Ragasa, D. R., and Glant, T. T., "Human Monocyte/Macrophage Response to Cobalt-Chromium Corrosion Products and Titanium Particles in Patients with Total Joint Replacements," *Journal of Orthopaedic Research*, Vol. 15, 1997, pp. 40-49.

[19]   Vermes, C., Chandrasekaran, R., Jacobs, J. J., Galante, J. O., Roebuck, K. A., and Glant, T. T., " The Effects of Particulate Wear Debris, Cytokines, and Growth Factors on the Functions of MG-63 Osteoblasts," *Journal of Bone Joint Surgery*, 83-A, 2001, pp. 201-211.

[20]   Case, C. P., Langkamer, V. G., James, C., Palmer, M. R., Kemp, A. J., Heap, P. F., and Solomon, L., Widespread Dissemination of Metal Debris from Implants," *Journal of Bone and Joint Surgery,* Vol. 76-B, 1994, pp. 701-712.

[21]   Urban, R. M., Jacobs, J. J., Tomlinson, M. J., Gavrilovic, J., Black, J., and Peoc'h, M., "Dissemination of Wear Particles to the Liver, Spleen and Abdominal Lymph Nodes of Patients with Hip or Knee Replacement," *Journal of Bone and Joint Surgery,* Vol. 82-A, 2000, pp. 457-477.

[22]   Jacobs, J. J., Skipor, A. S., Patterson, L. M., Hallab, N. J., Paprosky, W. G., Black, J., and Galante, J. O., "Metal Release in Patients Who Have a Primary Total Hip Arthroplasty," *Journal of Bone and Joint Surgery*, Vol. 80-A, 1998, pp. 1447-1458.

[23]   Hallab, N. J., Jacobs, J. J., Skipor, A. S., Black, J., Mikecz, K., and Galante, J. O., "Systemic Metal Binding Associated with Total Joint Replacement Arthroplasty," *Journal of Biomedical Materials Research*, Vol. 49(3), 2000, pp. 353-361.

Author Index

A

Agonstinho, Silvia M. L., 168

B

Barbosa, Celso A., 168
Berli, Bernhard, 249
Bigolin, Gianni, 93
Bingmann, Dieter, 119
Bogan, Jay-Anthony, 107, 154, 194
Boucher, Bruno, 13
Brauer, Holger, 119
Bullard, Sophie J., 176
Bumgardner, Joel D., 137

C

Covino, Bernard S., Jr., 176
Cowen, Stephen, 3
Craig, Charles H., 28, 61, 176
Cramer, Stephen D., 176

D

de Andrade, Arnaldo H. P., 168
Dennis, J. Zachary, 61
Dichtel, Jean-Paul, 13
Disegi, John A., 50

E

Edwards, Michael R., 28, 61, 176
Elke, Reinhard, 249
Eschbach, Lukas, 93

F

Fischer, Alfons, 119
Frick, Willi, 222
Friend, Clifford M., 28, 61, 176

G

Galante, Jorge O., 262
Gasser, Beat, 93
Gilbert, Jeremy L., 262
Glant, Tibor T., 262
Gokcen, Nev A., 28, 61, 176
Göpfert, Beat, 222
Govier, R. Dale, 28

H

Hallab, Nadim J., 262
Haraldsson, Christina, 3
Hicks, Albert G., 61
Hirsiger, Werner, 93

J

Jablonski, Paul D., 176
Jacobs, Joshua J., 262
Jenusaitis, Matthew, 61

L

Li, Feng, 222
Lin, Hsin-Yi, 137
MacDougall, Julie E., 209

M

Marsh, J. Lawrence, 262
Mikecz, Katalin, 262
Moölders, Martina, 119
Moraux, Jean-Yves, 13
Morscher, Erwin W., 222, 249

P

Pannek, Edward J., Jr., 61
Parker, Suzanne H., 137
Perot, Nicolas, 13

R

Radisch, Herbert R., Jr., 28, 61, 176
Roach, Michael, 107, 154, 194

S

Schenk, Rolf, 211
Skipor, Anastasia K., 262
Sokolowski, Alexandre, 168
Steger, Rainer, 39, 72

T

Tikhovski, Ilia, 119
Trozera, Thomas A., 28
Turner, Paul C., 28, 61, 176

U

Urban, Robert M., 262

V

Vesely, Edward J., Jr., 28
Villamil, Ruth F. V., 168

W

Wiemann, Martin, 119
Williamson, Scott, 107, 154, 194
Windler, Markus, 39, 72, 211, 235
Winters, Gary L., 72

Wirz, Dieter, 222
Woods, Terry O., 82

Z

Zardiackas, Lyle D., 50, 107, 137, 154,
  194
Zhu, Mengke, 235
Ziomek-Moroz, Margaret, 176
Zurfluh, Bruno, 222

Subject Index

316L stainless steel, 50, 194, 211
    macrophage cells and corrosion, 137

A

AISI 630, 13
Alloy, 176
Anodic polarization, 107
Arthroplasty, 222
ASTM A 262E, 176
ASTM F 138, 168
ASTM F 746, 176
ASTM F 1314, 3
ASTM F 1586, 3, 39, 168
ASTM F 1801, 194
ASTM F 1875, 235
ASTM F 2129, 176
ASTM F 2180, 50
ASTM G 5, 107
ASTM G 71, 107
Austenitic stainless steel, 119, 168, 194

B

Bending properties, 93
Biocompatibility, 119, 137
BioDur 108, 107, 154, 194
BioDur 316LS, 176
Biomechanics, 222
Bone plate, fatigue, 93
Bone resorption, 222
Bone screw, 93
Breakdown potentials, 168, 176

C

Cable systems, 50
Cell culture, 137
Cement fixation, 249
Chromium, 262
CoCr alloy, 211, 235
Compatibility, MRI, 82
Coronary stent, 28, 61, 176
Corrosion, 107, 176
    crevice, 176, 222, 262
    fatigue, 154, 194
    fretting, 222, 235, 262
    galvanic, 107

    intergranular, 176
    macrophage cells and, 137
    pitting, 3, 176
    properties, 39, 72
    resistance, 13, 119, 176
    wear-induced, 211
Crevice corrosion, 176, 222, 262
Cutting, 13
Cyclic fatigue, 119
Cytokines, 262
Cytotoxicity, 119

D

Dilation-balloon expandable coronary
    stents, 176

E

Electrochemical studies, 168
Electron microscopy, 222
Elongation, 39

F

Fatigue, 119, 194
    resistance, 93
    testing, 154, 194
Femoral head, 235
Femoral stem, 39, 249
Foreign-body reaction, 222
Forged hip stems, 39
Fretting corrosion, 222, 235, 262

G

Galvanic corrosion, 107

H

Hardness, 13, 39
High cycle fatigue tests, 93
High-nitrogen stainless steel, 39, 72, 119,
    211, 235
Hip prosthesis, 222
Hip stems, 39, 235

I

Implant materials, 3, 194, 211
Implant surface, 249

Inclusions, 72
Intergranular corrosion, 176
Intergranular crack initiation, 93
ISO 5832–9, 39

L

Low-nickel stainless steel, 93, 107
    notch sensitivity and stress
        corrosion, 154

M

Macrophage cells, stainless steel
    corrosion and, 137
Macrophages, 222
Magnetic resonance imaging, 82
Martensitic steel, 13
Mechanical properties, 3, 39, 72
Medical instruments, 13
Metal ions, 262
Metals, 222
Microstructure, 3, 39, 50, 72
Modularity, 262

N

New PHACOMP, 28
Nickel-free stainless steel, 119
Nitrogen alloyed steel, 13
Nonmetallic inclusions, 3, 50
Notch sensitivity, 154

O

Orthopedic implants, 168
Osteolysis, 262

P

P2000, 119
Particle size, 222
Particulate debris, 222, 262
Pitting corrosion, 3, 176
Platinum, 176
Platinum-enhanced radiopaque stainless
    steel, 28, 61, 176
Polymethylmethacrylate, 222
Potentiodynamic polarization, 176

R

Radiopacity, 28, 176
Repassivation, 211
Ringers solution, 176

S

Safety, MRI, 82
Sandvik Bioline High-N, 3
Sendzimir mill, 61
Serum proteins, 262
Sliding wear, 211
Stem-cement interface, wear, 222
Stress corrosion cracking, 154
Surface analysis, 137
Surgical implants, 50
Systemic dissemination, 262

T

Tapered stem, 249
Taper interface, 235
Tensile strength, 39
Titanium alloy, 211, 235
Total hip replacement, 222, 249

U

UNS S31683 alloys, 28, 61, 176

V

Vacuum arc remelting, 61
Vacuum induction melting, 61
Vickers hardness, 39

W

Wear, mechanism, 222
Wear-induced corrosion, 211
Wear resistance, 13
Wire, 50

X

XM 16, 13
X-rays, 176

Y

Yield strength, 39

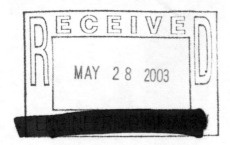